MAINSTREAM ME

Communicable and Tropical Diseases

G. C. COOK, MD, DSc (Lond.), FRCP, FRACP
Overseas Development Administration (ODA)
Lecturer, London School of Hygiene and Tropical Medicine.
Honorary Physician, Hospital for Tropical Diseases and University College Hospital, London.
Formerly, Professor of Medicine in the Universities of Zambia; Riyadh, Saudi Arabia; and Papua New Guinea.

HEINEMANN MEDICAL BOOKS
London

Heinemann Medical Books
22 Bedford Square
London WC1B 3HH

ISBN 0-433-00029-5

© G. C. Cook, 1988

First published 1988

British Library Cataloguing-in-Publication Data
Cook, G. C.
　Communicable and Tropical diseases.—
　(Mainstream medicine).
　1. Communicable diseases
　I. Title　II. Series
　616.9　　RC111

ISBN 0-433-00029-5

Titles in the series:
Cardiology
Endocrinology
Gastroenterology
Haematology
The Liver and Biliary System
Nephrology
Neurology
Respiratory Medicine
Rheumatology

Typeset by Latimer Trend & Company Ltd, Plymouth
and printed and bound in Great Britain by Biddles Ltd, Guildford

Contents

		Series Preface	vi
		Preface	vii
Chapter	1.	General Principles	1
	2.	Childhood Infections	31
	3.	Tuberculosis	43
	4.	Malaria	60
	5.	Gastrointestinal Infections	72
	6.	Infections Involving the Liver and Biliary System	99
	7.	Respiratory Infections (Excluding Tuberculosis)	119
	8.	Infections of the Cardiovascular System	138
	9.	Infections of the Central Nervous System	152
	10.	Renal and Urinary Tract Infections	174
	11.	Acquired Immune Deficiency Syndrome (AIDS)	185
	12.	Sexually Transmitted Diseases (Excluding AIDS)	195
	13.	Skin Infections	210
	14.	Leprosy	225
	15.	Systemic Infections	232
	16.	Antibiotics and Other Antimicrobial Agents	279
	17.	Diseases Affecting Travellers	299
	18.	Prevention and Control of Communicable Diseases	311
		Index	317

Series Preface

This is one of a series of small books with two objectives. The main aim is to help postgraduates both from the United Kingdom and overseas who are preparing for higher medical examinations; the MRCP (UK) is the primary target, but we believe that trainee surgeons will also find it useful. The second is to provide assistance in the clinical situation by summarising relevant information at rather more length than is possible in a general textbook of medicine.

The books are short, with only the essential diagrams and references, and the series seeks to cover comprehensively the field of internal medicine. The authors and editors are all experienced teachers. The approach is similar in each book, and the series will provide a valuable basis of factual knowledge for higher medical examinations. It is assumed that the examination candidate is already an experienced and conscientious physician—these books cannot, of course, compensate for clinical deficiencies.

Each book provides a factual and up-to-date review of clinical information and underlying concepts, avoiding complex discussion of matters where there is uncertainty or difference of opinion. Some material is tabulated for ease of scanning and learning. References are to review articles rather than to original data.

We have no qualms about producing a series of books with examination candidates in mind. The postgraduate has the greatest difficulty in keeping up with advances in the many specialties that make up internal medicine, and examinations may require knowledge of areas where postgraduate experience has been minimal. Our sympathy is with the candidates.

Series Editors:
P. W. Brunt
Consultant Physician, Woodend Hospital, Aberdeen
M. S. Losowsky
Professor of Medicine, University of Leeds
A. E. Read
Professor of Medicine, University of Bristol

Preface

This book should really be entitled simply *'Communicable Diseases'*, thus covering those diseases which are capable of being transmitted from one organism to another. However, within the UK, the subspecialty widely known as Tropical Medicine has over the last century developed separately from that involving the other Infectious Diseases. It is therefore necessary to expand the title to encompass all relevant infections. Although certain of these diseases have specific geographical distributions, this book attempts to cover them in a world context. In the latter years of the 20th century, travel is so rapid and frequent that almost any disease known to man can appear at any time in any geographical location. It is vital, therefore, that everyone who practises the art and science of medicine is able to recognise and furthermore, deal with every one of these problems; a high 'index of suspicion' is required, otherwise important diseases will be missed.

The various infections are arranged under the principal system involved (a clinical rather than a toxonomic grouping); however, because certain diseases—notably tuberculosis, malaria and intestinal infections cause such an enormous amount of morbidity and mortality in the world as a whole, and are so intimately intertwined with malnutrition, I have given early prominence to them.

Like the other books in this series, this one sets out to be of particular value to postgraduates preparing for the MRCP (UK) and other postgraduate examinations in medicine. However, it should also be of interest to senior undergraduates (whose training in this group of diseases is frequently painfully inadequate), those preparing for the DTM&H diplomas, and also other health personnel (including members of the nursing profession) intending to spend time in areas of the world where infectious diseases abound. It is in no way intended to replace standard texts on infectious diseases and tropical medicine; these will of necessity be required as a supplement to fill in detailed information.

Preface

I am grateful to the publishers for their forbearance and to Beryle Amerasinghe for interpreting and typing the whole text from my largely illegible longhand.

G. C. Cook

Chapter One

General Principles

Throughout the animal kingdom, and man is no exception, a delicate balance exists between the host and the multiplicity of potentially harmful agents in the environment; among them are viruses, rickettsia, bacteria, fungi, protozoa and helminths, organisms which are responsible for the whole range of communicable (including 'tropical') diseases. Although transmission of the infective agent may be from person-to-person (originating in either a sick patient or a carrier), one or more vectors may be involved and/or an animal reservoir may exist. These latter diseases are termed *zoonoses* (*see* p. 9), and those involved in certain occupations, e.g. farm workers, veterinary surgeons and abattoir workers, are especially affected.

The importance of *carriers* cannot be overstated. They can constitute the main reservoir of infection in which the organisms maintain themselves in a population in non-epidemic periods. Furthermore, they can constitute the origin for an epidemic.

The pattern of infective disease varies in different geographical locations, and also from time-to-time historically. Since the introduction of antibacterial chemotherapy, major changes in the incidence of some diseases have occurred. However in some cases, e.g. 'scarlet fever' and tuberculosis there is evidence that in the 'Western World' a decline in incidence was already taking place; the same probably applied to the world distribution of smallpox before the major campaign launched by the World Health Organisation (WHO) led to its final extinction in 1977.

Intimately involved in this subject is a knowledge of the pathogen itself, the reservoir or other source of infection, mode of transmission (contact, air, water, milk, food or insect) and the impact of the disease on population groups—this involves natural and acquired herd immunity and programmes of vaccination and immunisation.

The main portals of entry to the human body are: the intestinal tract (via ingestion), the skin (insect bites, scratches, etc) and the respiratory tract (inhalation) from a contaminated environment. Any non-pathogenic substance or inanimate object, other than food, which is capable of harbouring or transmitting pathogenic organisms is termed a *fomite*.

The *incubation period* (IC) is: the time between the entry of a critical mass of infecting (pathogenic) organisms and the onset of prodromal symptoms; this is influenced by the natural or acquired resistance of the host (the patient). In general, the IC is short where there is a massive infecting dose, in the young and elderly, and when there is little or no acquired immunity. It is important to recognise that the IC is not synonymous with the latent period between the initial infection, and the infectious stage of the disease; neither does the symptomatic stage correspond exactly with the infectious stage.

The practical impact of a communicable disease is described under several headings:

(i) *Sporadic*. This applies to a single episode of infection either in an individual or a small group (e.g. a family); it is a potential source of an epidemic.

(ii) *Endemic*. This indicates that the infection is habitually present in the geographical area under consideration; because the population has been exposed to this agent from birth onwards, a natural balance exists between the organism and the host. War and/or famine can disturb this state of equilibrium.

(iii) *Epidemic*. This implies the occurrence of a group of illnesses (or an outbreak) of similar nature which is in excess of the normal expectancy for that population group and which is derived from a common source.

(iv) *Pandemic*. This refers to the worldwide spread of a disease throughout continents—influenza and cholera provide good examples.

Epidemiology is: the study of the frequency, distribution and causation of disease in a population, taking into account factors in the physical and social environment. *Clinical epidemiology* is therefore based on observations made in clinical (bed-side) practice in contrast to those made on population groups. Investigation of an epidemic should proceed along certain lines. The 'originator' of the method was the anaesthetist Dr John Snow who in 1855 localised the epidemic of cholera in Soho, London, to infected water that was obtained by the local inhabitants from the Broad Street pump. As well as plotting the geographical location of infected persons with details of their age and sex, the background of occupation and travel must also be analysed; likewise, secondary cases and likely mode of spread must be recorded. Having established the source of infection, adequate control measures must then be outlined.

Under the *Infectious Diseases (Notification) Act* of 1889, the reporting of certain communicable diseases to the local Medical Officer of Health (MOH) by medical practitioners was required; 10 years later this became compulsory throughout Britain. The current list of notifiable diseases in England and Wales is summarised in Table 1.1. Responsibility for notification lies with the general practitioner or hospital doctor who originally makes the diagnosis; notification on a special form (for which a fee is payable) should be forwarded to the Medical Officer for Environmental Health (MOEH) at the local health authority. In the case of typhoid and paratyphoid fever, and poliomyelitis, the MOEH, or the alternative proper officer, visits the patient's home to arrange admission to an appropriate hospital with due arrangement for surveillance of contacts and disinfection of the premises. Failure to notify a diagnosed case carries a fine and is a legal offence. Each week, the MOEH informs the Registrar General of

Table 1.1

A LIST OF NOTIFIABLE DISEASES IN ENGLAND AND WALES

Anthrax	Paratyphoid fever
Cholera	Plague
Diphtheria	Poliomyelitis (acute)
Dysentery (amoebic or bacillary)	Rabies
Encephalitis (acute)	Relapsing fever
Infective jaundice	'Scarlet fever'
Lassa fever	Tetanus
Leprosy	Tuberculosis
Leptospirosis	Typhoid fever
Malaria	Typhus fever
Marburg virus disease	Viral haemorrhagic fever
Measles	Whooping cough
Meningitis (acute)	Yellow fever
Ophthalmia neonatorum	

the numbers of the different diseases notified in his or her area and this is copied to the Area Medical Officer (AMO); information collected from all over England and Wales is collated and published by the Registrar General in his or her weekly report, the *OPCS Monitor* (Office of Population Censuses and Surveys Report). In the light of new information these may be subsequently changed for the sake of accuracy; these figures are published in the Registrar General's quarterly report. Every year, the Chief Medical Officer (CMO) of the Department of Health and Social Security publishes his or her annual report on the state of the public health.

The Communicable Disease Surveillance Centre (CDSC) was set up in 1974 to help coordinate the investigation and control of communicable diseases in England and Wales. The CDSC has three main areas of activity:

(i) Communicable diseases surveillance—the Communicable Disease Report (CDR) is published weekly.
(ii) Advice and assistance in the investigation and control of communicable disease.
(iii) Assistance with teaching of the epidemiology of communicable disease.

FACTORS PREDISPOSING AN INDIVIDUAL TO INFECTION

Infections—viral, rickettsial, bacterial, fungal and parasitic—are present throughout the world. Incidence rates, however, have wide geographical variations. Furthermore, this is not a static but a dynamic state; most infections which are now common in developing 'Third World' countries were, for example, very common in the UK and north America during the 19th century. Cholera and typhoid were major health risks in Britain until the late 19th century, while malaria was present in southern England until the 1920s. Underlying standards of sanitation and socioeconomic conditions therefore have much to do with the overall incidence of communicable disease. The concept of 'tropical disease' is unsatisfactory; although certain diseases do require a relatively high ambient temperature for survival of the parasite and/or the vector, this only applies to a small minority (the 'exotic' diseases). Underlying standards of hygiene and sanitation, etc are far more important predisposing factors.

Genetic Factors

With all communicable diseases, a finely balanced equilibrium exists between the infective agent concerned and the defence mechanisms of the host (and these are in turn related to the host's genetic constitution); hepatitis B infections are a case in point—the likely clinical sequelae differ vastly between neonatal and adult infections. Similarly, good evidence exists that susceptibility to tuberculosis has an ethnic basis; it is especially common in people of Asian origin in the UK compared with the other minor ethnic groups. Good evidence also exists for differing susceptibility to infection in different individuals; this forms the basis for *ecogenetics* which can be applied to other environmental factors also, including foodstuffs, drugs and inhalants. The relationship is complex and in few cases is there a polarisation to genetic or environmental bases; the majority of communicable diseases involve a background of multifactorial origin involving both genetic and environmental factors.

Since mankind originated, adaptation to infections, including epidemics, has been necessary and this has undoubtedly been important in Darwinian evolution. The position of various genes on the chromosomes is perhaps of little consequence; it is what they contribute to the prevention of disease which really matters! An excellent example of the influence of genetic intervention in the control of survival comes from a study of the descendants of former Dutch colonists in Surinam, who emigrated there in the mid 19th century. Soon after arrival they were exposed to epidemics of typhoid and yellow fever (which they had not previously encountered); this resulted in a total mortality rate of around 60%. Gene frequencies in their descendants now living in Surinam have been compared with those in a large control sample in a population in Holland; significant difference was observed in the frequencies of C3, Gm, HLA–B and GLO which was not due to drift. These data strongly suggest selection through genetic control resulting from survival from these epidemics. Blood group A apparently protects against cholera and it seems likely that B and O groups were associated with a lower incidence of smallpox. Evidence exists also that a deficiency of complement components

C5–9 is associated with susceptibility to meningococcal meningitis. There is a suggestion that selection for malaria acts through the HLA system. Selection via communicable diseases might in fact form a parallel with the spread of the sickle-cell gene in relation to *Plasmodium falciparum* malaria.

Environmental Factors

Environmental factors are difficult to delineate. There is evidence that the sharp fall in the overall incidence of communicable disease in the UK during the 19th century coincided with the rise in cotton imports; because cotton clothes are more easily washed than woollen ones, it has been suggested that the explanation might lie here. One fact is clear and that is that whereas the incidence of *genetically* determined diseases in the UK has remained virtually unchanged for the last 100 years, infections have become far less common. In the developing countries of the 'Third World' however, infections of all types remain exceedingly common, and underlying these is a less obvious mass of non-communicable disease.*

WORLD DISTRIBUTION OF INFECTION

The prevalence of infections depends first and foremost on the underlying state of the public health and sanitation; as these improve, the overall incidence of infectious disease declines. Lindow man, who was discovered in 1984 in Cheshire, England, having been submerged in a peat bog for some 2000 years, was shown to be infected with *Ascaris lumbricoides* and *Trichuris trichiura*, parasites now unusual in the UK. Tuberculosis is another example. Cholera, typhoid and malaria were also commonplace infections in the UK during the 19th century (*see* p. 4). A few diseases are more common where ambient temperatures are high. However, in the latter 20th century, any disease can occur anywhere in the world; air transport is now so rapid that exotic diseases from a tropical country can present in a temperate one which has high standards of hygiene and sanitation.

Of viral diseases, the viral hepatitides and rabies are examples

*Hutt M. S. R., Burkitt D. P. (1986). *The Geography of Non-infectious Disease*, p. 164. Oxford: Oxford University Press.

which are more prevalent throughout tropical and subtropical countries; many of the viral encephalitides, however, have limited areas of distribution—the viral haemorrhagic fevers are more common in equatorial Africa (and to a lesser extent south America), while dengue fever tends to be predominantly a southeast Asian problem. Whereas many rickettsial diseases occur worldwide (e.g. Q fever, and flea- and louse-borne typhus), others, such as tick typhus are more common in Africa, while the mite-borne variety (Tsutsugamushi fever) is more common in south-east Asia and the Pacific. Many bacterial infections also are overall more common in tropical and subtropical countries, e.g. anthrax, tetanus, typhoid fever, cholera, shigellosis, brucellosis, diphtheria, leptospirosis and leprosy. Meningococcal disease, relapsing fever and plague, however, have limited areas of distribution. Superficial fungal infections are especially common in the humid tropics, while histoplasmosis and the deep mycoses have limited geographical distributions. Protozoan diseases too can be either widespread (e.g. amoebiasis), or they may have specific areas of distribution (e.g. African and south American trypanosomiasis, and visceral and cutaneous leishmaniasis). Helminthic diseases have their own characteristic distribution: whereas hookworm, *Ascaris lumbricoides* and *Trichuris trichiura* infections occur in all parts of the tropics and subtropics, various species of schistosomes and filariae, as well as clonorchiasis and opisthorchiasis, have their own well delineated geographical areas.

SOME EPIDEMIOLOGICAL ASPECTS OF COMMUNICABLE DISEASE IN THE UK

Table 1.2 summarises some diseases which in the UK have shown significant change or have remained constant in incidence rate over the last few decades. With some of them, introduction of vaccination has contributed to a decline. Poliomyelitis can still be contracted overseas; approximately 20 cases have occurred in the UK over the last 15 years. Measles has been reduced to about 20% compared with the prevaccination level. Viral hepatitis showed a great decline but increased sharply during the early 1980s; this was to some extent associated with transmission of HAV by shellfish. A marked increase in HBV in drug abusers was also an important factor; however, there is now good evidence that this has begun to decline (in 1985–86), probably as a result of

Table 1.2

EXAMPLES OF COMMUNICABLE DISEASES WHICH HAVE CHANGED IN PREVALENCE IN THE UK DURING THE LAST FEW DECADES

Prevalence	Communicable disease
Declined	Poliomyelitis Measles Viral hepatitis 'Scarlet fever' Diphtheria Tetanus Tuberculosis
Constant	Rubella Chickenpox Mumps Respiratory infections Typhoid Meningococcal meningitis Pneumococcal meningitis

Increased	Food-poisoning
	  Salmonellae
	  Rotavirus (<2 years old)
	  Campylobacter jejuni
	  Cryptosporidium spp.
	Acute haemorrhagic conjunctivitis
	Chlamydia trachomatis
	Delta hepatitis (HDV) (see p. 102)
	Dengue
	Pertussis
	Hantaan virus (muroid nephropathy)
	Fifth disease (see p. 42)
	Haemophilus influenzae (including meningitis)
	Botulism
	Legionella pneumophila
	Lyme disease (see p. 256)
	Group B streptococcus
	'Toxic shock syndrome'
	Malaria
	AIDS

publicity given to the high incidence of HIV infection in drug abusers. The reason for the sharp decline in incidence of 'scarlet fever' is unclear; it was to some extent influenced by the introduction of antibiotics. Tuberculosis continues to be present in the elderly and immigrant population; a focus for childhood infection still exists, therefore.

Of the infections which have increased significantly, many are of a gastrointestinal nature; many factors in addition to travel are important. *Campylobacter* is often associated with contaminated milk and water; *Cryptosporidium spp.* infection is largely a zoonotic disease but in addition, water transmission might be important. Zoonotic salmonellae, especially *Salmonella spp.* (e.g. *S. typhimurium*) have recently increased as causes of food poisoning. Of those not primarily involving the gastrointestinal tract, HIV (and the acquired immune deficiency syndrome (AIDS)) is becoming a major problem. Malaria is running at its highest rate in the UK since the 1920s!

ZOONOTIC DISEASES

Zoonotic diseases can be defined as: those diseases and infections for which the causative agent(s) is naturally transmitted between other vertebrates and man. Table 1.3 summarises some of the important human diseases. Domestic pets are a significant source of disease. Although more than 100 zoonotic diseases can be acquired from pets, only about 10–20 occur in the UK.

Of the viral zoonoses, rabies undoubtedly causes the most severe disease; this is transmitted not only by dog bites but a whole range of mammals. *Herpes simiae* is transmitted by bites from macaques, which are often asymptomatic. Psittacosis (ornithosis) is caused by *Chlamydia psittaci*, present in a whole range of birds and mammals. In birds it causes a range of illnesses from conjunctivitis to a severe disease with respiratory signs, diarrhoea and weakness. In man, the clinical disease varies from an atypical pneumonia to a non-specific fever—a 'flu'-like illness; tetracycline is effective in its treatment. Between 1975–84, 2561 cases were reported in England and Wales, and only 20% had had contact with birds. *Salmonella spp.*, *Shigella spp.* and *Campylobacter spp.* can all be transmitted by animals; they are usually acquired by eating infected foodstuffs and cause enteritis in man. *Yersinia pseudotuberculosis* is a rare disease in man, but can be acquired from captive

Table 1.3

SOME ZOONOTIC DISEASES WHICH CAN BE TRANSMITTED BY DOMESTIC PETS

Infective agent	Organism/disease (source of infection)	Clinical manifestation(s)
Virus	Rabies, *Herpes simiae* (dogs, other mammals)	Rabies (hydrophobia)
Rickettsia	Psittacosis (birds, mammals)	Atypical pneumonia; non-specific 'flu'-like illness
Bacteria	*Salmonella spp.* *Shigella spp.* *Campylobacter spp.*	Acute gastroenteritis
	Yersinia pseudotuberculosis	Mesenteric lymphadenitis
Fungus	Ringworm (dogs)	
Parasite	Toxocariasis (dogs, cats)	Choroidoretinitis, systemic illness
	Toxoplasmosis (cats, etc)	Lymphadenopathy, choroidoretinitis, general malaise, congenital abnormalities
	Hydatidosis (dogs)	Hydatid cysts in many organs
	Cryptosporidium spp. (calves, etc)	Acute gastroenteritis
Arthropod	Fleas (dogs, cats, etc)	Pruritus (Black death)
'Allergic'	Fur, feathers, scurf	Asthma, rhinitis, urticaria, bird breeders' or bird fanciers' lung

birds, rodents and small primates which are exposed to infection from wild birds and rats; this bacterium causes mesenteric lymphadenitis, usually in young children. Ringworm is usually caused by *Microsporum canis*. Although in England and Wales only 300 cases are reported annually, it has been estimated that more than 9000 cases per year are probably caused by dogs alone.

Larvae of *Toxocara canis* and *Toxocara spp.* are responsible for toxocariasis. Eggs, which are excreted in dog faeces, can survive in soil for several years. Infection can take place directly from dogs and cats, or via contaminated soil. Human disease is caused by migration of second-stage larvae through the liver, mesenteric lymph-nodes, lung and most importantly the eye and brain. Blindness, especially in children, is the most serious sequel of infection: between 1975–84, 107 cases were reported in England and Wales, but this is undoubtedly an underestimate. Prevention is by exclusion of dogs and cats from children's playgrounds, together with rigorous anthelmintic treatment of dogs. Serological studies indicate that almost half the adult UK population has been in contact with the protozoan *Toxoplasma gondii*. The definitive hosts of *T. gondii* are the genera *Felis* and *Lynx*; intermediate stages occur in a wide range of animals and man. Cats become infected by eating flesh infected with *T. gondii* and they excrete oocysts for up to 5 weeks; these form sporocysts which can survive in soil for 18 months. Man is infected by accidental ingestion of oocysts or by eating raw meat. Clinically, it causes lymphadenopathy, choroidoretinitis and general malaise (*see* Chapter 15); infection during pregnancy may cause neonatal death, hydrocephalus, and CNS and ocular disease. Prevention is by thorough cooking of meat, the prevention of cats eating vermin and raw meat, and avoidance of contact with oocyst-excreting cats during pregnancy. Between 1975–84, 7239 cases of this zoonosis were reported in England and Wales.

Hydatidosis is acquired by ingesting eggs of the tapeworm *Echinococcus granulosus*: the host is the dog which acquires infection by ingesting meat (from sheep, cattle and horses) containing the larval cysts. In man, hydatid cysts can form in any organ. Prevention is by careful disposal of infected meat and offal, elimination of stray dogs, and the administration of praziquantel to pet dogs. Between 1975–84, 42 deaths were reported in England and Wales.

Cryptosporidium spp. usually causes an acute gastroenteritis. As well as being a zoonosis, person-to-person transmission is now known to be important. The importance of a canine reservoir for *Giardia lamblia* is to date unclear.

Although fleas can cause significant disease, this is rarely of a serious nature in the UK. Unlike the human flea, *Pulex irritans*, few animal fleas can survive on man for more than a few days. Although mange mites (*Sarcoptes spp.* and *Notoedres cati*) can infect man, they usually fail to establish themselves permanently.

Many of these diseases (e.g. *Cryptosporidium spp.* and *T. gondii*) can be especially severe in immunosuppressed and immunodepressed patients including those with AIDS (*see* Chapter 11).

VECTORS IN THE TRANSMISSION OF INFECTION

Molluscs

When eaten, some molluscs produce human infection because bacteria and viruses are concentrated in them by filter feeding; bivalves, oysters, mussels and clams are examples. Some parasites (e.g. schistosomes) utilise the snail as a first and/or second intermediate host for their larval stages; usually, the parasite enters the human host by skin penetration. Alternatively transmission can occur through raw or poorly cooked snails. Table 1.4 summarises some human diseases which are conveyed by molluscs. Prevention of human contact with infected molluscs is the obvious way of breaking the life-cycle; however, few of these measures can be forcibly brought about and they are therefore largely ineffective. Four main mechanisms exist for snail control:

(i) *Snail removal.* This may be either mechanical or manual.
(ii) *Snail control.* This may be achieved by manipulation of the environment.
(iii) *Molluscicides.* These include: copper sulphate, sodium pen-

Table 1.4

SOME MOLLUSC-TRANSMITTED DISEASES OF MAN

Disease	*Common parasite*	*Mollusc (genus)*
Schistosomiasis	*Schistosoma haematobium*	*Bulinus spp.*
	S. mansoni	*Biomphalaria spp.*
	S. japonicum	*Oncomelania spp.*
Clonorchiasis	*Clonorchis sinensis*	*Bithynia spp.*
Opisthorchiasis	*Opisthorchis spp.*	*Bithynia spp.*
Fascioliasis	*Fasciola hepatica*	*Lymnaea spp.*
	F. gigantica	
Paragonimiasis	*Paragonimus westermani*	*Semisulcospira spp.*
		Thiara spp.
Fasciolopsiasis	*Fasciolopsis buski*	*Hippeutis spp.*
Gastrodisciasis	*Gastrodiscoides hominis*	*Helicorbis spp.*
Heterophyiasis	*Heterophyes heterophyes*	*Pirenella conica*
Metagonimiasis	*Metagonimus yokogawai*	*Thiara granifera*

tachlorophenate, niclosamide, N-tritylmorpholine and preparations of plant origin.
(iv) *Biological control.* Competitive or predator species can be utilised.

Ticks and Mites

Ticks

Approximately 100 of over 800 tick species are known to transmit infectious agents to man or to cause toxin-induced irritation after a bite. Transovarial survival of infective agents is a relatively common occurrence in ticks. In most cases the infective agents normally circulate among ticks, livestock and/or wildlife; humans are occasional hosts. Many organisms produce benign infections in wildlife, but more serious disease in livestock and humans. The relapsing fevers, Colorado tick fever, Q fever, Rocky Mountain spotted fever, Kyasanur forest disease, and Lyme disease are some of the diseases transmitted by soft ticks. African tick typhus, Crimean-Congo haemorrhagic fever, yellow fever, together with Colorado tick fever are transmitted by hard ticks.

Mites

More than 30 000 species of mite have been described. Those of medical importance are responsible for the transmission of: scrub and murine typhus, rickettsialpox, Q fever, tularaemia, plague and several arboviruses, dermatitis, and house dust allergy. Chigger bites too are a widespread problem in tropical countries.

Insects

The importance of insects in the transmission of disease was first recognised by Manson in 1877; he demonstrated the developmental stage of *Wuchereria bancrofti* (one of the nematodes responsible for lymphatic filariasis) in the mosquito. Since then, many infective agents—viruses, rickettsiae, bacteria and protozoa as well as nematodes have been shown to be transmitted by insects. Table 1.5 summarises some diseases which are transmitted by insects. Transmission of disease to man can be by mechanical or

Table 1.5

SOME EXAMPLES OF INSECT-TRANSMITTED DISEASES

Pathogen	Organism	Disease	Vector
Viruses	HBV	Hepatitis B	Bed bugs
	Phlebovirus	Sandfly fever	Fly
	Flavivirus	Yellow fever	Mosquito
	Dengue virus	Dengue	Mosquito
Rickettsiae	*Rickettsia typhi*	Murine typhus	Flea
	R. prowazekii	Epidemic typhus	Lice
	R. quintana	Trench fever	Lice
	Borrelia recurrentis	Epidemic relapsing fever	Lice
Bacteria	*Yersinia pestis*	Plague	Flea
	Bartonella bacilliformis	Bartonellosis	Fly
	Bacillus anthracis	Anthrax	Fly
Protozoa	*Plasmodium spp.*	Malaria	Mosquito
	Trypanosoma cruzi	Chagas' disease	Reduviid bug
	T. rhodesiense	Sleeping sickness	Tsetse fly
	Leishmania donovani	Kala azar	Fly
	L. tropica	Oriental sore	Fly
	L. brasiliensis	Mucocutaneous leishmaniasis	Fly
Helminths	*Wuchereria bancrofti*	Lymphatic filariasis	Mosquito
	Brugia malayi	Lymphatic filariasis	Mosquito
	Mansonella ozzardi	Filariasis	Fly
	M. perstans	Filariasis	Fly
	Onchocerca volvulus	River blindness	Black fly
	Dipylidium caninum	Dog tapeworm	Flea

biological means; spread by house flies is an example of the former, and malaria (in which the parasite undergoes development within the mosquito vector) of the latter. Resurgence of malaria, leishmaniasis, yellow fever and dengue haemorrhagic fever is largely attributable to increased insect propagation of the infective agents. In a tropical context, therefore, elimination of insects which are important vectors of disease would reduce significantly the incidence of many diseases. In practice, this is difficult; of methods used, collecting and trapping, environmental control, insecticides, and biological and genetic control have been used. Only on rare occasions have such preventive programmes been successful; elimination of malaria from Sri Lanka was one such success (albeit only temporarily). Unfortunately insects show no respect for international frontiers!

INFECTIONS IN SPECIAL GROUPS AND CIRCUMSTANCES

Hospital Acquired Infection

Hospital infections include those:

(i) acquired while in hospital—*nosocomial* (*see* Table 1.6);
(ii) introduced into a hospital, having been acquired in the 'community'.

In Britain, about half of all infections occurring in in-patients fall into group (ii); furthermore, from 8–16% of hospital patients acquire infections while in hospital. In orthopaedic and cardiac surgery such infections may have especially disastrous consequences. Gram-negative infections have greatly increased in

Table 1.6

SOME NOSOCOMIAL INFECTIONS AND THEIR CAUSES

Bacteria	
Gram-positive	
Staph. aureus	Surgical/skin sepsis
Strep. pneumoniae	Lower respiratory infections (e.g. postoperative pneumonias)
Gram-negative	
Escherichia coli	
Bacteroides spp.	Disease, surgery or instrumentation of
Klebsiella spp.	gastrointestinal or genitourinary tracts
Proteus spp.	
Pseudomonas spp.	
Legionella pneumophila	Unusual in presence of intact immunity
Mycobacterium tuberculosis	
Fungi and viruses	Unusual (e.g. HBV)
Protozoa	Rare

recent years; they may give rise to 'septicaemic shock'. Legionnaire's disease also can be a major problem (*see* Chapter 7). Members of hospital staff also are occasionally at risk from infection, e.g. tuberculosis and viral hepatitis (HBV).

Fig. 1.1 summarises some of the factors which determine whether a patient will acquire a nosocomial infection. Fig. 1.2 summarises the main routes of infection; self-, cross- and environmental-infection. As well as the common pathogens, opportunistic infections (*see* p. 21) can cause problems. Impairment of *local* defence mechanisms includes breaking of skin and mucosal surfaces, e.g. surgery, trauma, burns, pressure sores, varicose ulcer, intravenous infusions, insertion of intravenous lines, and instrumentation of gastrointestinal, genitourinary and respiratory tracts. (Local immunoglobulin A, and inhibitory factors—fatty acids and lysozymes—normally contribute to an effective local barrier.) Impairment in *general* host defences can result from extremes of age, nature of the disease process (e.g. immunosuppression in lymphomas, or immunodepression in AIDS sufferers) and chemotherapy (e.g. immunosuppression, cytotoxic therapy).

Many procedures and policies to attempt to reduce the likelihood of hospital acquired infection exist. Careful sterilisation and disinfection of contaminated items, disposal of infected rubbish

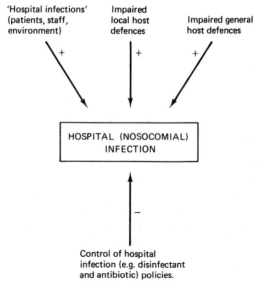

Fig. 1.1. A summary of the main routes of infection.

General Principles 17

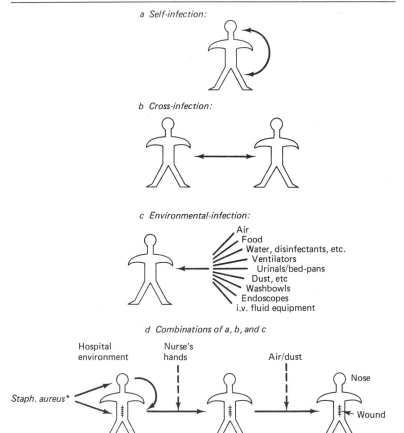

Staph. aureus is the most common cause of Gram-positive hospital infections, and is usually associated with skin sepsis.

Fig. 1.2. Some of the factors determining whether a patient will acquire a nosocomial infection.

and linen, aseptic operating techniques, ward procedures for wound dressing, urinary catheterisation, the setting-up of an intravenous 'drip' or line, and various biopsy procedures are all important. Source isolation of infected and protective isolation of highly susceptible patients, administration of appropriate antibiotics for certain surgical procedures, and the use of an agreed policy (usually in conjunction with a microbiologist) for treating certain infections are other lines of control. Education of staff in hospital hygiene, good staff health facilities, and a microbiology department of excellence in order to make an exact diagnosis are essential. These procedures must all be coordinated by the Control or Infection Officer with the assistance of a trained Infection Control Nurse; full cooperation from junior medical microbiology staff is also essential. A Control of Infection Committee is of great value in designing and implementing hospital policies.

Urinary catheterisation accounts for a very high rate of nosocomial infections; this is especially so when carried out on a long-term basis, e.g. in paraplegic patients. Wound infections are a major problem after surgery on the mouth, colon, gall bladder and vagina. Where the operation site is already infected at the time of surgery (e.g. incision of an abscess), infection rates are especially high. Appropriate antibiotic therapy before operation is of value, e.g. metronidazole preceding colonic surgery, and benzyl penicillin + cloxacillin (to reduce *Clostridium perfringens* infections) before lower limb amputation and major hip surgery. Careful surveillance is necessary to recognise wound sepsis early. Phage-typing of *Staphylococcus aureus* by the microbiologist is essential in management; if a carrier of an epidemic strain is identified among hospital staff, he or she may have to cease work with surgical patients temporarily until the infection has cleared. Where *Staph. aureus* strains are resistant to methicillin and gentamicin, temporary closure of surgical wards is occasionally necessary as part of the control programme.

Hospital acquired infections are a special problem in intensive care units. Gram-positive (e.g. pneumococci and staphylococci) and Gram-negative (e.g. coliforms, *Haemophilus*, *Pseudomonas* and *Bacteroides spp.*) infections of the respiratory tract are a major problem. Widespread use of antibiotics such as ampicillin + cloxacillin tends to select out *Klebsiella, Pseudomonas* and *Serratia*. Infections of intravenous infusion sites and central venous lines which are potentially life-threatening can also be a major problem; there are numerous routes for infection. Skilled setting-up and maintenance of 'drips' by trained 'i.v. teams' reduces significantly the incidence of infection.

Tuberculosis

Before starting hospital employment, staff should be given BCG when tuberculin-negative, as well as undergoing chest radiography. Despite this, staff in close contact with 'open' cases of tuberculosis should receive adequate follow-up; this applies also to patient contacts.

Viral hepatitis

Hepatitis B (HBV) infections have occurred from time-to-time in renal dialysis units. Staff who have negative serology for HBV infections should be vaccinated; they are included in the list of priority groups for HBV vaccination (*see* Chapter 6). Care in avoidance of skin or eye contact with blood from any patient, especially HB_sAg carriers, is essential.

Acquired immune deficiency syndrome (AIDS)

Evidence that the transmission of HIV infection has occurred from needle-stick injury within hospitals is scanty; however, extreme care when dealing with blood and other tissue fluids, which are likely to be infected, is essential (*see* Chapter 11).

Infection in Pregnancy

Risks from communicable disease to the pregnant woman are now much less in the developed world than they were in the preantibiotic era; puerperal sepsis, which carried a high mortality rate well into the 20th century, and infections such as pyelonephritis are now rare. Puerperal sepsis is usually caused by a Lancefield group A haemolytic streptococcus which spreads rapidly within the soft tissues of the genital tract causing a fatal septicaemia and frequently death within 24–48 h; *Clostridium perfringens*, *Bacteroides spp.* and *Escherichia coli* may also be responsible. However, these hazards are still present in developing countries; spontaneous abortion, premature labour, still-birth and congenital and perinatal infections are all common. Maternal endocarditis can complicate cardiac disease, most frequently during or shortly after labour. Septic abortion, following criminal interference may still be followed by a *Clostridium perfringens* infection.

Many infections are more likely to produce fetal abnormalities if they occur during the first trimester of pregnancy; the earlier infection occurs in pregnancy the higher the risk of *multiple* congenital defects. Some of these infections are summarised in Table 1.7. When infection is acquired during the first trimester, termination of pregnancy (with all of the ethical issues which it involves) should be considered.

Neonatal (Perinatal) Infection

Low birth-weight babies are especially vulnerable to infection as a result of their immature phagocytic, humoral and cellular

Table 1.7

SOME IMPORTANT CONGENITAL INFECTIONS

Organism	Result of infection	Route of infection*
Viruses		
Rubella	Congenital rubella	P
Herpes simplex (type II)	Neonatal herpes simplex	N
Varicella zoster	Congenital varicella	N; P
CMV	Congenital cytomegalovirus disease	P
HBV	Congenital HBV infection	N; ? P
Chlamydiae		
Chlamydia trachomatis (TRIC agent)	Ophthalmia neonatorum, Neonatal pneumonia	N
Bacteria		
Neisseria gonorrhoeae	Ophthalmia neonatorum	N
Treponema pallidum	Congenital syphilis	P
Listeria monocytogenes	Listeriosis	N
Fungi		
Candida albicans	Neonatal oral thrush	N
Protozoa		
Toxoplasma gondii	Congenital toxoplasmosis (retinopathy)	P

*P = transplacental infection; N = neonatal infection acquired before or during delivery.

immune defence mechanisms. IgM production begins only at about 20 weeks into fetal life; IgG is derived entirely from the maternal circulation, via the transplacental route. The risk of neonatal infection is therefore greatest when the pregnancy has not reached full term. The most common organisms are Lancefield B haemolytic streptococci and Gram-negative bacilli, including *E. coli*, *Klebsiella aerogenes* and *Pseudomonas aeruginosa*. *Staph. aureus* (usually penicillin resistant) is a frequent cause of minor neonatal sepsis, and can occasionally produce more serious infection; an infected umbilical stump can give rise both to portal venous thrombosis and tetanus—relatively common events in most developing countries. Neonatal gastroenteritis can be a major problem in maternity and neonatal units; enteropathogenic or enterotoxigenic *E. coli*, *Salmonella spp.* and *Campylobacter* have been implicated. Necrotising enterocolitis (which carries a high mortality rate) is a rare complication in low birth-weight neonates.

Table 1.7 also summarises some of the perinatally transmitted infections which can produce congenital abnormalities. Specific preventive measures can be used in the neonate against HBV, gonococcal ophthalmia neonatorum, herpes simplex (type II) and varicella zoster infections.

Opportunistic Infection in the Immunocompromised Patient

The group of infections frequently termed 'opportunistic', constitutes a major source of illness in immunocompromised individuals; several may be present simultaneously. Those affected include: individuals on immunosuppressive drugs or receiving radiotherapy, and those with reticuloses, lymphomas, etc, but the major disease entity now affected is AIDS (*see* Chapter 11). These organisms are usually of low pathogenicity and can produce severe disease only in the presence of immunosuppression; the illness produced in the immunosuppressed patient is atypical when compared to that in an individual with intact immunity. Furthermore, these infections are often exceedingly difficult (and sometimes impossible) to treat in the immunosuppressed patient. Many are summarised in Chapter 11; although treatment is basically the same as that used in the otherwise healthy individual (if required at all), prolonged courses are frequently ineffective.

Anaerobic Infections

Predisposing factors to anaerobic infection include: trauma, presence of a foreign body, ischaemia (and/or gangrene) and presence of other organisms which lower the oxidation–reduction potential, e.g. *E. coli*. Bacteria involved can only grow under *anaerobic* conditions, and can be divided into non-sporing and spore-forming anaerobes.

Non-sporing anaerobes

This group includes: *Bacteroides fragilis*, *Bacteroides melaninogenicus* and *Fusiformis spp.* (Gram-negative), anaerobic cocci and *Actinomycetes israelii* (Gram-positive). They form an important component of the normal flora of the mouth, colon, lower female genital tract and skin. In addition to factors already mentioned, impaired immunity and debilitating conditions, broad-spectrum antibiotic therapy, and damaged tissue in the presence of a prosthesis, predispose to infection. Laboratory isolation of the organism is difficult if metronidazole has previously been given. *Bacteroides fragilis* infections can give rise to: endotoxic shock, renal failure, endocarditis, jaundice, suppurative thrombophlebitis and embolism, and metastatic abscesses. Treatment (*see* Chapter 16) consists of surgical drainage of pus, and either metronidazole or clindamycin; penicillin is active against *Actinomycetes*.

Spore-forming anaerobes

There are many species of clostridia, e.g. *Clostridium perfringens*, *Clostridium tetani* (which causes tetanus) and *Clostridium difficile* (the main cause of pseudomembranous colitis). They are found amongst faecal flora of man and other mammals and are also common in the environment, especially soil and dust, etc. The spores are highly resistant and can survive for many years; they resist drying, many chemical disinfectants and are not always killed by boiling water at 100°C. *Clostridium perfringens* can be responsible for gas-gangrene, food-poisoning, necrotising jejunitis and clostridial septic abortion. Gas-gangrene is a complication of war injuries and other traumas in which spores enter a deep wound; spores from the patient's own faecal flora may also enter surgical wounds. Untreated, this condition is associated with a high mortality rate. Treatment consists of hyperbaric oxygen, removal of dead and infected tissue by surgery, and penicillin (gentamicin and cloxacillin are often given to cover accompanying organisms). Administration of antitoxin is probably of value also.

NUTRITION–INFECTION INTERACTIONS: A VICIOUS CYCLE

In most developing countries, the interaction of malnutrition, malabsorption and infection constitutes the leading cause of morbidity and mortality; frequently 50% or more are dead before 5 years of age. Apart from young children, pregnant and lactating women are particularly vulnerable; the outcome of pregnancy and subsequent physical and mental development of the fetus and infant may be jeopardised. All infections impart a nutritional cost to the host; fever, anorexia, tachypnoea, congested nasal passages and cough lead either to excessive energy utilisation (and catabolism), or to reduced food intake. Intestinal infections can lead to malabsorption; parasites are often involved. Accompanying the malabsorption, loss of nutrients may result from vomiting and excessive perspiration. Protein requirement is also increased during infection; therefore, gradual depletion of muscle occurs due to a 'stress reaction' mediated via adrenocortical hormones.

Malnutrition also has an adverse effect on the host's *response* to infection. Physical barriers to infection, e.g. mucosal surfaces of the gums and oral cavity, and epithelial coverings of the eye and respiratory and gastrointestinal tracts, are compromised. Antibody response to some infections can be depressed, e.g. in typhoid, diphtheria and yellow fever. Leucocyte function may be compromised. Cell-mediated immunity (CMI) is depressed by depletion of lymphoid tissue (in severe protein/energy malnutrition); this can affect tuberculosis and certain fungal, viral and bacterial infections. Furthermore, depressed CMI prevents a satisfactory response to immunisations, e.g. BCG against tuberculosis; the tuberculin test is often negative. Zinc, folic acid and pyridoxine deficiencies can also depress by CMI. Some serum proteins, e.g. transferrin and lactoferrin are markedly reduced by malnutrition; *free* iron promotes bacterial growth, resulting in sepsis. The complement system can be deleted, leading to worsening of some viral and bacterial infections.

Childhood measles is an excellent example in which this vicious cycle operates. Diarrhoea occurring at the time of weaning is a further example. Borderline nutritional status may be accompanied by malabsorption and frank malnutrition may ensue. On the contrary, some data indicate a relative suppression of infection by malnutrition; this applies to malaria and ascariasis.

Therefore, in developing countries, nutritional status must be improved by continued attention to environmental sanitation, immunisation programmes and early treatment of infection; similarly, underlying nutritional status must be improved in order to obtain control of infection and optimal vaccination responses. More overall joint effort is required therefore to improve nutrition and to eliminate infection.

PYREXIA OF UNDETERMINED ORIGIN (PUO)

An undiagnosed fever of 10 days or more is frequently referred to as a PUO; if present for a few days only it is sometimes called an 'acute' PUO, and after 3 weeks this becomes a 'chronic' PUO! Infections account for three-quarters of acute and approximately one-quarter of chronic PUOs. Table 1.8 summarises many of the overall causes, and Table 1.9 causes of chronic PUO.

When a PUO is present, a history of overseas travel must always be sought; furthermore, the exact location of visits must be documented. A precise record of malaria prophylaxis (if any) is essential. Ethnic status should be recorded. Other information of relevance includes: occupation, possible contact with animals (including pets) and individuals with infectious diseases, and a dietary history including consumption of uncooked fish, meat and unpasteurised milk (or milk products). Recent antibiotic usage is important. A detailed history of hetero- and homosexual contacts and hardline drugs is now mandatory. A full and careful clinical examination—which includes oral, genital and rectal examination—is also essential.

The extent to which laboratory investigation can aid a definitive diagnosis varies enormously; in developing countries few tests can be carried out. The value of bone marrow culture should not be underestimated; liver and lymph-node biopsy (with culture) can also give valuable results. Occasionally, a therapeutic trial of a specific antimicrobial agent is justified in a sick patient in whom

Table 1.8

SOME INFECTIVE CAUSES OF PYREXIA OF UNDETERMINED ORIGIN

Non-specific causes
Hidden abscess ('sepsis')	Liver and biliary tract, abdomen, pelvis, retroperitoneal or mediastinal
Endocarditis	
Urinary tract infection	
Dental, ear or nasal sinus infections	

Specific causes
Viral	Myxoviruses, adenoviruses, enteroviruses, EBV, CMV, HAV, HBV, sandfly fever, yellow fever, Lassa fever
Bacterial	Typhoid and paratyphoid, brucellosis, Legionnaire's disease, secondary syphilis, tuberculosis, leptospirosis, relapsing fever, nocardiosis, Q fever
Rickettsial	Typhus
Chlamydial	Psittacosis, cat-scratch fever
Fungal	Candidiasis, cryptococcosis, histoplasmosis, aspergillosis
Protozoan	Malaria, amoebiasis, toxoplasmosis, visceral leishmaniasis, trypanosomiasis, pneumocystosis
Helminthic	Toxocariasis, filariasis, fascioliasis

a definitive diagnosis has not been made, but in whom there is suggestive evidence of a particular infection. Examples are: tuberculosis (usually extrapulmonary), typhoid, typhus and endocarditis. Occasionally, malaria and visceral leishmaniasis fall into this category. Only very rarely should corticosteroids be administered to a patient suffering from a PUO.

DIAGNOSTIC TECHNIQUES

In the majority of cases infective (including tropical) diseases can be diagnosed from a well-obtained history (*see* p. 24) and careful physical examination; however, good laboratory back-up is more

Table 1.9

INFECTIVE CAUSES OF CHRONIC PYREXIA OF UNDETERMINED ORIGIN

Non-specific causes
  Endocarditis (*see* Chapter 8) ⎫
  Hepato-biliary sepsis ⎬ Pyogenic sepsis
  Intra-abdominal abscess(es) ⎬
  Pyelonephritis (*see* Chapter 10) ⎭

Specific causes
Bacterial	Brucellosis
	Tuberculosis
	Gonorrhoea
Chlamydial	Psittacosis
Parasitic	Malaria

important here than in most areas within clinical medicine. Molecular biology has not yet proved of great value; however, it is likely to improve the speed and accuracy of diagnosis by detecting microbial antigen and nucleic acids in clinical specimens by the use of monoclonal antibodies and DNA probes, respectively.

Microbiological

Satisfactory safeguards are essential when dealing with dangerous pathogens; where there is a likelihood of HBV or HIV infections, laboratory techniques must be exceptionally rigid. In patients from west Africa in whom blood films prove negative for malaria parasites, the possibility of Lassa fever should always be considered. Multiple blood cultures are essential when dealing with a febrile illness of undiagnosed cause, e.g. typhoid and brucellosis. Bone marrow culture is often of value when a diagnosis of *Salmonella typhi* is being considered; this is also a valuable technique in several other infections. Liver biopsy is of value not only histologically, but also when miliary tuberculosis is under consideration; culture may reveal *Mycobacterium tuberculosis*. Lumbar puncture (cerebrospinal fluid examination) is crucial for the accurate diagnosis of bacterial meningitis. However, this should only be undertaken when there is certainty that the intracranial pressure is normal. When a *Cryptococcus neoformans* infection is suspected, cerebrospinal fluid should be stained with Indian ink.

Parasitological

In searching for malaria parasites, thick and thin blood films should be stained with Giemsa. Other peripheral blood parasites include: trypanosomes (also in cerebrospinal fluid), filariae and *Borrelia spp.* (relapsing fever). Day and night blood films should be examined for microfilariae; *Wuchereria bancrofti* is nocturnal, and *Loa loa* diurnal. Bone marrow examination and/or splenic fluid (from puncture) are crucial in the diagnosis of visceral leishmaniasis.

Faecal samples should be examined in the fresh state; only then will active motile trophozoites of *Entamoeba histolytica* be recognised. Cysts tend to be excreted in a cyclical pattern; therefore, at least 3 and preferably 6 samples should be examined to exclude an infection. Concentration techniques are of value when searching for protozoan cysts and eggs and larvae of helminths. Quantitative egg counts may give valuable information. Both a rectal swab and the 'Sellotape' technique (in which a strip of adhesive tape is placed over the anus, subsequently removed and stuck to a microscope slide) are of value in searching for *Enterobius vermicularis*. Small intestinal aspirates (mucus gives the highest yield) can reveal parasites—especially *Giardia lamblia*, *Strongyloides stercoralis* and hookworms. The 'Enterotest' (string test) is also of value. After an overnight fast, a nylon thread, to which a gelatin capsule is attached, is swallowed by the patient and withdrawn after 4–5 h; the distal end of the thread is then smeared on to a microscope slide and the mucus examined for parasites.

In searching for *Schistosoma haematobium* an end-stream urine specimen (preferably the first of the day) gives the best chance of a positive result. *S. mansoni* and *S. japonicum* eggs are most often found in a rectal biopsy or a colonic polyp.

In cutaneous leishmaniasis, an aspirate or biopsy from the periphery of the lesion often reveals leishmania organisms. Skin snips for *Onchocerca volvulus* should be examined in the fresh state after being taken from sites most likely to be affected: buttocks and lower legs (Africa), and head, shoulders and trunk (central America).

Sputum may be examined for *Paragonimus westermani* eggs. Lymph node fluid is of value in the diagnosis of trypanosomiasis and lymphatic filariasis. In trichinosis (trichinellosis) infection, muscle biopsy may be of value. In *Trypanosoma cruzi* infection, xenodiagnosis is sometimes diagnostic.

Serological

In the diagnosis of an acute febrile illness, a serum sample at admission should be obtained, paired with a further sample after 10 days or so, and a 'rising titre' sought; serological diagnosis of cytomegalovirus (CMV) and Epstein-Barr virus (EBV) infections, Q fever and brucellosis is usually clear-cut. Typhoid serology (Widal) is only rarely of value diagnostically.

Various serological reactions are used to detect antibody and/or antigen from a present or past parasitic infection: complement fixation (CF), agglutination, indirect immunofluorescence (IIF) and agar gel tests have been used for many years. Recently, the enzyme-linked immunosorbent assay (ELISA) and radioimmunoassay (RIA) have been developed for use in parasitic infections. Table 1.10 summarises some of the serological tests currently in use. The ELISA in particular gives a high degree of sensitivity and specificity; however, some cross-reaction between different parasitic antigens still exists—filariasis and strongyloidiasis is a case in point. Tests with a relatively low level of reactivity, e.g. immunoelectrophoresis (IE) and counter-current immunoelectrophoresis (CIE) are sometimes of value in the diagnosis of a current infection in which other tests are 'oversensitive' and remain positive for long periods of time. For example, when invasive hepatic amoebiasis is suspected, the CIE or CAP are often of greater value than the IIF or ELISA.

These tests do not become positive immediately after infection. Therefore, an amoebic liver 'abscess' or acute schistosomiasis (Katayama fever) may be present before the test becomes positive. In a proportion of cases where there is only mild tissue invasion, results are negative; thus, amoebic colitis is accompanied by positive serology in only some 70% of cases, and in the remainder diagnosis can only be made from the presence of *Entamoeba histolytica* trophozoites in faecal samples.

Serological tests should not replace parasitological techniques in diagnosis; a parasitological (or tissue) diagnosis is the only definitive technique. The schistosomal or filarial ELISA tests do not, for example, differentiate between the various species of parasite.

Table 1.10

SOME SEROLOGICAL TESTS CURRENTLY IN USE FOR THE DIAGNOSIS OF PARASITIC INFECTIONS
(These tests are not usually species specific)

Disease	Test
Malaria *	ELISA; IIF
Amoebiasis	ELISA; CIE; CAP; IIF
Toxoplasmosis	Dye-test
Trypanosomiasis	
African	ELISA; IIF
South American	ELISA; IIF
Leishmaniasis	ELISA; IIF
Schistosomiasis	ELISA; IIF
Filariasis†	ELISA; IIF
Cysticercosis	ELISA; IIF
Fascioliasis	IIF
Trichinosis	IIF
Hydatidosis	ELISA; CF
Toxocariasis	ELISA
Pneumocystosis	IIF

CAP = Cellulose acetate precipitin; CF = Complement fixation; ELISA = Enzyme-linked immunosorbent assay; CIE = Countercurrent immunoelectrophoresis; IIF = Indirect immunofluorescence; *This is of no value in the diagnosis of an acute infection; † Cross-reaction with strongyloidiasis.

FURTHER READING

Brock J. H. (1986). Iron and the outcome of infection. *Brit. Med. J*; **293**: 518–20.
Coates A. R. M. (1986). The impact of molecular biology on the diagnosis and treatment of infection. *J. Infect*; **13**: 217–33.
Cook G. C. (1987). Opportunistic parasitic infections associated with acquired immune deficiency syndrome (AIDS): parasitology, clinical presentation, diagnosis and management. *Q. J. Med*; **65**: (in press).
De Vries R. R. P., Khan P. M., Bernini L. F., Loghem E. van, Rood J. J. van (1979). Genetic control of survival in epidemics. *J. Immunogenet*; **6**: 271–87.
Editorial. (1985). Decline in rheumatic fever. *Lancet*; **2**: 647–8.
Editorial. (1985). Defences against meningococcal infections. *Lancet*; **2**: 929–30.
Editorial. (1985). Splenectomy—a long-term risk of infection. *Lancet*; **2**: 928–9.
Fallon R. J. (1980). Nosocomial infections with *Legionella pneumophila*. *J. Hosp. Infect*; **1**: 299-305.
Kirkwood J. K. (1987). Animals at home—pets as pests: a review. *J. Roy. Soc. Med*; **80**: 97–100.
Relier J. P. (1979). Listeriosis. *J. Antimicrob. Chemother*; **5(A)**: 51–7.

Shepherd J. J. (1983). Tropical myositis: is it an entity and what is its cause? *Lancet*; **2:** 1240–2.
Southwood T. R. E. (1987). The natural environment and disease: an evolutionary perspective. *Brit. Med. J*; **294:** 1086–9.
Valman H. B. (1980). Bacterial infection in the newborn. *Brit. Med. J*; **1:** 772–5.
Wainscoat J. S., Hill A. V. S., Boyce A. L., *et al.* (1985). Evolutionary relationships of human populations from an analysis of nuclear DNA polymorphisms. *Nature*; **319:** 491–3.
Zimran A., Rudensky B., Kramer M. R., *et al.* (1987). Hereditary complement deficiency in survivors of meningococcal disease: high prevalence of C7/C8 deficiency in Sephardic (Moroccan) Jews. *Q. J. Med*; **63:** 349–58.

Chapter Two

Childhood Infections

Although most infections can involve individuals at any age, some assume special importance in the causation of morbidity and mortality in infancy and childhood. Of the diseases covered in this section all can occur in both temperate and tropical areas; however, immunisation programmes have made some of them, e.g. poliomyelitis and diphtheria, unusual in the former. Also, 'scarlet fever', and its sequel rheumatic fever, have become unusual diseases in developed countries but are still extremely common in the developing 'Third World'. The reason(s) for the sharp decline during the last 3–4 decades is complex and although connected with the introduction of antibacterial agents and antibiotics, the overall incidence was declining before these agents were widely used; other factors, such as improved living standards, are clearly relevant.

Vaccination campaigns in developed, and to a lesser extent developing countries have given encouraging results; in the latter, this must be carried out in younger children to be effective, because exposure to infection is significantly earlier in life.

MEASLES

Measles (rubeola) is an acute viral illness characterised by fever, a generalised maculopapular rash, cough, coryza and conjunctivitis. In tropical countries, high fatality rates occur in children under 5 years old; the disease is more common in some areas than others, west Africa being an example of the former.

The causative agent, a *paramyxovirus*, is the same throughout the world (there is no evidence for increased virulence in Africa) and was first cultured in 1954. Infection is spread in respiratory droplets. Humans form the sole reservoir and vector. The disease is highly contagious especially in the pre-eruptive phase; approximately 90% of susceptible individuals who come into close contact with a patient during the infectious phase will develop the disease. In tropical countries, epidemics usually occur in the dry season; in the UK, the peak incidence is in late winter or early spring.

Maternal antibody is protective until late in the first year of life; children who develop the disease at less than 1 year are especially vulnerable to complications. In unvaccinated populations in Africa, the mean age at infection is 2–4 years in rural areas, and 1–3 years in large cities; however, in 'westernised' countries this is around 5 years—which coincides with the beginning of schooling.

Virus particles initially enter lymphoid tissue in the respiratory tract; this event is followed by reticuloendothelial hyperplasia, viral replication and haematogenous dissemination. During the incubation period (Table 2.1) there is a lymphopenia and general anergy which is associated with lymphocyte destruction; pre-existing tuberculosis is sometimes reactivated. At the time of appearance of the rash, IgG and IgM antibodies become detectable; IgM reaches a peak at about 10 days after the rash appears, and IgG at about 30 days. The immunopathology of the rash is difficult to classify and may constitute a type II, III or IV sensitivity reaction, or possibly a combination of these. Cellular

Table 2.1

INCUBATION PERIODS OF SOME INFECTIONS WITH A PREDILECTION FOR CHILDHOOD

Disease	Days	Portal of entry
Measles	8–14	URT
Poliomyelitis	9–12	Faecal–oral; URT
Mumps	12–35	Oral
Pertussis	5–20	URT
Diphtheria	1–7	URT; skin
Varicella	12–16	URT
Scarlet fever	approx. 3	URT; oral

URT = Upper respiratory tract.

immunity plays a part in clearing the viraemia, and immunity is life-long.

Cough, conjunctivitis and coryza appear simultaneously with pyrexia (38–40°C). Koplik's spots appear on the buccal mucous membrane after 2–3 days. The maculopapular (morbilliform) rash begins after 1–7 (mean 3) days of illness; it first appears on the upper face and head, then becomes generalised and subsequently desquamates. Diarrhoea can be a prominent symptom (especially in developing countries) and an infection–malnutrition cycle is frequently set up. In a severe case there may be generalised lymphadenopathy. The entire illness lasts from 10–14 days. Case fatality rate depends on age, nutritional status and type and severity of any intercurrent infection; while in developed countries, the mortality rate is about 0.001%, in Africa, Asia and southern America it is overall 1–5% but a rate as high as 25% has been recorded in west Africa. Otitis media, acute mastoiditis, laryngotracheitis and acute encephalitis are major complications; stomatitis may interfere with eating, and hence with nutritional status. Cancrum oris rarely occurs. Vitamin A deficiency and its consequences may ensue. A rare and late complication is subacute sclerosing panencephalitis (SSPE) (*see* Chapter 9).

Diagnosis is usually straightforward, but other viral infections, drug eruptions, meningococcal infection, scarlet fever, typhus and tick fevers, and infectious mononucleosis (EBV) should be considered. Serology shows a rising titre of measles antibody; virus can be isolated from blood or nasopharyngeal secretions early in the course of infection. In the presence of measles encephalitis, a raised CSF protein, with up to 1000 mononuclear cells $\times 10^6/l$ is recorded.

Treatment of an attack is supportive with special attention directed at care of conjunctivae and prevention of secondary infection. Pre-exposure γ-globulin is effective if given at least 5 days before exposure. Measles vaccine is safe and effective; antibody titre falls after 2 years but persists for more than 15 years after vaccination. In 'Third World' countries, young children should be vaccinated at 9 months old; in developed countries, this is usually carried out at 12–15 months. Vaccine trials started in Upper Volta in the early 1960s, and mass vaccination has since been carried out in both west and central Africa.

POLIOMYELITIS

The importance of this acute viral infection lies in the fact that neurological sequelae, causing asymmetrical paralyses and acute mortality, occasionally occur. Following the advent of vaccination (introduced by Salk in 1953, and Sabin in 1955) the disease has become rare in the developed countries, but both the acute illness and its long-term sequelae are still very common in most 'Third World' countries. Where it exists in developed countries, incidence is highest in the summer months; in the tropics it occurs throughout the year.

Poliomyelitis is caused by an RNA virus of the family *Picornaviridae*; there are three antigenic types—1, 2 and 3. Following ingestion of the virus, replication takes place in the oropharyngeal and intestinal mucosa; this is usually followed by a transitory viraemia, which in a minority attains a high concentration and it is then that CNS invasion occurs, presumably resulting from haematogenous spread. The anterior horn cells of the spinal cord constitute the main site of attack, and a lower motor neuron lesion may develop.

Transmission is usually by the faecal–oral route, although respiratory spread also occurs; underlying standards of sanitation are therefore important. In unvaccinated populations, the disease has a peak prevalence (up to 95%) in children between 6 months and 5 years old. Although subsequent paralysis can occur following childhood infections ('infantile paralysis') this complication is more common with infection in later life.

Clinically, infections range from a subclinical one to fatal bulbar palsy; up to 95% of infections are either subclinical, or are accompanied by a brief fever, sore throat and myalgia. About 1% of those infected develop an aseptic meningitis, with meningismus, myalgia and headache (non-paralytic poliomyelitis). A small minority however develops *paralytic* poliomyelitis following the acute illness. Paralysis is asymmetrical, more often proximal than distal, and affects the leg more often than the arm. Cranial nerve involvement may give rise to various clinical syndromes (bulbar palsy). Paralytic poliomyelitis is more common after tonsillectomy, during pregnancy, following severe fatigue and exercise, in children with an immunodeficiency state and after injections and other local traumas. Malnutrition might also be important.

Diagnosis is basically a clinical one; paralytic disease should be differentiated from the Guillain–Barré syndrome (*see* Chapter 9). The virus can be isolated from pharyngeal secretions or faecal samples; a rise in neutralising antibody can be demonstrated against one of the three polio viruses in paired serum samples.

Management is symptomatic and supportive. Initially, bed-rest is essential. Physiotherapy should be initiated 3–4 days after the fever has abated, and the progression of paralysis (when present) has ceased. A respirator may be required if intercostal function is seriously impaired. Bulbar paralysis requires special facilities; repeated aspiration, causing pneumonia, is common. In prophylaxis, vaccination (live attenuated) (Sabin) should be begun at 2 months of age, with a 'booster' at 18 months. Very rarely (perhaps once in 10 million) paralysis and/or bulbar disease is a complication in the immunised person or contact; this vaccine should not be given to an immunosuppressed individual. Formalin-inactivated vaccine (Salk) is more heat-stable and can be given simultaneously with DPT* vaccine; it is however considerably more expensive.

The long-term results of paralytic poliomyelitis are still relatively common in most 'Third World' countries; various types of appliance, crutches, etc are of value provided the local health budget can afford them.

MUMPS

This very common communicable disease is caused by the mumps virus (90–140 nm in size). It is characterised by non-suppurative enlargement of the parotid and other salivary glands. Infection is by direct passage from the mouth into the parotid ducts; haematogenous spread subsequently results in other organ involvement; this is more common in later life. In generalised infections, the pancreas, testes, ovaries and brain are also affected; involvement of these organs can result in significant morbidity. Above the age of 10 years approximately one-third of men and boys develop orchitis, and approximately half of them have bilateral testicular involvement; up to 50% of adults suffer from CNS involvement.

Incubation period is usually between 18 and 21 days. Approximately one-third of infections are subclinical. Fever and malaise may precede the parotid symptoms and signs (which are usually

---

*Diptheria/pertussis/tetanus toxoid, which should be given at 3–6 months then 6–8 weeks later, and after a further 4–6 months.

bilateral); enlargement of the gland(s) lasts from 4–10 days; sublingual and submaxillary glands may also be enlarged and tender. CNS involvement is rarely serious; cranial nerve palsies, transverse myelitis and fatal demyelinating encephalitis have been reported. Aseptic meningitis occurs in up to 10% of infections. Deafness can be a major problem. Orchitis rarely leads to sterility, or pancreatitis to diabetes mellitus. Myocarditis has also been reported.

The diagnosis is essentially a clinical one. The virus can however be detected in saliva, CSF and urine; there is also a rise in haemagglutinins. After about 2 weeks, a rise in serum antibody is detectable.

Routine immunisation is not carried out although a live attenuated mumps vaccine has been used in the USA and USSR with some degree of success; immunity lasting up to 3 years has been reported.

PERTUSSIS (WHOOPING COUGH)

Pertussis, a bacterial infection of the respiratory tract, is caused by *Bordetella pertussis* (there are three serotypes) and is characterised by severe paroxysms of coughing. Other bacteria, including other *Bordetella spp.* can cause a similar clinical syndrome. The disease exists worldwide, in both developed and developing countries; infants less than 6 months who have not received maternal antibody (and consequent protection) are especially vulnerable. Transmission is by the air-borne route from respiratory droplets, or by objects (fomites) freshly contaminated with nasopharyngeal secretions. It is one of the most readily transmitted diseases of man and exerts an attack rate of up to 100% in susceptible contacts; the most contagious phase is the early preparoxysmal stage. Infection renders life-long immunity.

B. pertussis adheres to the cilia of respiratory tract epithelial cells from the nasopharynx to the bronchioles; it is non-invasive, but its presence is associated with tenacious mucus secretion. Impairment of cilial function allows secondary infection to supervene; pneumococcus, *Haemophilus influenzae* type B, *Staphylococcus aureus* and Group A haemolytic streptococci can all be involved. Necrosis of epithelial surfaces occurs. There is patchy perihilar atelectasis. Some degree of bronchitis and bronchospasm are usual. An encephalopathy occasionally occurs; however, pathogenesis of this is not understood.

The incubation period is usually about 7–10 days. There are three clinical stages:

(i) Catarrhal, prodromal or pre-paroxysmal.
(ii) Acute paroxysmal, or spasmodic cough.
(iii) Convalescent.

During the first of these (the most infectious stage) the disease is virtually identical with a common cold (*see* Chapter 7) although the cough may be more severe and persistent, especially at night. During stage (ii), violent attacks of paroxysmal coughing last up to several minutes; the inspiratory 'whoop' is characteristic. Vomiting may occur and venous engorgement of the head and neck, with production of petechiae and scleral haemorrhages is common. Exhaustion, apnoea, cyanosis and loss of consciousness may ensue; anoxic cerebral damage and death may follow. In stage (iii) a chronic cough replaces the paroxysms and this usually continues for 3–4 weeks but sometimes much longer. Complications include: secondary infections, otitis media, bronchopneumonia and segmental or lobar atelectasis. Subarachnoid and subdural haemorrhages can be produced during the coughing paroxysms; transient hemiplegia (Todd's paralysis), encephalopathy and coma may supervene. Pneumothorax, hernias and rectal prolapse are less common complications. Continuous vomiting rarely produces a metabolic acidosis and tetany.

Numerous other respiratory tract infections should be considered in the differential diagnosis, but they do not usually produce the characteristic 'whoop'. The possibility of a foreign body in the larynx and mucoviscidosis must be excluded. Diagnosis is by identification of *B. pertussis* in respiratory tract secretion; Bordet–Gengou medium should be used. Serology is of very limited value. A peripheral lymphocytosis (20–$100 \times 10^9/l$), which is brought about by a lymphocyte-promoting factor, should lead to differentiation from other diseases associated with a lymphocytosis, including acute leukaemia.

Treatment is supportive. Young infants should be admitted to hospital because good nursing care is essential, Cough suppressants, expectorants, bronchodilators and sedatives are unhelpful. Erythromycin, and to a lesser extent tetracycline and chloramphenicol, are of value if started early in the illness, but they are ineffective after the onset of stage (ii). Corticosteroids are of proven efficacy in severe cases. Hyperimmune pertussis globulin is of little or no value. In uncomplicated cases, the prognosis is good. In the malnourished child in a tropical country the outcome is however less favourable, but few data on this are currently available.

Partial protection is obtained from active immunisation; as well as modifying the severity of disease, the attack rate is reduced to approximately 20%. Protection lasts for about 3 years and then gradually declines until 12 years; booster doses should be given up to 6 years. However, vaccine protects against *B. pertussis* only; incidence of infection by other organisms producing a similar illness is not influenced. Changes in prevalence of pertussis in Britain have followed changes in vaccination status of the community; epidemics occurred in 1977–79, 1981–3 and 1985–7.

DIPHTHERIA

Diphtheria is an acute bacterial infection caused by virulent strains of *Corynebacterium diphtheriae*. A membrane involving the throat is characteristic; myocardial and neurological problems are caused by an exotoxin; localised skin infection also occurs. The disease is most common in children of 1–6 years old.

C. diphtheriae is a pleomorphic, Gram-positive, non-motile, non-sporulating, clavate bacillus; colony morphology and biochemical characteristics allow differentiation into: *mitis*, *gravis* and *intermedius*. The toxin which is extremely potent, is an acidic globular protein (molecular weight 62 000) with a cellular site of action; after a latent period, inhibition of protein synthesis occurs.

The disease occurs worldwide being endemic in many developing countries. In developed countries, mass vaccination campaigns (introduced in England and Wales in 1940) have produced satisfactory population immunity. Man is the main reservoir; droplet and occasionally fomite transmission is important. Skin infections are a major potential reservoir of infection. It can also be transmitted by contaminated milk.

Infants are protected until 6 months by maternal antitoxins. Following this, protection depends on the presence of antitoxin (acquired either naturally or by immunisation). The Schick test is of some value in assessing immunity in older children and adults (a positive result indicates lack of antitoxin required to neutralise injected toxin), but the correlation between the test result and antitoxin concentration is inexact.

Infection is usually acquired via the upper respiratory tract; invasion of pharyngeal epithelial cells results in the formation of an adherent membrane composed of bacteria, necrotic cells, phagocytes and fibrin. Other sites of infection, especially in developing 'Third World' countries are: skin, genitalia, umbilical cord, eyes and middle ear.

In *pharyngeal* disease, the incubation period is relatively short (1-7 days). Low-grade fever, sore throat and malaise are the usual presenting features; sometimes these are accompanied by nausea, vomiting, headache and dysphagia. The diphtheritic membrane (greyish-green) then forms; attempts to remove it cause bleeding. Ultimately the entire throat and mouth can be covered by membrane. Cervical lymphadenopathy and local oedema give rise to a 'bull-neck' appearance. Airway obstruction, with cough and laryngeal stridor, may follow. Pallor, tachycardia and weakness may also supervene. Alternatively, diphtheria can be localised to nasal mucosa giving rise to a unilateral, serosanguineous or thick mucopurulent nasal discharge. *Cutaneous* disease is more common in developing countries; it can be primary (a characteristic diphtheritic ulcer is usually confined to an extremity) or secondary (to wounds, burns or infected insect bites). The ulcer is shallow with rolled edges, and covered by a hard, adherent membrane. Genital involvement is a rare event.

The course of the disease depends on:

(i)   The degree of immunity.
(ii) The amount of toxin absorbed.
(iii) The location and extent of the membrane.

Spread of the membrane to involve the pharynx, trachea and bronchioles gives rise to severe respiratory symptoms including obstruction. The exotoxin causes a myocarditis, cardiac arrhythmias (e.g. arteriovenous block and left bundle-branch block) and rarely cardiac failure. Peripheral neuropathy with paralysis, usually affecting the lower limbs, and occasionally cranial nerve involvement (with resultant paralysis of the soft palate, blurred vision, or loss of accommodation) are most likely to occur between 1-4 weeks after onset of the illness.

Diagnosis is by detecting *C. diphtheriae* in stained smears from either the exudate or skin. Aerobic growth on Loeffler's medium is the most effective diagnostic technique. Significant ECG changes usually occur during the first week which are associated with increased mortality.

When possible patients should be isolated and admitted to hospital. The essential requirement is to start antitoxin administration as soon as possible (certainly within the first 48 h), without awaiting laboratory confirmation; however, this should be preceded by conjunctival and intradermal sensitivity testing to serum antitoxin; if either is positive, desensitisation is necessary. Antitoxin dose depends on site, extent and severity of the infection; where involvement is merely tonsillar, 10 000–20 000 U (by the intramuscular or intravenous route) are given and in more severe disease (e.g. nasopharyngeal involvement) 50 000–100 000 U (equal intramuscular and intravenous doses). Procaine penicillin (600 mg intramuscularly 12-hourly), or erythromycin (250 mg orally 6-hourly) should be given for 10 days. In severely ill patients, prednisolone 5 mg/kg daily may be added. Laryngeal obstruction may necessitate intubation or tracheostomy; excellent nursing is required to prevent secondary bacterial pneumonia and other infections.

Immunised patients have fewer complications and experience a much lower mortality rate than the non-immunised. At least two successive nasal and throat swabs should be negative for *C. diphtheriae* before discharge from hospital. Infected contacts should receive 1000–2000 U antitoxin, and penicillin or erythromycin for 10 days; active immunisation should be started later. Carriers of *C. diphtheriae* should also be given penicillin or erythromycin.

Diphtheria immunisation is usually given to children less than 1 year old at specified intervals, with booster doses at 1 and 5 years of age, and is combined with pertussis vaccine, tetanus toxoid and oral poliomyelitis vaccine. Primary immunisation after 6 years of age (which includes adults) should comprise 3 doses of diphtheria toxoid, combined with purified tetanus toxoid; booster doses are recommended every 10 years.

OTHER INFECTIONS WITH A PREDILECTION FOR CHILDHOOD

Some bacterial (e.g. 'scarlet fever' and rheumatic fever (*see* Chapter 8)) and viral (e.g. varicella and rubella) infections tend to occur more commonly in children than adults. Although 'scarlet fever' (usually caused by *Streptococcus pyogenes*, Lancefield group A) is no longer a serious problem in developed countries, it continues to be a significant cause of illness. Following a sore throat and generalised erythematous punctate rash, rheumatic fever, glomerulonephritis and erysipelas are occasional complications. Following the decline in 'scarlet fever' in developed countries, acute rheumatic fever (*see* Chapter 8) has become an unusual disease in the UK; however it remains the commonest cause of cardiac disease in developing countries.

Varicella (Chickenpox)

Varicella is usually a trivial virus infection of nuisance value only, but both in children (especially infants) and adults, serious complications can sometimes arise. The characteristic vesicular rash occurs some 24 h after the beginning of the initial febrile illness; the rash had formerly to be differentiated from that of smallpox. In central and west Africa, it should, however, be distinguished from that of monkeypox (*see* p. 239) (clinically similar to smallpox with the exception that lymphadenopathy is much more common). Herpes zoster is probably a second clinical manifestation of infection with the same virus, which has remained latent since the chickenpox infection. Immunoglobulin has no part to play in prophylaxis. Antivaricella zoster immunoglobulin (ZIg) is available for 'high risk' patients without a history of chickenpox who have recently been in contact with this disease (e.g. pregnant women, where fetal risk is a possible sequel). Although it does not prevent infection, ZIg reduces severity of disease and presumably the degree of viraemia. In the neonate and immunosuppressed patient the disease can sometimes pursue an aggressive course; chickenpox pneumonia is occasionally a serious problem (but only rarely with mortality); years after recovery, calcified foci can often be detected throughout both lung fields on chest radiography. Immunity after an attack is permanent. There is no specific treatment; however, antibiotics can be used to minimise secondary infection of chickenpox vesicles.

Rubella

This mild febrile illness (incubation period: 10–21 days) which is often accompanied by a faint macular rash, is only of importance because fetal damage can result when it is acquired during pregnancy, especially the first trimester. A live attenuated vaccine is available.

Erythema infectiosum

Outbreaks of erythema infectiosum (fifth disease) have recently increased in frequency in children in the UK. This trivial disease which is most common between the ages of 4 and 10 years is caused by a *parvovirus*. An erythematous rash usually begins on the cheeks ('slapped-cheek appearance') and subsequently involves the trunk and limbs; it has a lacy or reticular appearance and fades and recrudesces alternately over the course of about a week. Arthralgias are common in adults with this infection, but unusual in children. During the disease, there is a temporary interruption of erythropoiesis; although this is of little significance in an otherwise healthy individual, it can precipitate a 'crisis' in those with underlying sickle-cell (SS) disease and other chronic haemolytic anaemias.

FURTHER READING

Anderson M. J., Lewis E., Kidd I. M., *et al.* (1984). An outbreak of erythema infectiosum associated with human parvovirus infection. *J. Hyg. Camb*; **93:** 85–93.

Cradock-Watson J. E., Ridehalgh M. K. S., Bourne M. S. (1979). Specific immunoglobulin responses after varicella and herpes zoster. *J. Hyg. Camb*; **82:** 319–36.

Dixon J. M. S. (1984). Diphtheria in North America. *J. Hyg. Camb*; **93:** 419–32.

Editorial. (1986). Late sequelae of poliomyelitis. *Lancet*; **2:** 1195–6.

Khanum S., Uddin N., Garelick H., *et al.* (1987). Comparison of Edmonston–Zagreb and Schwarz strains of measles vaccine given by aerosol or subcutaneous injection. *Lancet*; **1:** 150–3.

Kjeldsen K., Simonsen O., Heron I. (1985). Immunity against diphtheria 25–30 years after primary vaccination in childhood. *Lancet*; **1:** 900–2.

Kwantes W. (1984). Diphtheria in Europe. *J. Hyg. Camb*; **93:** 433–7.

Lambert H. P. (1985). The enigma of pertussis. *J. Roy. Col. Phycns*; **19:** 67–71.

McCloskey R. V., Green M. J., Eller J., Smilack J. (1974). Treatment of diphtheria carriers: benzathine penicillin, erythromycin, and clindamycin. *Ann. Intern. Med*; **81:** 788–91.

McIntosh K. (1984). Varicella vaccine: decisions a little nearer. *New Engl. J. Med*; **310:** 1456–7.

Mortimer J., Melville-Smith M., Sheffield F. (1986) Diphtheria vaccine for adults. *Lancet*; **2:** 1182–3.

Chapter Three

Tuberculosis

'The captain of all these men of death that came against him to take him away was the consumption; for it was that that brought him down to the grave.'

John Bunyan (1628–88)

Tuberculosis is an infection caused by *Mycobacterium tuberculosis* or *M. bovis*. It has a long and tragic history and among the very many distinguished people who have died from the disease are: John Keats, Frédéric Chopin and D. H. Lawrence. Whereas in 'developed countries' incidence rates have declined markedly over the last half century (they were in fact declining *before* the advent of antituberculosis chemotherapy), the disease is still very common in countries of the 'Third World', and in a world context it is still responsible for more deaths than any other bacterial disease. WHO estimates are that approximately 10 million people develop the disease, and at least 3 million die of it annually. This is associated with: undernutrition, overcrowding, lack of diagnostic facilities and an overall shortage of funding so that effective chemotherapy is outside the reach of the national health budget. In developed countries the disease is still a major problem in members of the minor ethnic groups, especially from the Indian subcontinent; there is also good evidence that it is increasing in prevalence in the elderly indigenous population of the UK— especially in men with an excessive alcohol intake. Therefore, a high 'index of suspicion' is required for both pulmonary and extrapulmonary disease in these groups. Tuberculosis is still a potential health hazard to doctors and other medical personnel. Although infection with *M. bovis* (acquired from ingestion of infected milk) is now unusual in the Western World, it is still extremely common in the developing countries where pasteurisation of milk is not compulsory and infected cattle are not destroyed.

Following a primary infection (portals of entry: tonsils, lung parenchyma, ileum and skin) (Fig. 3.1), the 'primary complex' arises. Clinical disease may or may not arise at this stage (and indeed the infection can be asymptomatic); after a period of latency, slowly destructive pulmonary lesions may appear with other organ involvement including: bones, joints, kidneys, gastrointestinal tract, lymph glands, meninges, etc (*see* p. 49).

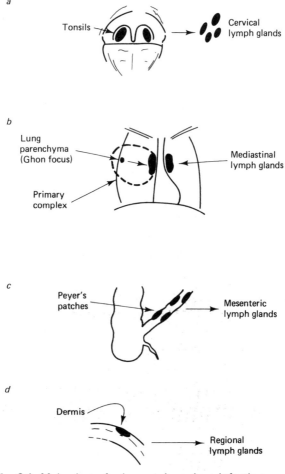

Fig. 3.1. Main sites of primary tuberculous infection.

Mycobacterium tuberculosis was first identified by Robert Koch in 1882. It is a non-motile slender rod (2–4 µm in length and 0·2–0·4 µm in width) and an obligate aerobe. It is *not* discoloured by acid–alcohol when stained with carbolfuchsin and is thus 'acid-fast'; Ziehl–Neelsen or Kinyoun staining techniques are usually used for identification. Fluorescence microscopy, after auramine rhodamine staining, is more sensitive but less specific. Guinea-pigs are especially susceptible, and rabbits unusually resistant to infection. Growth is slow and 3 weeks or more are required for colonies to develop on solid media; the usual culture medium is the Löwenstein–Jensen medium; growth is accelerated by adding 5% carbon dioxide in the local atmosphere. Colonies are non-pigmented, grow at 33–39°C and with maximal growth occurring at pH 6·6–6·8 and a Po_2 of 120 mmHg. Although easily killed by ultraviolet light, they are resistant to heat and disinfectants. Various biochemical tests are of value in identification of *M. tuberculosis*; it produces nicotinic acid (niacin), reduces nitrate to nitrite, and has weak catalase activity which is destroyed by heating. *In vivo*, the organism grows best where the Po_2 is highest, e.g. in the lung apices, and to a lesser extent kidneys and growing epiphyses. Where the Po_2 is low, e.g. in spleen and liver, growth is poor and disease is confined to the disseminated 'miliary' form. *M. tuberculosis* can replicate extracellularly and also within phagocytic cells; the generation time is 16–24 h.

Infection can be identified *in vivo* by an intradermal skin test using purified protein derivative (PPD). After the administration of 5 U PPD, an area of induration measuring more than 10 mm after 48–72 h constitutes a positive response. Modifications are contained in the Mantoux and Heaf tests. A positive response depends on the number of circulating sensitised T lymphocytes; in 15–20% of patients with active tuberculosis, negative results are obtained because sensitised T cells are depleted or non-functional—this may result from old age, general debilitation, fever, an acute overwhelming infection, or a large pleural effusion. A positive reaction can also be obtained after BCG (bacille Calmette–Guérin) vaccination. This vaccine (which only rarely produces side-effects) was originally produced in 1921 from *M. bovis*. In the UK, long-term studies carried out by the Medical Research Council have clearly shown that BCG vaccination exerts a significant protective effect against *M. tuberculosis* infection. However, in south India evidence presented within the last decade suggests that the same degree of protection is not forthcoming, especially during the first 5 years—possibly due to impaired underlying nutritional status. The role of BCG vaccination in indigenous populations in developing 'Third World' countries must therefore remain *sub judice*. Despite this conflicting evidence the vaccine is still widely used in 'Third World' countries.

In countries where BCG is not administered, the tuberculin test is thus of value in identification of prevalence of infection in the community. Furthermore, early demonstration of 'conversion' from a negative to a positive reaction, with prompt initiation of isoniazid therapy can prevent development of disease in more than 90% of individuals. *M. tuberculosis* can remain dormant for many years in apical pulmonary scars and may reactivate years or decades later, with production of 'secondary' tuberculosis; other sites with a high Po_2 concentration may also be affected: kidneys, vertebral column, long bones, meninges, lymph nodes and fallopian tubes.

With regard to immunity, natural resistance seems to be greater in Europids, Jews and Mongolians than in Indians, Africans and Eskimos; in the latter groups, infection tends to be more acute and rapidly progressive. These ethnic differences probably result from genetic factors operating via natural selection (*see* Chapter 1). Immunity is mediated by sensitised T lymphocytes; they release lymphokines (after stimulation by tuberculin antigen) which in turn activate macrophages to lyse ingested mycobacteria. Although specific IgA may be increased in actively infected individuals, the role of immunoglobulins is unclear. It is likely, but not proved, that recrudescence of infection in the elderly, malnourished and debilitated is associated with waning of cellular immune surveillance. The tuberculin test (*see* p. 45) when positive, indicates delayed hypersensitivity to tubercle bacilli. In an individual with intact immunity, primary infection (or BCG vaccination) renders some degree of protection. Therefore, subsequent inhalation or ingestion of *M. tuberculosis* mobilises the cellular immune response with elimination of bacteria. In such a patient, therefore, the risk is from 'within' rather than 'without'!

After entry to the body (*see* Fig. 3.1), (the pulmonary route is most common) *M. tuberculosis* multiplies locally before reaching the lymphatics and blood circulation; organisms are engulfed by macrophages but remain viable for 3–6 weeks; sensitised T cells are initially absent. In the majority of cases disease remains localised at the initial lesion (the *primary* or *Ghon focus*) where the characteristic *granuloma* (the hallmark of the disease) develops, together with the local lymphadenopathy. The basic lesion (which consists of epithelioid cells, multinucleated (Langerhan's) giant cells, and caseating necrosis) results from delayed hypersensitivity to the invading bacilli and is a 'dynamic' event in which macrophages from the peripheral blood are recruited; cell division, activation and death occur simultaneously. As the granuloma regresses (the normal course) resolution, fibrosis and subsequent calcification occur. If the immune response fails, infection may overwhelm the patient, with the production of various quantities of tuberculous disease, which is often widely disseminated (miliary).

During the initial phase of infection, a bacteraemia may be accompanied by a mild febrile illness. During this period, *M. tuberculosis* is disseminated to many organs and may establish itself wherever Po_2 is high (*see* p. 45); although these foci usually become quiescent (dormant) they may 'flare-up' in later life. Clinical disease, which may take many forms, can result at any time after the primary infection. In possibly 5–10% of infected individuals, disease occurs within 1–2 years; this is, however, hastened and exacerbated by malnutrition and is hence common in children in developing countries. In a further 5–10%, a late recrudescence of a dormant lesion occurs, often at the lung apices (*see* p. 48). Bacteraemia, resulting in miliary (disseminated) tuberculosis, may result at any stage.

Any organ can be affected by this disease at any age. In developing 'Third World' countries, initial infection usually occurs in childhood, and widespread dissemination is common. However, in developed countries, infection is more often in young adult life, and lungs and pleura are most commonly affected. Primary infection produces either a mild disease with malaise and low grade fever, or it may be entirely asymptomatic (*see* p. 44). Occasionally, hilar lymphadenopathy produces collapse of a lobe or segment (usually the right middle lobe (Brock's syndrome)) by compression of a bronchus; this occurs in children especially, and if inadequately treated, results in bronchiectasis of this lobe. A primary pulmonary parenchymal lesion can proceed to tuberculous pneumonia or to pleurisy, with or without effusion. Haematogenous spread occasionally occurs: this can produce miliary disease and tuberculous meningitis; these sequelae are most common in children older than 5 years and especially in the presence of malnutrition. Manifestations of 'allergy' during the initial infection include: erythema nodosum and phlyctenular conjunctivitis.

PULMONARY TUBERCULOSIS

Where transmission of infection is airborne the source of infection in an adult is most often a pulmonary lesion (not necessarily symptomatic); respiratory droplets remain suspended in the air and are potentially infectious; inhaled into the bronchioles and alveoli they can establish a new infection. Household contacts of a person with 'smear-positive' disease (an 'open case') are at the greatest risk of infection, but even then only 25–50% are likely to be infected. Infected individuals with negative smears ('closed' cases) are a threat to others only when contact with them is close and prolonged; this situation is similar to that in leprosy (*see* Chapter 14). Airborne transmission of *M. bovis* from man to animals is also possible. The lungs may be severely affected in the primary (initial) infection—especially in childhood; collapse of a lobe, and tuberculous pneumonia and/or pleurisy (with or without effusion) may occur (*see* p. 47). After a variable period, recrudescence of a dormant lesion, usually at the apex of a lung (often bilateral), produces a fibrocaseous lesion with cavitation. *M. tuberculosis* is abundant in caseous fluid within the cavitating lesions; organisms spread rapidly throughout the lungs and into the air in droplets.

Clinically, illness usually starts insidiously—with a mild cough. As the disease progresses, malaise, anorexia, a low-grade fever and weight-loss dominate the picture. Night sweats, fatigue and depression are common. The cough may be dry or productive; sputum is often green or yellowish-green and may be bloodstained. Massive haemoptyses, caused by rupture of a pulmonary artery within a cavity can produce severe exsanguination and may even prove fatal; this is a difficult medical emergency to manage and one which is not uncommon in adults in developing countries. Dyspnoea results from widespread destruction of lung parenchyma, tuberculous pneumonia or pleural effusion.

Although absent or minimal early on, physical signs may be gross in advanced cases; evidence of cavitation, fibrosis, pleural effusion, pneumothorax or collapse may be clinically apparent. Finger and toe clubbing is unusual; when present other diseases or superadded pyogenic infections should be suspected. Anaemia and amenorrhoea are common. Involvement of the larynx, trachea and bronchi can be associated with advanced cavitating disease; hoarseness may be present. Lymph-node compression of bronchi by granulomatous inflammation can give rise to an expiratory wheeze. Rupture of a mediastinal node into a bronchus may produce a tuberculous pneumonia, with dyspnoea and pyrexia. Pleurisy, with or without effusion, can occur soon after the initial infection or at the time of recrudescence. The latter results from pleural involvement by a subpleural focus. Pleuritic pain and severe dyspnoea (with a large effusion) are common clinical manifestations. Rupture of a large caseous lesion and contamination of the pleural space may produce a bronchopleural fistula and tuberculous empyema; a severe illness with fever, cough and expectoration is often present and this requires urgent medical and frequently surgical management also (*see* p. 53 and 56).

Investigation involves a sputum smear. This is always positive in severe pulmonary disease (at least 3 early-morning specimens should be examined); in mild infections, the concentration of *M. tuberculosis* may be too low for a positive smear result. Pharyngeal suction, bronchial washing, or fasting gastric juice are alternative techniques to establish a definitive diagnosis. Pleural fluid usually contains more than 40 g/l protein, a lymphocytosis, an elevated lactic dehydrogenase (LDH) concentration, and a pH of 7·0–7·25; due to a low concentration of *M. tuberculosis*, smear and culture are often negative. Pleural biopsy (using an Abram's needle) may reveal granulomas on histological examination and *M. tuberculosis* on culture. Radiology (when available) is of enormous value in diagnosis and in the assessment of the extent, severity and progress of pulmonary disease. Tomography can detect cavitation within lesions.

EXTRAPULMONARY TUBERCULOSIS

Disease in organs other than the lungs can form part of the primary infection or result from secondary disease (*see* p. 44 and 47). Gastrointestinal infection with *M. bovis* is still common in developing countries, where drinking milk from infected cows is common. Tuberculomas can present as a 'space-occupying' lesion in almost any organ, including the brain (*see* Chapter 9). Overall, extrapulmonary disease is more common in 'Third World' countries than Western ones, although it is now a significant problem in the minor ethnic groups within the UK.

Lymphadenitis

Lymphadenitis is common in developing countries and is often caused by *M. bovis*; systemic manifestations may or may not be present. The cervical glands are most often affected, but mesenteric node involvement can cause abdominal pain and an inflammatory mass.

Gastrointestinal Disease

Gastrointestinal disease is a major clinical problem in developing countries, where *M. bovis* infection involves the ileum and mesenteric lymph glands. Infection can take place via haematogenous spread or directly via the intestinal wall; the peritoneum may also be involved. The ileocaecal region is often the site of infection (hypertrophic ileocaecal disease) sometimes with stricture formation; however peritonitis (with or without ascites), mesenteric adenitis and hepatic involvement are also common. Abdominal pain, fever, night sweats, diarrhoea, malabsorption (*see* Chapter 5) and weight-loss are important presenting features; the caecum and/or mesenteric glands may be palpable and ascites detected. Ileocaecal disease can usually be detected by barium studies; ascitic fluid, when present, has a high protein content (>40 g/l), a raised LDH and a lymphocytosis. Peritoneal biopsy (percutaneous) is sometimes of value diagnostically.

Genitourinary Disease

Renal involvement results from haematogenous dissemination; tissue necrosis is accompanied by bacteriuria. This is not a common form of tuberculosis, even in developing countries. The entire genitourinary system may also be infected. Urinary frequency, dysuria, pain and/or swelling of the epididymis, or amenorrhoea, vaginal discharge and sterility may be accompanied by fever, malaise and loin pains. Urinalysis may reveal: gross or microscopic haematuria or pyuria with 'sterile' urine; early morning specimens should be cultured for *M. tuberculosis*. Intravenous urogram and retrograde pyelography are of value in locating the lesion anatomically. In women, endometrial curettage, laparoscopy or laparotomy may give diagnostic results.

Osteomyelitis/Arthritis

While the epiphyses are growing they may be infected via haematogenous spread; later, reactivation of a dormant lesion can occur. This form of disease is therefore most common in children and young adults; the vertebral column is a frequent site of infection (Pott's disease), but the hip, knee, wrist, elbow and shoulder joints are also vulnerable. A monoarticular arthritis with effusion, should always raise the possibility of tuberculosis. Accumulation of caseous material around affected bones and joints or along fascial plains (paravertebral or psoas abscess) can result. Radiology reveals areas of rarefaction with sclerosis; narrowing of a disc space is common with vertebral involvement after the first few weeks of illness, and this later progresses to collapse of a vertebral body and formation of an angular kyphosis. Paraparesis or paraplegia may ensue. Biopsy and culture confirm the diagnosis.

Pericarditis

A granulomatous reaction is subsequently followed by fibrosis (constrictive pericarditis). Constrictive pericarditis caused by tuberculosis must be differentiated from that of other aetiologies. Chronic pericardial tamponade with resulting symptoms and signs may occur; pericardial biopsy and culture of fluid confirm the diagnosis—numerous lymphocytes with or without red cells may be present. Pericardiocentesis is an emergency procedure in relieving a life-threatening tamponade.

Meningitis (*see* p. 166)

Meningitis results either from miliary dissemination or discharge from a caseous cerebral lesion into the subarachnoid space; it can occur either in the initial (overwhelming) infection, or during recrudescence of a dormant lesion(s). Headache, irritability and restlessness are followed by neck stiffness, localising neurological signs and coma; fever, malaise, night sweats and weight-loss may also be present. Hydrocephalus and permanent neurological damage are complications which occur when treatment is delayed. Cerebrospinal fluid characteristically shows a lymphocytosis with a low glucose concentration; protein and pressure are usually elevated, but direct smears for *M. tuberculosis* are often negative. Other aetiological agents in chronic meningitis (e.g. cryptococcosis and histoplasmosis) (*see* Chapter 15) should be differentiated. Treatment must be started urgently.

Adrenal Involvement

Caseous necrosis resulting from haematogenous spread can result in Addison's disease; corticosteroid replacement therapy is then necessary.

Disseminated ('Miliary') Disease

This results from an overwhelming initial infection (which is haematogenous) or from recrudescence of a dormant lesion. A caseous focus may erode a vein, also producing a bacteraemia. Whereas this event can lead to a rapid downhill course, especially in infancy, in adults it may be a chronic process which is diagnosed by liver biopsy or bone-marrow in a pyrexial adult (a 'PUO'; Chapter 1, p. 24). Symptoms result from multiorgan involvement. Occasionally retinal tubercles are visible. Chest radiography reveals a 'snow shower' effect consisting of soft opacities throughout both lung fields; the diameter of the lesions varies with their density—the list of differential diagnoses is long. Biopsy and culture of liver, bone-marrow or lung parenchyma usually confirm the diagnosis. The tuberculin test is frequently negative. Chemotherapy should be instituted immediately.

MANAGEMENT OF TUBERCULOSIS

Chemotherapy of tuberculosis dates from 1944 with the introduction of streptomycin. Assuming that the organism is sensitive to chemotherapeutic agents and furthermore that the nutritional status is reasonable, cure of disease is dependent on a prolonged course of antituberculous agents. However, in the presence of severe disease with widespread tissue involvement, sudden deterioration and sudden death is a relatively common sequel. The mechanism for this is unclear, but an 'immunological' basis seems probable. Similar regimens are used in pulmonary and extrapulmonary disease. The usual causes of a lack of success are: a wrongly chosen regimen or a failure of compliance. There is no longer an indication for the formerly used regimens: artificial pneumothorax, artificial peritoneum, thoracoplasty, 'plombage', etc; these procedures were designed to 'collapse' a lung temporarily or permanently, and thus to allow more rapid recovery of the tuberculous lesion.

Individuals are no longer infectious after 2 weeks of antituberculous chemotherapy even though the sputum may still be 'positive'; infectivity begins declining immediately chemotherapy is initiated. Prolonged isolation is thus no longer indicated; indeed, if admission to hospital is necessary, patients can be treated in general wards. Although a positive smear or culture for *M. tuberculosis* should ideally be obtained before starting chemotherapy, in practice this is sometimes started on the basis of a *clinical* diagnosis; a 'therapeutic trial' must then be closely supervised, and if adequate evidence for the diagnosis was initially forthcoming, it should be continued for the full course. Whereas formerly, treatment had to continue for 18–24 months, with present chemotherapy, 9 months or even less is usually adequate (*see* p. 56); however, the appropriate agents are often unobtainable in developing countries.

Antituberculous agents are either *bactericidal* or *bacteriostatic*; Table 3.1 summarises the agents currently in use. *Isoniazid* (*INAH*) is active against both intra- and extracellular organisms; it is inactivated by hepatic acetylation which is under genetic control—the proportion of rapid and slow inactivators varies in different ethnic groups. It diffuses widely into all tissues, including the CNS. Because it competes with pyridoxine which can result in anaemia and peripheral neuropathy, pyridoxine supplements should be given. *Rifampicin* is also active against intra- and extracellular organisms and also diffuses into all tissues. Urine appears red after administration. It is however expensive and this limits its use in 'Third World' countries. *Streptomycin* is active

Table 3.1

AGENTS COMMONLY USED IN ANTITUBERCULOUS CHEMOTHERAPY

	Adult dose Daily	Adult dose Twice weekly	Side-effects
Bactericidal			
Isoniazid (INAH)	300 mg*† (+ pyridoxine 50 mg)	900 mg*	Peripheral neuritis, hepatotoxicity (idiosyncratic), allergic fever and rash, DLE phenomenon
Rifampicin	450–600 mg*	450–600 mg*	Hepatotoxicity, nausea and vomiting, allergic fever and rash, influenza-like syndrome, petechiae and thrombocytopenia, acute renal failure
Streptomycin	0·5–1·0 g†	1·0–1·5 g†	VIII nerve damage, nephrotoxicity, allergic fever, rash
Pyrazinamide	1·5–2·5 g*	3·0–3·5 g*	Hyperuricaemia, hepatotoxicity, allergic fever and rash
Bacteriostatic			
Ethambutol	0·8–1·6 g*		Optic neuritis, rash
Ethionamide	500–750 mg*		Nausea, vomiting, anorexia, hepatotoxicity, allergic fever and rash
Cycloserine	0·75–1·0 g* (+ pyridoxine 100 mg)*		Personality change, psychosis, convulsions, rash

continued

	Adult dose		Side-effects
	Daily	Twice weekly	
Para-aminosalicylic acid (PAS)	12 g*		Nausea, vomiting, diarrhoea, hepatotoxicity, allergic fever and rash, goitre
Thiacetazone	150 mg*		Allergic rash and fever, Stevens–Johnson syndrome, haematological disorders, nausea and vomiting

* = oral; † = intramuscular.

extracellularly only and does not cross the blood–brain barrier. *Pyrazinamide*, although effective within macrophages has little effect against extracellular organisms; its main use is in 'drug-resistant' cases and in short-course regimens. Like rifampicin it is relatively expensive. *Ethambutol* is active both intra- and extracellularly; it is frequently used with INAH because it inhibits the multiplication of mutants resistant to that agent. It is also relatively expensive. *Ethionamide* is largely reserved for drug-resistant infections. *Cycloserine* is largely kept for complicated cases requiring retreatment. *Para-aminosalicylic acid (PAS)* has the great advantage of low cost; it is, however, of limited value and is only a bacteriostatic agent. *Thiacetazone*, in common with PAS, is inexpensive, dermatological side-effects can however be severe and seem to have ethnic differences in incidence rate.

Chemotherapeutic agents are most active against rapidly dividing organisms; this applies especially therefore to those present in apical lung cavities. In 'closed' lesions, organisms replicate less frequently and longer courses of treatment tend to be necessary. Infections acquired in south-east Asia, Mexico and some other 'Third World' countries are often resistant to multiple therapeutic agents.

Treatment regimens must ideally utilise two bactericidal agents in their major thrust (this rapidly reduces the extracellular bacterial population and avoids selection of drug-resistant mutants); therefore, in developed countries, INAH and rifampicin are usually administered for 9 months, but in 'Third World' countries the latter agent is frequently too expensive. A regimen utilising four bactericidal agents (INAH + rifampicin + pyrazinamide + streptomycin (or ethambutol)) given for 6 months seems to give very satisfactory results. Other regimens must be given for longer periods, which is often necessary in 'Third World' countries where cost is such an important factor; a commonly used combination is: INAH + thiacetazone (+ streptomycin during the first 2–3 months only). Compliance over this long period is often poor and cure of the disease incomplete; this results in frequent exacerbations and infection of other individuals.

Rarely corticosteroids are indicated in the management of tuberculosis. Surgery is occasionally indicated for complications which include constrictive pericarditis, hydrocephalus, etc.

Follow-up is extremely important, but often exceedingly difficult in 'Third World' countries, even where primary health care, with Aid-posts, etc are well developed.

In the USA, several groups are advised to receive INAH (300 mg daily) for 1 year:

(i) Household contacts of patients with active disease.
(ii) Those with an abnormal chest radiograph (which is not worsening), a positive tuberculin reaction, and negative sputum, who have not previously received a full course of antituberculous chemotherapy.
(iii) Tuberculin 'converters' within the previous 2 years, who have a 5–10% risk of progression to active disease.
(iv) Tuberculin-positive individuals on long-term immunosuppressive and corticosteroid therapy, and those with reticuloses, diabetes mellitus, silicosis and previous gastrectomy.
(v) Individuals less than 5 years old with a positive tuberculin test and normal chest radiograph.

ATYPICAL MYCOBACTERIA

Several species of mycobacteria can cause pulmonary and extrapulmonary disease; *M. kansasii* and *M. intracellulare* are examples.

As well as *M. tuberculosis*, *M. avium intracellulare* is a frequent pathogen in AIDS (*see* Chapter 11). Identification of these organisms is based on morphological and chemical testing; they are niacin-negative. Division is into:

(i) Photochromogens.
(ii) Scotochromogens.
(iii) Non-photochromogens.
(iv) A 'variable' group and 'others'.

Skin-testing has not proved of value for clinical differentiation within the group. Person-to-person transmission is low; response to the usual antituberculous chemotherapeutic agents tends to be poor (especially with *M. intracellulare*); *M. kansasii* usually responds however.

Around 10% of all patients initially diagnosed as suffering from 'tuberculosis' are probably infected with one of these organisms. These mycobacteria have been recognised for very many years but it was only when the incidence of *M. tuberculosis* infection declined in developed countries that their true clinical importance became clear. They have been isolated from soil, milk, tap water, fresh water, coastal water, etc. *M. kansasii* has been demonstrated in tap water. They are present worldwide but the incidence of each of them varies geographically. Not all mycobacteria isolated from human tissue are actually pathogenic to man; however, 17 species are known to infect and produce significant disease.

Mode of transmission is largely unknown; some atypical mycobacteria are not infrequently isolated from sputum and gastric contents of normal healthy people. The respiratory tract is probably the main route of infection. They are found more frequently in individuals with lungs previously damaged by bronchitis, emphysema, silicosis, etc. Some evidence suggests that *M. avium intracellulare* infects man via droplet aerosol from coastal and inland water. Some (e.g. *M. ulcerans*) can produce local granulomatous disease by entering skin abrasions (*see* Chapter 13); subcutaneous tissues also can be involved. Others can produce disseminated disease involving several organs.

Clinical, radiological and pathological features are indistinguishable from those of *M. tuberculosis*. However, they can also be present as saprophytic colonisers of the respiratory tract, or non-pathogenic or low-grade pathogens. When affecting the lung (*see* above) they produce disease which can be identical to that caused by *M. tuberculosis*; *M. kansasii* and *M. intracellulare* are examples. The tuberculin reaction is usually weakly positive. The disease is usually slowly but occasionally rapidly progressive, with widely disseminated disease. Lymphadenitis can occur in children; in the USA this more often results from these agents than from *M. tuberculosis*; it is clinically and pathogenically identical. In immunocompromised hosts (e.g. AIDS sufferers) disseminated disease can also occur (especially with *M. avium intracellulare*); skin and subcutaneous tissue, bone, joints, tendon sheaths, kidneys and meninges can all be affected; surgical incision and prosthetic heart valves have also been infected.

M. ulcerans which produces skin (and occasionally bone) lesions was first described in Uganda by Sir Albert Cook in 1897; the disease, acquired by skin inoculation from the environment, is known as Buruli ulcer. Distribution is: central Africa, south-east Asia, Papua New Guinea, Australia, and central and south America. Wide excision is the treatment of choice, but in addition grafting is usually necessary. *M. marinum* also produces dermatological lesions, often known as 'swimming pool granulomas'; these organisms were first isolated in 1954 from a group of individuals who had used a swimming pool in Sweden. Most lesions heal spontaneously. Skin lesions can also be produced by *M. kansasii*, *M. fortuitum* and *M. chelonei*; the latter organisms are commonly found in soil and water. *M. avium intracellulare* and *M. scrofulaceum* (known as the MAIS complex) produce lymphadenitis and scrofuloderma in children.

Although this group of infections is overall of borderline virulence, management is unsatisfactory; all atypical mycobacteria display either relative or complete *in vitro* resistance to standard antituberculous agents. With *M. intracellulare* infections, a complex regimen consisting of up to 6 antituberculous agents sometimes achieves relative success. When amenable to surgical resection, this should be combined with chemotherapy for up to 24 months. *M. kansasii* usually responds to a regimen containing isoniazid and rifampicin despite relative *in vitro* resistance. Other chemotherapeutic agents—amikacin, doxycycline, and sulphamethoxazole—have given reasonable results with other atypical mycobacteria, including *M. ulcerans*, especially when used in conjunction with resection of affected tissue and local lymph glands.

FURTHER READING

Bhargava D. K., Shriniwas, Tandon B. N., *et al.* (1986). Serodiagnosis of intestinal tuberculosis by the soluble antigen fluorescent antibody test (SAFA test). *J. Trop. Med. Hyg*; **89:** 61–5.

Cook G. C. (1985). Tuberculosis—certainly not a disease of the past! *Q. J. Med*; **56:** 519–21.

Editorial (1986). Management of non-respiratory tuberculosis. *Lancet*; **1:** 1423–4.

Fox W. (1981). Whither short-course chemotherapy? *Brit. J. Dis. Chest*; **75:** 331–57.

Goldman K. P. (1987). AIDS and tuberculosis. *Brit. Med. J.*; **295:** 511–12.

Holm J. (1984). Tuberculosis control in the developing world : it's time for a change. *Wld. Hlth. Forum*; **5:** 103–19.

Schofield P. F. (1985). Abdominal tuberculosis. *Gut*; **26:** 1275–8.

Strole W. E., Compton C. C. (1986). A 28-year-old Cambodian immigrant woman with recent fever and abdominal distension. *New Engl. J. Med*; **315:** 952–6.

Traub M., Colchester A. C. F., Kingsley D. P. E., Swash M. (1984). Tuberculosis of the central nervous system. *Q. J. Med*; **53:** 81–100.

Chapter Four

Malaria

'He is so shak'd of a burning quotidian tertian that it is most lamentable to behold.'
William Shakespeare (1564–1616), Henry V, II, i, 123

Although largely and most importantly a disease of the tropics and subtropics, it should not be forgotten that malaria was a significant medical problem in the UK until the 1920s; the last focus was on the Isle of Dogs in south-east England. Nevertheless, malaria *transmission* is overall influenced by ambient temperature; optimal conditions are a temperature of 20–30°C, and mean relative humidity of more than 60%. Many classical and historical descriptions of 'ague' probably referred to this infection (*see* above). It is a disease of great antiquity and probably originated in Africa, being adapted from enterocytic coccidia; transmission by bloodsucking arthropods is considered to have occurred at least 30 million years ago.

It was described in ancient Hindu, Chinese, Assyrian, Babylonian, Egyptian and Greek writings; the term *mal aria* (foul air) probably originated in Italy in the 18th century. Few diseases have had a greater impact on world history; many wars have been lost as a result of decimation of armies by this major scourge. The malaria parasite was first visualised by Laveran in 1880 in Algeria, and was identified in the gut of a mosquito by Sir Ronald Ross in India in 1897.

Indigenous people in 'Third World' countries are usually exposed to this infection from the moment of birth; assuming survival occurs, some degree of humoral immunity (serum IgG concentration is raised) is slowly built up. Genetic and nutritional factors are clearly important in the development of immunity. Non-immunes entering a malarious area are 'wide open' to this infection and may succumb very rapidly to an overwhelming parasitaemia. WHO estimates for incidence rates are 200 million infected with 2 million deaths annually—frequently in childhood. Fig. 4.1 indicates areas with known malaria transmission at the present time. Attempts to control the disease in 'Third World' countries have usually failed; these include vector control programmes, improved health education, government drug-control programmes and attempts to raise living standards. The disease thus ranks with malnutrition, diarrhoeal disease and tuberculosis as one of the world's most important 'killers'. In the UK, the majority of imported cases are contracted in the Indian subcontinent and are caused by *Plasmodium vivax*; most of the remainder, caused by *P. falciparum* are from tropical Africa. Overall, some 1500–2000 'imported' cases are diagnosed annually in the UK and of those around 10 die because diagnosis is either late or even missed.

Transmission via contaminated blood transfusion and blood products should always be suspected, and this applies to temperate as well as 'Third World' countries. The possibility of congenital transmission should not be forgotten. Although an epidemiological association between hyperendemic and holoendemic (i.e. a prevalence of spleen and parasite rate of $>50\%$ and $>75\%$, respectively, in 2–9 year-old children) malaria, Epstein–Barr virus (EBV) infection, and Burkitt's (B cell) lymphoma has been documented, further work is required.

The various species of *Plasmodium* produce very different clinical syndromes and should be considered under separate headings.

PLASMODIUM FALCIPARUM MALARIA

Of the four species of malaria parasite to infect man, *P. falciparum* is the most serious by far; unlike the other species it carries a high mortality rate, especially in non-immune people.

Parasitology

The mosquito, a species of *Anopheles*, is the vector; the mosquito (sexual) and human (non-sexual) cycles occur with all four species. Fig. 4.2 shows these in diagrammatic form. With *P. falciparum* infections, the presence of fetal and S haemoglobin

62 Communicable and Tropical Diseases

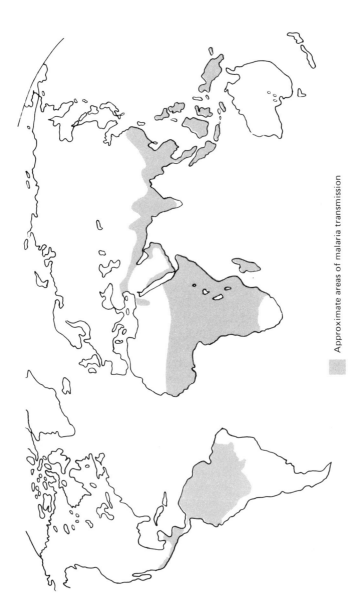

Fig. 4.1. Areas of malaria transmission at the present time.

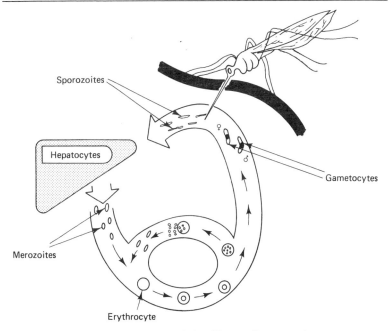

Fig. 4.2. Life-cycle of the *Plasmodium* parasite.

significantly reduces the risk of infection; the high incidence rate of S haemoglobin in some parts of Africa is attributed to the selective advantage of this balanced polymorphism. Low iron status is probably also protective. Following a mosquito bite— usually between dusk and dawn—sporozoites are released into the human circulation, and within 30 min are taken up by hepatocytes. Following maturation (incubation period 9–14 days), merozoites are released from the liver into the circulation, and an attack of fever with other clinical manifestations occurs (*see* p. 64). Thereafter, reinfection and maturation of merozoites within erythrocytes occurs in cycles (every 48 h) and is followed by their periodic release into the circulation, causing further symptoms. Gametocytes (sexual forms) are later produced and these are taken into a mosquito at a subsequent bite; the cycle is thus completed.

Several methods are available for determining resistance to the various chemoprophylactic and chemotherapeutic agents. The WHO clinical method grades resistance into RI, RII and RIII. *In vitro* cultivation of *P. falciparum* parasites was first made possible by Trager and Jensen in 1976.

Clinical Aspects and Complications

Following the incubation period, headaches, mild confusion, limb pains, nausea and vomiting herald an attack. Diarrhoea is a common symptom—especially in children. Fever, often accompanied by rigors then becomes prominent; an entire paroxysm averages 9–10 h. It is important however not to look for a classical fever chart before making a diagnosis. The degree of prostration varies in different individuals. Splenomegaly, jaundice and anaemia may all be present. The pathogenesis of the anaemia is complex; immunological factors are clearly involved and IgG and complement components are present on the erythrocyte membrane—this might facilitate uptake by phagocytic cells. Herpes labialis (see Chapter 13) is a common complication. Differential diagnosis is from other causes of fever and splenomegaly; viral (including Lassa fever, if the patient has come from west Africa—especially from a rural area), bacterial (including salmonellosis) and parasitic (e.g. visceral leishmaniasis, which can also present with fever and splenomegaly) diseases must all be considered. The complete list of differential diagnoses is a very long one.

As the disease progresses, cerebral involvement and acute haemolysis, proceeding to acute tubular necrosis and 'blackwater fever', are serious complications (Table 4.1). Other sequelae are acute pulmonary oedema, hypoglycaemia (frequently associated with quinine treatment) and complications in pregnancy. Retinal haemorrhages may also be present. It is also important to

Table 4.1

COMPLICATIONS OF *PLASMODIUM FALCIPARUM* MALARIA

Cerebral involvement
Acute renal failure
Intravascular haemolysis ('blackwater fever')
Acute pulmonary oedema
Peripheral circulatory failure
Algid malaria
Complications of pregnancy
Hypoglycaemia (worsened by quinine)
Retinal haemorrhage
DEATH
---

recognise the algid form of the disease, in which there is often profound peripheral vasoconstriction and hypotension.

Diagnostically, the demonstration of parasites in thick and thin blood films is the only acceptable method. Although there is an approximate correlation between the level of parasitaemia and the clinical severity, this is by no means absolute; cerebral malaria can in fact be present in the presence of a very low peripheral blood *P. falciparum* parasitaemia. Serology (elevated malarial antibodies using the ELISA technique) is of no value in the diagnosis of an acute case; it is only of value retrospectively, and in the attribution of a chronic complication to the disease (*see* p. 70). It is conceivable that in the future, DNA probes might replace blood smear examination in diagnosis. Anaemia, leucopenia and thrombocytopenia are usual and there is often evidence of haemolysis. Hepatic enzymes and serum bilirubin are frequently elevated, sometimes markedly. Serum albumin is often depressed and total globulin elevated. The prothrombin time may be prolonged. Urine examination reveals albuminuria, together with urobilinogen and sometimes conjugated bilirubin.

Prophylaxis

Obviously, if mosquito bites can be prevented, no other form of prophylaxis is necessary. Suitable clothing between dusk and dawn and mosquito nets are thus of value. In many major towns and cities in infected areas, the risk to the traveller is either low or non-existent. All chemotherapeutic agents must be taken regularly, beginning 1 week before possible exposure and completing 4 to 6 weeks after departure from the infected area. It is important to appreciate that no prophylactic regimen *prevents* infection occurring, or is 100% effective; all fevers must therefore be taken seriously.

Until a decade ago, chloroquine, proguanil and pyrimethamine were acceptable and reliable prophylactics (*see* Table 4.2). Since then, resistance of the *P. falciparum* parasite to these and other chemoprophylactic agents has occurred. Fig. 4.3 illustrates the geographical areas where chloroquine resistance is a major problem. Second-line chemoprophylactic regimens often utilise combination tablets—'Fansidar' or 'Maloprim'. These have been combined with chloroquine in areas where *P. vivax* is also a problem (*see* p. 69). However, serious toxic effects have been

Table 4.2

PROPHYLAXIS IN *Plasmodium falciparum* MALARIA*

Recommended drug	Adult dose
Recommendations until 1986	
Chloroquine	300 mg weekly
Proguanil ('Paludrine')	100–200 mg daily
Pyrimethamine ('Daraprim')	25 mg weekly
Pyrimethamine (25 mg) + Sulfadoxine (500 mg) ('Fansidar')	i tab weekly
Pyrimethamine (12·5 mg) + Dapsone (100 mg) ('Maloprim')	i tab weekly
Amodiaquine	400 mg weekly
Current recommendations	
Areas with no chloroquine resistance:	
Proguanil	100–200 mg daily
Areas with chloroquine resistance:	
Most areas of the world	
Proguanil	200 mg daily
+ Chloroquine	300 mg weekly
South-east Asia and Papua New Guinea	
'Maloprim'	i tab weekly
+ Chloroquine	300 mg weekly

*If further information for any given area, or advice in infancy and pregnancy is required, the following should be contacted: London School of Hygiene and Tropical Medicine (01 636 8636); Liverpool School of Tropical Medicine (051 708 9393) or East Birmingham Hospital (021 772 4311).

reported using 'Fansidar' (especially when combined with chloroquine), and to a lesser extent with 'Maloprim' (only rarely with i tablet weekly). With the former agent, rashes, Stevens–Johnson syndrome, jaundice, renal failure, blood dyscrasias and death have been reported; 'Maloprim' (usually with ii tablets weekly) has been associated with blood dyscrasias (marrow depression), liver damage and death. More recently, amodiaquine was used, especially in east Africa; however, marrow depression and

Malaria 67

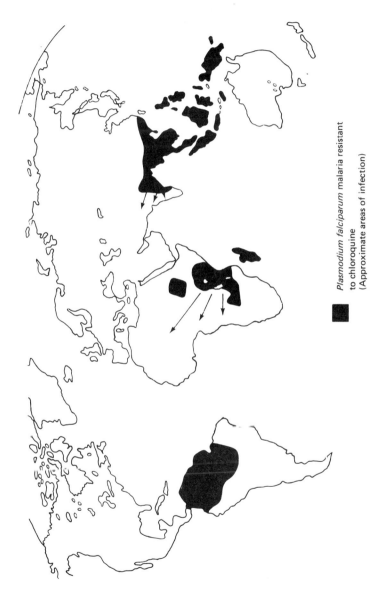

Fig. 4.3. Geographical distribution of areas where chloroquine resistance in *Plasmodium falciparum* malaria is a major problem.

hepatocellular damage—especially when given with proguanil—have forced it to be abandoned. Current recommendations for chemoprophylaxis are summarised in Table 4.2.

A large amount of work using recombinant DNA technology is in progress in an attempt to produce a satisfactory vaccine—aimed at either sporozoite, merozoite or gametocyte (or possibly a combination of two or three of these) stages: there is no cross-protection because the antigens are 'stage specific'. Whether such a vaccine will solve this major world problem is however open to serious doubt (*see* Chapter 18).

Treatment

The first form of treatment used against this infection was the bark of the Peruvian guina-guina (cinchona) tree in the early 17th century (it was included in the London Pharmacopoeia in 1677 as *Cortex peruanus*); the alkaloid, quinine, was subsequently isolated in France in 1820. Between 1920–50 a number of antimalarial compounds were synthesised. In 1955, the WHO adopted a policy of 'global eradication' which was based on insecticide control of mosquitoes; however, resistance to dichloro-diphenyl-trichloroethane (DDT) by the vector rapidly led to the failure of this project. Unfortunately, the search for new antimalarial compounds largely ceased at the introduction of this ambitious eradication programme. Whereas until recently chloroquine was the therapeutic agent of choice, with progressive resistance to this agent it is now of very limited value in most of the geographical areas involved (*see* Fig. 4.3). Similar problems face 'Fansidar' which was also widely used therapeutically (Table 4.3). Quinine is therefore the usual therapeutic agent against *P. falciparum*—however, hyperinsulinism and hypoglycaemia, especially in late pregnancy, are important side-effects. Quinidine is also effective but has a similar effect on insulin production. Quinine followed by 'Fansidar' has proved to be a successful regimen. It is extremely important that chemotherapy is started immediately after diagnosis; deterioration can occur very rapidly. In all except straightforward cases (who are fully conscious), quinine administration should be initially by the intravenous route. Agents 'waiting in the wings' are mefloquine and qinghaosu (prepared from the Chinese herb *Artemisia annua*); phenanthrene

Table 4.3

DRUG REGIMENS USED IN THE TREATMENT OF *PLASMODIUM FALCIPARUM* MALARIA

Drug	Adult dose
Chloroquine	600 mg initially followed by 300 mg at 6, 24 and 48 h
'Fansidar'	iii tab stat
Quinine	600 mg b.d. or t.d.s. for 5 or 7 days
Quinidine	
Other regimens	
Quinine, followed by 'Fansidar'	(Doses as above)
Quinine + tetracycline	(Not widely used)
Mefloquine (1·5 g as a single dose)	
Qinghaosu	Not yet in routine use
Phenanthrene methanol compounds	

methanol compounds are also effective in clearing parasitaemia.

Treatment of complications is even more important. When cerebral involvement is present, dexamethasone has in the past been widely used; however, a controlled trial in Thailand produced no evidence that it is effective—probably because cerebral oedema is an inconsistent manifestation in *P. falciparum* malaria with coma. Renal failure must be treated on its merits by peritoneal or haemodialysis. Exchange blood transfusion has occasionally proved of value in patients with a heavy parasitaemia; indications for its use are so far not clearly delineated, a few physicians suggest that any ill patient with a parasitaemia of more than 10% should be treated by this means. Pulmonary oedema may benefit from prostacyclin.

PLASMODIUM VIVAX AND *PLASMODIUM OVALE* MALARIA

These two infections can be considered together. They both have an exo-erythrocytic cycle in the liver, and this was first described by Shortt and Garnham in 1948. Late relapses are caused by a dormant liver stage—the hypnozoite—first described by Krotoski and Garnham in 1980. Absence of Duffy blood group determinants renders resistance to *P. vivax* infection. Both infections, especially that caused by *P. ovale*, can occur simultaneously with *P. falciparum*. Incubation periods are varied, being usually 12–17 days but occasionally longer, especially in the case of *P. vivax* (9 months or even more). Fevers occur characteristically every third day (i.e. every 48 h), and can cause considerable morbidity but very rarely mortality. Anaemia (of haemolytic type), and splenomegaly are common accompaniments. Haemolysis can continue for several weeks after successful treatment of this infection; immunological mechanisms are involved. Treatment is with a 3-day chloroquine course as formerly used in *P. falciparum* infections (Table 4.3, p. 69); this must be followed by primaquine to eliminate the exo-erythrocytic cycle (a so-called 'radical cure'); the dose is 7·5 mg b.d. for 14 days, except in south-east Asia and the Pacific where twice this dose should be used due to partial resistance of the *P. vivax* parasite. Glucose-6-phosphate dehydrogenase (G–6–PD) status should be assayed before primaquine is administered; if the concentration of this enzyme is very low, acute haemolysis can be a serious complication. There is no satisfactory alternative to primaquine; however, in the G–6–PD deficient individual a longer course at low concentration has been used with success.

PLASMODIUM MALARIAE MALARIA

This is the most chronic form of malaria. *P. malariae* was in fact the first of the malaria parasites to be described. Incubation period is more than 18 days. Characteristically, fevers occur every fourth day (i.e. every 72 h). Infection can persist for up to 50 years and even more, producing occasional febrile episodes. More important, however, are two major complications. First, the *nephrotic syndrome of 'quartan' malaria* (*see* Chapter 10), which does not respond to antimalarial or immunosuppressive agents. This complication is particularly common in tropical Africa, especially Uganda. Granular deposits of IgG and IgM can be demonstrated by immunofluorescence in all of the glomerulae, with C3 and *P. malariae* antigen in some of them. Second, the *tropical splenomegaly syndrome* (TSS) was initially associated with this infection; however, recent evidence suggests that all four malaria species can cause this complication; host genetic factors are clearly involved also. TSS is considered to be an aberrant immune response to malaria infection; the main clinical manifestation is gross splenomegaly occurring in someone in a highly malarious area, and the laboratory abnormalities are: a raised malarial antibody titre, elevated serum IgM (caused by enhanced synthesis), and sinusoidal lymphocytosis (with T lymphocytes) in a liver biopsy specimen; Kupffer cells contain a heavy IgM deposition. Anaemia, with an increased reticulocyte count and thrombocytopenia, is usual; neutropenia may also be present. Severe haemolytic episodes are especially common in pregnancy. Bone marrow is hypercellular.

Long-term malaria prophylaxis (which should be life-long) has been shown to produce a reduction in splenic size, but only after many months or years of continuous treatment. Splenectomy should be avoided if possible because this leaves the patient highly vulnerable not only to recurrent malaria but also to bacterial infections—especially those of pneumococcal origin. *P. malariae* infections are treated with chloroquine. Because there is no clear evidence of an exo-erythrocytic cycle, primaquine is not indicated.

FURTHER READING

Bruce-Chwatt L. J. (1985). *Essential Malariology*, 2nd edn, p. 452. London: William Heinemann Medical Books.

Cook G. C. (1980). The tropical splenomegaly syndrome. In *Tropical Gastroenterology*, p. 205–15. Oxford: Oxford University Press.

Cook G. C. (1986). *Plasmodium falciparum* infection: problems in prophylaxis and treatment in 1986. *Q. J. Med*; **61:** 1091–1115.

Cook G. C. (1986). Serious problems with antimalarial drugs *J. Infect*; **13:** 1–4.

Peters W. (1982). Antimalarial drug resistance: an increasing problem. *Brit. Med. Bull*; **38:** 187-92.

White N. J., Warrell D. A., Chanthavanich P., *et al.*(1983). Severe hypoglycemia and hyperinsulinemia in falciparum malaria. *N. Engl. J. Med*; **309:** 61–6.

Whitfield D., Curtis C. F., White G. B., *et al.* (1984). Two cases of falciparum malaria acquired in Britain. *Brit. Med. J*; **289:** 1607–9.

Warrell D. A., Looareesuwan S., Warrell M. J., *et al.* (1982). Dexamethazone proves deleterious in cerebral malaria: a double-blind trial in 100 comatose patients. *New Engl. J. Med*; **306:** 313–19.

Chapter Five

Gastrointestinal Infections

'A dirty cook gives diarrhoea quicker than rhubarb.'
Tung-su Pai
(Wang Chi Min. (1926). *Rep. Northern Manchurian Plague Prev. Service, Tientsin,* **v:** 300–15).

During the last decade, *Campylobacter pylori (pyloridis)* has been repeatedly demonstrated in the stomach and duodenum of patients with gastritis and peptic ulcer. While claims have been made that this organism is aetiologically important in these two diseases, not all of Koch's postulates have yet been fulfilled, and a cause–effect relationship has not therefore been established.

With all acute gastrointestinal infections (whether they are viral, bacterial or parasitic in origin) several possible sequelae exist:

(i)   Rapid resolution (fortunately the usual course).
(ii) Rapid death (caused usually by severe dehydration and electrolyte disturbance).
(iii) A subacute course with subsequent resolution.
(iv) A chronic course (an arbitrary length of illness is 2 months)—postinfective malabsorption (PIM) (*see* p. 92).

TRAVELLERS' DIARRHOEA (TD)

This trivial clinical syndrome which afflicts the vast majority of travellers at one time or another, is known by many colloquial names: turista, Montezuma's revenge, Aztec two-step, GI trots, gyppi tummy, Spanish flux, Casablanca crud, Aden gut, Bassah belly, Turkey trot, Poona poohs, Malta dog, Rangoon runs, Tokyo trots, Trotsky's, Bombay runs, Ho Chi Minhs, Hong Kong dog and emporiatric enteritis to name but only a few.

Aetiologically, little was known about this clinical syndrome until 1970, when Rowe and his coworkers reported that a high proportion of British soldiers afflicted soon after arrival in Aden had 'foreign' serotypes of *Escherichia coli* in faecal samples. Enterotoxigenic *E. coli* (both heat-labile and heat-stable toxin-producing strains, and some with enter-adherent properties also) are now known to be responsible for a high proportion of cases—perhaps 40–70%. However, many other infective agents are also involved, and they vary in different geographical locations. Table 5.1 summarises some of the more important organisms. It is clear, therefore, that the syndrome is caused by a 'mixed bag' of infective agents, and furthermore, that this mix varies from area to area; the predominant agent(s) in Mexico are, for example, likely to be different from those in south-east Asia or east Africa. Also, these often differ from those causing similar syndromes in temperate (westernised) parts of the world. Furthermore, several different organisms may be responsible for a single attack; in a study in Thailand, for example, one-third of cases were shown to have from 2 to 4 potential pathogens in a faecal sample. Clearly, host factors also are important—not least gastric acidity which can be significantly influenced by life-style; whereas moderate alcohol consumption is known to stimulate gastric-acid secretion, cannabis has a reverse action. The importance of H_2-receptor

Table 5.1

SOME OF THE CAUSATIVE ORGANISMS RESPONSIBLE FOR THE CLINICAL SYNDROME OF TRAVELLERS' DIARRHOEA

Bacteria
  Escherichia coli (heat-labile and heat-stable toxigenic strains)
  Campylobacter spp.
  Salmonella spp.
  Shigella spp.

Viruses
  Rotavirus
  Norwalk agent

Parasites
  Giardia lamblia
  Cryptosporidium spp.
  Entamoeba histolytica (?)

antagonists as predisposing factors is unclear and requires elucidation. The eminent British gastroenterologist Sir Arthur Hurst wrote in 1934 that 'the services would save much more invaliding if men with achlorhydria were not sent to the tropics'. In this, as well as many other matters, he was ahead of his time!

Clinically the syndrome is dominated by self-limiting diarrhoea which usually, but not always, begins within the first week of arrival to a new 'heavily contaminated' environment; peak incidence is at 3–4 days with a secondary (lesser) one at about 10 days. Some travel resorts, Tunisia is one example, have a bad reputation and this has been confirmed in an epidemiological study. The disease is usually mild—4–5 stools daily at most, and the course usually lasts no more than 3–4 days. Vomiting is unusual (although anorexia and nausea are common); bloody diarrhoea is rare. Although pyrexia is very unusual, generalised aches and pains and headache are common. Mortality rate is close to zero; it is a serious illness only in the elderly and debilitated.

Until recently few facts were available on the effect of antibiotics given prophylactically. Studies in Mexico by DuPont and his colleagues have now confirmed that prophylactic antibiotics will statistically reduce the overall incidence; Table 5.2 summarises several agents which have been used prophylactically. However, antibiotics should be used cautiously because they all carry side-effects; therefore, certain 'high risk' groups only should be delineated for such treatment:

achlorhydrics and hypochlorhydrics (including those receiving H_2-receptor antagonists);
patients with known inflammatory bowel disease;
individuals in whom electrolyte imbalance can be exacerbated by TD (e.g. those receiving diuretics);
miscellaneous group (those on important business trips, military populations, airline pilots, etc).

Efficacy of bismuth subsalicylate has also been established, but the sheer bulk of suspension which must be carried around by the traveller limits its value. Antiperistaltic agents also should be used cautiously (*see* p. 75).

In treatment, recent controlled trials from Mexico have shown that the length of an attack of TD can be shortened significantly by antibiotics; Table 5.3 summarises some agents used. Co-trimoxazole (TMP–SMZ) is probably the most successful; how-

Table 5.2

AGENTS WHICH HAVE BEEN USED FOR PROPHYLAXIS OF TRAVELLERS' DIARRHOEA

Agent	Dose
Antibiotics	
Doxycycline	100 mg daily
Trimethoprim (TMP)	200 mg daily
Trimethoprim + sulphamethoxazole (TMP + SMZ)	2 tab b.d.
Furazolidone	100 mg b.d.
(Also phthalylsulphathiazole, neomycin, 'Streptotriad')	
Other agents	
Bismuth subsalicylate	
Antiperistaltics	
Diphenoxylate	
Loperamide	
Codeine phosphate	

Table 5.3

AGENTS WHICH HAVE BEEN USED IN THE TREATMENT OF TRAVELLERS' DIARRHOEA

Agent	Dose
Antibiotics	
Trimethoprim (TMP)	200 mg b.d. (3–5 days)
Trimethoprim + sulphamethoxazole (TMP + SMZ)	1 tab b.d. (3–5 days)
Bicozamycin	500 mg 6 hourly (3 days)
Other agents	
Kaolin	
Pectin	
Hydrated aluminium silicate	
Tincture of opium	
(Also, starches, talcs, chalks, gums, other absorbents)	
Antiperistaltic agents	
(*See* Table 5.2)	

ever, as in prophylaxis, all antibiotics carry side-effects (Table 5.4 summarises some of them) and should be used sparingly. Antiperistaltic agents (some have antisecretory properties also) should be used sparingly; acting unphysiologically, excretion of pathogenic organisms can be prolonged. The basis for management of an attack of TD must always be rehydration (*see* p. 95): all travellers should carry sachets of an appropriate glucose-electrolyte mixture (e.g. Dioralyte (Armour Laboratories), Rehidrat (Searle), or UNICEF 15–611–00).

Many principles of management, and also problems associated with antibiotics which apply to TD, are also relevant to most other acute intestinal infections (certainly in relation to medicine in the tropics and subtropics).

VIRAL CAUSES OF DIARRHOEA

Twenty years ago, very little was known about viral causes of diarrhoea. In the developing 'Third World', viruses are now known to be important aetiological agents in diarrhoea, especially in infants and children. The role of rotaviruses, caliciviruses and Norwalk agent is now clear. They are also important in diarrhoeal outbreaks in developed temperate countries.

Undoubtedly many viruses causing diarrhoea are still unidentified. An effect on mucosal integrity is important in the pathogenesis of diarrhoea; rotavirus destroys villus morphology (as demonstrated in scanning electron micrographs). Important questions regard the number of serotypes, and whether protection against animal viruses should be carried out also. Vaccines against rotavirus will eventually become available; however, they must be acid stable so that they can be given to infants in a formula feed.

BACTERIAL CAUSES OF DIARRHOEA

Cholera

Of the secretory (or watery) diarrhoeas of *small intestinal* origin, cholera is the archetypal infection. This disease is now localised in tropical and subtropical countries, where standards of sanitation, etc leave much to be desired. This was formerly, however, a

Table 5.4

SOME SIDE-EFFECTS AND OTHER PROBLEMS ATTRIBUTED TO ANTIBIOTICS USED IN PROPHYLAXIS AND TREATMENT OF TRAVELLERS' DIARRHOEA

Drug rashes

Stevens–Johnson syndrome

Antibiotic-associated colitis

Increased risk of superinfection by other pathogens (e.g. zoonotic salmonellae)

Masking of more serious gastrointestinal infections with resulting difficulty in diagnosis

Development of bacterial resistance; enteropathogenicity and antibiotic-resistance are often transferred together

Ineffective in many infections, e.g. certain bacterial (e.g. *Campylobacter*), viruses, parasites

---

worldwide disease, and epidemics in northern Europe (including the UK) and north America were major problems up to the latter years of the 19th century. Major pandemics usually originate from south-east Asia; they have swept across Asia, the Middle-east, and more recently, parts of Africa. A major contribution to the understanding of the causation of cholera epidemics was made by the anaesthetist Dr John Snow, who during an epidemic at Soho, London in 1854, was able to delineate a high concentration of cases in the immediate vicinity of the Broad Street pump. Following his removal of the handle of the pump, the epidemic subsided; this is rightly claimed as one of the greatest of epidemiological discoveries; it is to this day commemorated by an 'oral rehydration' centre on the site which goes by the name of the 'Doctor John Snow'. A more recent cholera epidemic was described by Somerset Maugham in his novel *The Painted Veil*.

The 'classical' organism is the *Vibrio cholerae*; however, around 1960, the *El tor* variant of this organism appeared and has since accounted for most cases, with reservoirs of *V. cholerae* confined to the Indian subcontinent—notably the Ganges and Brahmaputra river deltas. There are three major subtypes of the organism: Ogawa, Inaba and Hikojima. The organisms are spread predominantly by infected water supplies; overcrowding is important. The annual Hadj to Mecca has for long been a major means of spread of the disease. The whereabouts of the *V. cholerae* organism between epidemics requires further study. In recent years, a few cases have been contracted from contaminated food supplies on aeroplanes. Host factors are important, e.g. blood group A is associated with infection and O with relative protection; moderate alcohol consumption stimulates gastric acid production (which is protective).

Although jejunal morphology remains normal, the enterotoxin produced by rapidly proliferating *V. cholerae* attaches to enterocyte receptors and results in a massive net water secretion into the lumen by reversing, via cyclic adenosine monophosphate (cAMP), the normal net flow across the mucosa. By introducing fluids of correct composition, which contain glucose and sodium chloride, into the lumen the net flow can, however, be reversed (*see* p. 97).

Clinically, torrential watery diarrhoea ('rice-water' stools) constitutes the dominant feature; up to 24 l may be lost in 24 h. This results in severe dehydration, which if untreated precipitates circulatory failure, acute tubular necrosis and uraemia. The *El tor* variant produces a rather milder illness compared with classical cholera, although in an individual case the two are clinically inseparable. In an unsophisticated environment, the 'cholera cot' is of value in management; the watery stool is collected via a circular hole in the middle of a canvas bed, into a bucket (or other container) in which the volume of fluid is monitored with a 'dip stick' at 2-hourly intervals; output volume can thus be assessed. Although in severe cases, intravenous rehydration is required in the early stage, thereafter, management is with oral rehydration using an appropriate fluid (oral rehydration therapy, ORT). An example of a suitable intravenous fluid is: NaCl 5, KCl 1, $NaHCO_3$ 4 g/l [$\approx$ Na^+ 133, K^+ 13, HCO_3^- 48, Cl^- 98 mEq/l]. Tetracyclines (250 mg t.d.s. for 4 days), are of value especially in *El tor* disease, in shortening the length of diarrhoea and should be started soon after oral rehydration has begun. However, resistance (often multiple) soon emerges, and antibiotic treatment cannot be recommended in epidemics. Cholera vaccines are presently of limited value and are no longer mandatory for entry to any country; although they diminish the severity of an attack and are of some value to the traveller they are virtually useless in limiting an epidemic.

Other bacterial causes of small intestinal diarrhoea

In the UK, the most common cause of acute diarrhoeal disease is now *Campylobacter spp.* infection; this infection has during the last decade overtaken the zoonotic salmonellae. The emergence of this pathogen is due to increased recognition of the organism consequent upon improved culture techniques, and a probable actual increased incidence. Other important organisms are: *Escherichia coli*, *Shigella spp.* and the rotavirus. This same mix of pathogens also applies to developing 'Third World' countries although the frequencies and relative ratios here are often different. There is an overlap between cases of acute diarrhoeal disease with a single cause, travellers' diarrhoea (*see* p. 72), 'food poisoning' and the various more exotic acute intestinal infections (*see* pp. 82 and 83) contracted by travellers and introduced into developed countries including the UK.

Campylobacter jejuni

Now the most common cause of acute gastroenteritis (and 'food poisoning') in England and Wales, this organism causes a systemic illness with headache and limb pains in addition to diarrhoea, after an incubation period of 16–48 h. Nearly all strains are sensitive to erythromycin but clinically this antibiotic is only of value in limiting the disease if started early.

Salmonella spp

These organisms are zoonotic being common in poultry, cattle and many other species of mammals and other animals. There are over 2000 different strains and of these at least 700 are known to produce 'food poisoning'. The incubation period is 16–48 h. A bacteraemia may ensue and bone and joint complications can result in patients with sickle-cell disease. A severe septicaemic illness can result in infants, elderly and debilitated individuals.

Escherichia coli

This form of gastroenteritis occurs worldwide; the greatest risk of dehydration is in small infants. Strains can be divided into:

(i) *Enteropathogenic* (adherence and colonising factors are important in pathogenicity).

(ii) *Enterotoxigenic* (heat-labile and heat-stable toxigenic).
(iii) *Enteroinvasive*, in which pathogenicity is similar to that of the shigellae.

Breast-feeding exerts a protective effect in infants. Treatment is with oral rehydration. Lactose intolerance may be a complication.

Clostridium perfringens

This organism produces outbreaks of food poisoning in institutions, usually where food is cooked in bulk. The reheating of food allows proliferation of these sporulating anaerobes. The incubation period is 12–24 h.

Clostridium botulinum

An enterotoxin which counteracts release of acetylcholine, interferes with neurotransmission. Although classified as a cause of 'food poisoning' the illness is a systemic one with neurological complications. The incubation period is 12–72 h. An antitoxin should be given as early as possible.

Staphylococcus aureus

A heat-stable enterotoxin is responsible for this acute disease which is usually dominated by severe vomiting after a short incubation period of 1–6 h. The toxin is resistant to heat and may survive cooking.

Bacterial Causes of Diarrhoea of Colorectal Origin

Although *Campylobacter spp.* and enteroinvasive strains of *E. coli* are sometimes pathogenic in the colon, the most classical group of organisms is the shigellae, headed by *Shigella dysenteriae-I* (Shiga's bacillus); *S. dysenteriae* (other serotypes), *S. flexneri*, *S. boydii* and *S. sonnei* constitute the remainder. Clinically, shigellosis presents with features of *invasive* colitis, i.e. bloody diarrhoea with mucus and often pus also. This group of organisms is invasive and enterotoxins are of relatively minor importance. In severe shigella infections, with for example *S. dysenteriae-I*, antibiotics are usually indicated, but the problem is that these organisms are frequently resistant to a wide range of antibiotics. Severe *Campylobacter* infections, especially when accompanied by septicaemia should be treated with erythromycin but this agent is of no value after the early phase of disease.

Yersinia enterocolitica, an organism widespread in wild and domestic animals, is a cause of ileocaecal disease; the terminal ileum is predominantly involved. Septicaemia, arthritis, mesenteric adenitis and erythema nodosum may occur. Appendicitis may be 'mimicked' by *Y. pseudotuberculosis* infection which also causes mesenteric adenitis.

Clostridium difficile is an important cause of antibiotic-associated (pseudomembranous) colitis. The toxin of this Gram-positive, anaerobic bacillus, which can become a problem in the presence of antibiotic exposure, is responsible for life-threatening colitis. Special facilities are required for tissue culture assay to detect the toxin. Treatment is with vancomycin or metronidazole.

The *Shigella* group of bacteria can be associated with Reiter's syndrome (*see* p. 201), in which a generalised arthropathy that sometimes persists for many months, occurs after the colorectal symptoms have subsided; treatment is with anti-inflammatory agents.

Inflammatory bowel disease

Although the *Shigella* group of bacilli and *Entamoeba histolytica* (i.e. invasive strains) (*see* p. 88) are generally considered to be responsible for acute bloody diarrhoea in travellers, this is not always true. In a retrospective study at The Hospital for Tropical Diseases, London, the most common single cause of 'dysentery' in returning UK residents was inflammatory bowel disease (IBD) (usually non-specific ulcerative colitis); this presented for the first time during or immediately after return from a tropical location. The reason for this is presumably connected with an alteration of colonic flora, which triggers the onset of symptoms of IBD for the first time.

Although many claims have been made for an infective aetiology of IBD (many organisms, including mycobacteria have been suggested) there are no conclusive data.

PARASITIC CAUSES OF DIARRHOEA

Small-Intestinal Parasites

Tables 5.5 and 5.6 summarise the more important organisms.

Protozoa

Giardia lamblia infections which can be completely asymptomatic and at the other extreme associated with gross malabsorption (indistinguishable from postinfective malabsorption (PIM)) (*see* p. 92), are the most common in the UK. Although considered by paediatricians for many years to be a significant cause of diarrhoea, weight-loss and failure to thrive, only during the last two decades has the true significance of *G. lamblia* in adult life been delineated. The organism was first demonstrated by van Leeuwenhoek at Delft, Holland, in 1681. Epidemiologically, giardiasis is associated with sudden outbreaks of acute diarrhoea, usually with marked flatus, in travellers. Although Leningrad has achieved considerable notoriety in this respect, the disease can afflict travellers to most parts of the world; contaminated water supplies often form the major reservoir of infection. Clinically the disease (incubation period approximately 14 days) can present as travellers' diarrhoea (*see* p. 72), or it can bear all the clinical and laboratory features of PIM; in the latter disease, the only distinguishing feature is the parasitological absence of a *G. lamblia* infection. Diagnosis is by demonstration of cysts (excretion of

Table 5.5

SMALL-INTESTINAL PROTOZOA

Giardia lamblia
Cryptosporidium spp.
Isospora belli
Sarcocystis spp.

Note: All of these parasites can be associated with significant intestinal malabsorption; with the latter three infections this is usually confined to immunosuppressed individuals.

Table 5.6

SMALL-INTESTINAL HELMINTHS

(i) *No malabsorption:* major *clinical significance*
Nematodes
   Ankylostoma duodenale
   Necator americanus
   Ascaris lumbricoides
   Anisakis spp.

Trematodes
   Heterophyes heterophyes
   Fasciolopsis buski

Cestodes
   Taenia solium (Cysticercus cellulosae)
   T. saginata

(ii) *No malabsorption:* minor *clinical significance*
Nematodes
   Gnathostoma spinigerum
   Angiostrongylus costaricensis
   Ternidens deminutus
   Trichinella spiralis
   Trichostrongylus spp.

Trematodes
   Echinostoma spp.
   Gastrodiscoides hominis

Cestodes
   Dipylidium caninum
   Hymenolepis diminuta
   H. nana

(iii) *Malabsorption*
   Strongyloides stercoralis
   Capillaria philippinensis
   Metagonimus yokogawai*
   Diphylobothrium latum*

*Evidence that these helminths can produce significant malabsorption is limited.

which is notoriously erratic) in faecal samples, or trophozoites in jejunal fluid, jejunal biopsy specimens or by the 'Enterotest' (string test) (*see* p. 27); the organism encysts as it progresses along the gastrointestinal tract. Absorptive function should be investigated in a severe case. Treatment is: metronidazole (2 g daily for 3 consecutive days), or tinidazole (a single dose of 2 g). Occasionally this treatment has to be repeated.

Cryptosporidium spp., *Isospora belli* and *Sarcocystis spp.* infections have only become widely appreciated over the last few years; this is largely because previously used staining techniques for *Cryptosporidium* were inadequate for their demonstration; a modified Ziehl–Neelsen technique is required. These organisms can also produce illnesses varying from an acute self-limiting travellers' diarrhoea syndrome to severe malabsorption. However, the latter clinical presentation is largely confined to immunosuppressed individuals including those with AIDS; severe intractable diarrhoea (sometimes of parasitic origin) is an important complication of this syndrome. Diagnosis is similar to that of *G. lamblia* infection; associated malabsorption should be investigated. Treatment, when required, is more difficult however; in an individual with intact immunity, this is not required. Spiramycin is of value in *Cryptosporidium* infection. *I. belli* and *Sarcocystis hominis* infections often respond to trimethoprim and furazolidone.

Several of these parasites have also assumed a greater importance in the context of male homosexuality.

Helminths

Table 5.6 (p. 83) summarises small intestinal helminthic infections. In a world context, they are extremely common; prevalence rates can be measured in millions if not billions! This applies especially to hookworm and roundworm infections. It is legitimate, therefore, to consider small-intestinal parasites as the normal state for *Homo sapiens* or to say in truth, that we live in a very wormy world! The factors determining individual infection rates are largely unknown; genetic factors in the host might well be at least as important as acquired immunity. The helminths which are not associated with an absorptive defect are covered first.

Helminths not associated with malabsorption

Hookworm

Two species infect man: *Ankylostoma duodenale* and *Necator americanus*. Because infection occurs through intact skin this is especially prevalent in countries with poor standards of hygiene and sanitation; use of night soil for fertilising crops for example, leads to numerous cases. The life-cycle is shown in Fig. 5.1. Skin penetration is sometimes accompanied by a local 'itchy' papulovesicular reaction ('ground itch'). This is probably an allergic response to the larvae; it rarely occurs in those living in areas of endemic infection, probably because blocking antibodies are present.

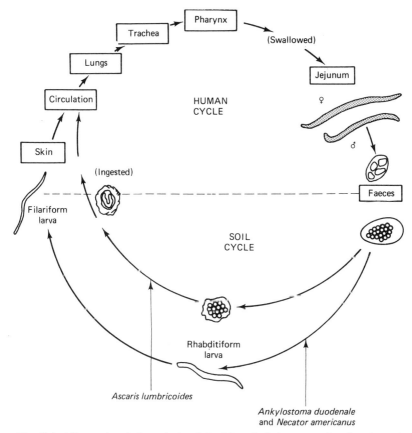

Fig. 5.1. Life cycle of *Ascaris lumbricoides, Ankylostoma duodenale* and *Necator americanus*.

During the migratory cycle following infection, various systemic manifestations including bronchospasm (less marked than with *Ascaris lumbricoides* infection (*see* below)) can be troublesome. Adult worms mature in the duodenum and jejunum, and by causing local mucosal trauma (with their hooks or teeth) produce blood-loss (up to 0·2 ml with *A. duodenale* and 0·05 ml/worm/day with *N. americanus*); however, because the small intestine has a substantial functional reserve much of this lost iron is reabsorbed before the caecum is reached! Severity of the resulting hypochromic, iron-deficiency anaemia depends on worm load; extreme symptoms, leading to cardiac decompensation, can occur with luminal loads of 500–1000 worms. Epigastric pain, hypoproteinaemia and resulting oedema may complicate heavy infections. Diagnosis is by demonstration of eggs in faecal samples, and adult worms in jejunal fluid or biopsy. Peripheral eosinophilia, raised serum IgE and reduced albumin concentration may coexist. Much of the IgE is non-specific and inactive against the parasite; its function is unknown but it might help to modulate IgE-mediated allergic reactions. Treatment is with mebendazole (100 mg b.d. for 3 days) or albendazole (400 mg stat); bephenium hydroxynaphthoate, pyrantel, levamisole and tetrachlorethylene (which is much cheaper) can also be used.

Roundworm

Ascaris lumbricoides is ingested in the form of eggs (derived from contaminated food or water); the subsequent life-cycle is similar to that of the hookworm. Infection has recently increased in the UK; this might be due to: increased holiday travel, infections acquired from immigrants or imported food and/or vegetables, or to contact with pigs (which harbour a similar worm). Bronchospasm and dyspnoea can be a major problem during pulmonary migration; this is often accompanied by patchy shadowing on the chest radiograph. It probably represents a type I allergic reaction to migrating larvae. Adult worms can reach a length of 40 cm, and usually live in the mid-jejunum. Although epigastric pain can occur with heavy infections, intestinal obstruction (mainly in children) and common bile-duct and pancreatic duct obstruction are more important complications; perforation and volvulus rarely occur. Growth retardation in the presence of heavy infection is confined to children. Ova are found in faecal samples, and adult worms in the duodenum and jejunum where they may be outlined during barium studies; an eosinophilia may be present. Treatment is with mebendazole or albendazole (as for hookworm), pyrantel, levamisole or one of the piperazine compounds (which are cheaper).

Anisakis spp. which is acquired from raw or poorly cooked fish (obtained in 'Sushi' bars) can produce an appendicitis-like syndrome in the ileocaecal region. *Trichinella spiralis* is not a true gastrointestinal nematode, but for part of its life-cycle resides here (*see* Chapter 15).

Small intestinal flukes, e.g. *Fasciolopsis buski*, can be associated with anorexia, diarrhoea, vomiting, allergic oedema and eosinophilia.

Tapeworm

The important cestodes of man are *Taenia solium* and *T. saginata*; they are acquired from infected pork and beef respectively, and have straightforward life-cycles, the adult tapeworm maturing in the small intestinal lumen. Symptoms in the absence of complications are few; segments may be noted in the stool—worm phobias may result. Treatment is with niclosamide (2 g for an adult), praziquantel (single dose of 25 mg/kg) or mepacrine (1 g stat). The important complication with *T. solium* is cysticercosis; cysts form in skeletal muscles, subcutaneous tissue, brain and other organs during an aberrant cycle in man. Cerebral cysts are the most important, and epileptic fits, psychiatric disturbances, etc can result; here they rarely calcify, unlike cysts in muscles. Treatment is with praziquantel (50 mg/kg for 15 days); good evidence is now available that cyst size and subsequent disappearance can usually be achieved with this regimen; whether dexamethasone (or another corticosteroid) should be given in addition, is unresolved. The freshwater fish tapeworm *Diphyllobothrium latum* can occasionally cause vitamin B12 deficiency and megaloblastic anaemia; this is however a rare event.

Helminths associated with malabsorption

Two helminths can be associated with an absorptive defect: *Strongyloides stercoralis* and *Capillaria philippinensis*. *S. stercoralis* has a similar life-cycle to that of *A. lumbricoides*; the exception is that there is an additional component, and autoinfection can occur;

larvae can re-enter the human cycle in the perianal region—the cycle can therefore continue for at least 40 years. Adult worms in the jejunum can cause epigastric pain (duodenitis), and by invading mucosa, they can produce malabsorption. A marked eosinophilia may be present during the migratory phase. More persistent pulmonary symptoms than those in ascariasis may occur and these follow aberrant multiplication of larvae in the lungs; they may be found in sputum samples. Ova and sometimes larvae can be found in faecal samples and adults in jejunal fluid, biopsy samples or in samples obtained by the 'Enterotest' (*see* p. 27). Barium meal and follow-through may show abnormalities in the small intestinal mucosal pattern, which reverse after treatment. Tests of absorption are abnormal in a severe infection. During the autoinfection cycle, intermittent urticarial rashes over the lower abdomen and buttocks prove troublesome: many men who were prisoners of war in south-east Asia during World War II (1939–45) in Japanese hands have experienced this problem. In immunosuppressed states, the risk of a hyperinfection syndrome must be borne in mind; all organs may be involved by invading organisms, a paralytic ileus may be present, and a Gram-negative septicaemia can be responsible for serious morbidity; unless treated promptly, death results. Treatment of strongyloidiasis is with thiabendazole (1·5 g b.d. on 3 consecutive days); side-effects are common and the cure rate with one course is around 70% only. Mebendazole and albendazole are inferior. In Papua New Guinea and Zambia, a related species, *S. fülleborni*, can cause severe malabsorption, pot-belly and malnutrition in children. *C. philippinensis* is of limited geographical importance, being confined to the northern Philippines and Thailand. Epidemics have been reported; a reservoir exists in fish and birds. Like *S. stercoralis* severe malabsorption (and protein-losing enteropathy) can occur. Treatment is with mebendazole.

Parasites of Colorectal Origin

Colorectal protozoa and helminths are summarised in Tables 5.7 and 5.8. respectively.

Colorectal protozoa

The protozoa are dominated by *Entamoeba histolytica*. The life-

Table 5.7

COLORECTAL PROTOZOA

Luminal
  Pathogenic
    Entamoeba histolytica
    Balantidium coli
    *Dientamoeba fragilis**
    *E. polecki**
    *Giardia lamblia**
  Non-pathogenic
    E. hartmanni
    E. coli
    Iodamoeba bütschlii
    Endolimax nana
    Chilomastix mesnili
    Trichomonas hominis
    Retortamonas intestinalis
    Enteromonas hominis

Non-luminal
  Pathogenic
    Trypanosoma cruzi (Chagas' disease)

*Although these organisms can at times produce colonic disease, this is probably unusual except in very heavy infections.

cycle is straightforward (Fig. 5.2); cysts are ingested in contaminated food or water and after the cyst-wall has been eroded by digestive enzymes the trophozoites emerge within the colonic lumen. A small epidemic resulting from colonic irrigation used for constipation has been described. By isoenzyme techniques, it is now possible to separate *E. histolytica* into two groups—there are 9 *invasive* and 13 *non-invasive* strains. Other characteristics, such as adherence, lysis etc are currently undergoing investigation. Amoebic colitis usually presents with chronic diarrhoea, often with blood and mucus. Diagnosis is by demonstration of trophozoites (containing ingested red blood cells) in faecal samples. Serological diagnosis is unreliable unless there is advanced invasive disease. It is important to distinguish this from inflammatory bowel disease; if this is erroneously diagnosed and corticosteroids and/or surgery instigated, results can be disastrous and mortality

Table 5.8

COLORECTAL HELMINTHS

Nematodes
  Trichuris trichiura
  Enterobius vermicularis
  Oesophagostomum spp.
  Anisakis spp.

  Ternidens deminutus ⎫ These are predominantly small
  Strongyloides stercoralis ⎬ intestinal helminths, but it is
   ⎭ possible that they can contribute to colonic pathology.

Trematodes
  Schistosoma mansoni ⎫ The schistosomes are not true
  S. intercalatum ⎪ colorectal parasites; adults live in
  S. mattheei ⎬ the portal system (*see* Chapter 6)
  S. japonicum ⎪ and it is the eggs which produce
  S. mekongi ⎭ colonic disease.

may ensue. Treatment is with metronidazole (800 mg t.d.s. for 5 days); this should be followed by diloxanide furoate (500 mg t.d.s. for 10 days) which is a far better luminal amoebicide than metronidazole. Hepatic amoebiasis is dealt with in Chapter 6 (p. 108). Balantidiasis consists of a similar infection; it is caused by *Balantidium coli* and is related to exposure to pigs in which it has a reservoir. The organism can be easily identified microscopically. Invasive disease involving other organs including the liver, is rare. Treatment is with tetracycline.

Colorectal helminths

Of the helminthic infections, *Trichuris trichiura* (whipworm) (a caecal parasite), and *Enterobius vermicularis* (threadworm) are especially important in children. With *T. trichiura*, colonic haemorrhage, iron deficiency anaemia and rectal prolapse occur in children with very heavy infections. Threadworm infections can affect whole families and may be difficult to eradicate—pruritus ani is the classical presenting symptom; appendicitis is an occasional complication. The benzimidazole compounds, mebendazole and albendazole, are the best chemotherapeutic agents for these infections.

Gastrointestinal Infections 91

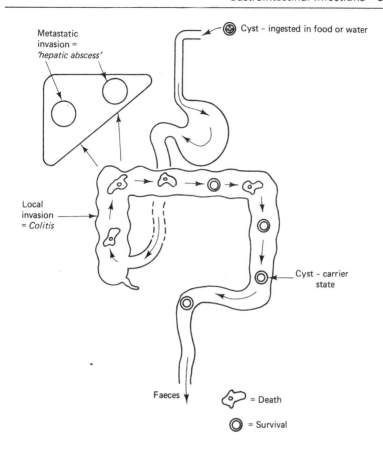

Fig. 5.2. Life cycle of *Entamoeba histolytica*.

Colonic schistosomiasis can present with intermittent diarrhoea, with or without bleeding. Typical mucosal lesions can be demonstrated and colonic polyposis may be present, often being associated with bloody diarrhoea, in Egypt and Sudan. Diagnosis is by detection of eggs of *Schistosoma mansoni* or *S. japonicum* (or a species of less numerical importance) in faecal samples or by the ELISA serological test, which is positive in approximately 95% of cases. Treatment is dealt with under hepatic schistosomiasis (*see* Chapter 6 and p. 109).

POSTINFECTIVE MALABSORPTION (PIM) (TROPICAL SPRUE)

For many centuries there has been an awareness in tropical and subtropical countries of a chronic form of (small intestinal) diarrhoea in which the stools are large, bulky, fatty and offensive, and weight-loss is common. This entity should be separated from a very common condition in tropical countries (especially among lower socioeconomic groups) in which there is mild malabsorption (*tropical enteropathy*); here jejunal morphology consists of leaf and ridged-shaped villi, finger-shaped villi being absent. Reports of severe malabsorption are to be found in ancient Indian writings; probably the earliest in the western literature is by William Hillary in Barbadoes in 1759. Various descriptions are given: the 'white flux', 'diarrhoea alba', 'psilosis', etc. It is therefore clear that malabsorption in tropical countries has for long been recognised, but it is now known that there are many causes of this; Table 5.9 summarises the major ones. It is clearly important to consider all of these in a given individual; in addition, travellers sometimes experience symptoms caused by gluten-induced enteropathy for the first time during or immediately after a tropical exposure. Sir Patrick Manson first drew attention to the importance of 'malabsorption in the tropics'; he first used the term *sprue* in the English language in 1880 while working in Amoy, China; the Dutch used the term *sprouw* to describe cases of malabsorption (with aphthous oral ulceration) in Indonesia.

A clearly delineated entity consisting of malabsorption following an acute gastrointestinal insult, which is more common in tropical and subtropical regions, but which exists albeit unusually in temperate areas also, is now well recognised. This entity— PIM, is often designated 'tropical sprue' (an all embracing term) and should be considered separately. PIM has an interesting geographical distribution which is shown in Fig. 5.3. Although it exists worldwide, the local prevalence rate depends on the incidence of underlying acute diarrhoeal disease, and hence indirectly the underlying standard of sanitation, etc. Epidemics have been reported, especially in south Indians. It was very common in the British Army in Asia during World War II. In the UK, the disease was formerly common in overlanders crossing Asia; however, political events in Afghanistan halted this, and because

Table 5.9

CAUSES OF MALABSORPTION IN TROPICAL AND SUBTROPICAL COUNTRIES

Extra-intestinal
Chronic calcific pancreatitis
Acute and chronic liver disease

Small intestinal causes
Postinfective malabsorption (tropical sprue)
Ileocaecal tuberculosis (*see* Chapter 3)
Mediterranean (α-chain) lymphoma
Intestinal resection (after intussusception, pig-bel disease, etc)
Severe malnutrition (Kwashiorkor)
Small intestinal parasites (*see* Table 5.4):
 Giardia lamblia
 Cryptosporidium spp.
 Isospora belli
 Sarcocystis spp.
 Strongyloides stercoralis
 Capillaria philippinensis
 Acute *Plasmodium falciparum* ⎫
 Visceral leishmaniasis (Kala ⎬ less common causes
 azar) ⎭

Specific malabsorption
Hypolactasia (either genetically determined, 'primary' or secondary to mucosal damage resulting from numerous different insults).

Note: Gluten-induced enteropathy seems to be very unusual in tropical and subtropical countries, but can occasionally present for the first time in travellers to those countries.

more travellers now traverse Africa instead (where less PIM exists) it is now less frequently seen.

Clinically, the disease presents with continuing chronic diarrhoea (with typical malabsorption stools) following an acute gastrointestinal infection; weight-loss is progressive. Tests of absorption are abnormal. As it progresses, serum folate concentration falls (it is often very low by 4 months), and megaloblastic anaemia ensues. Hypoalbuminaemia and vitamin B12 deficiency occur later. In a few extremely chronic cases studied in London

94 Communicable and Tropical Diseases

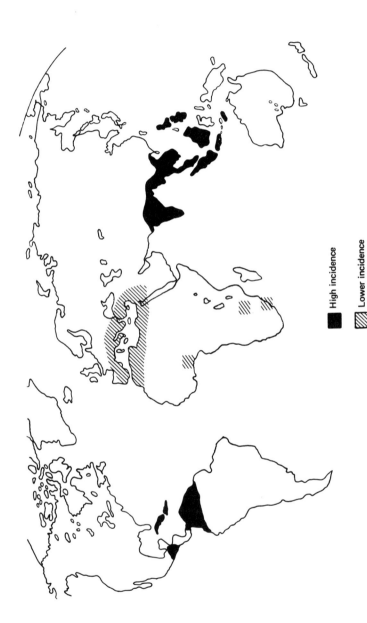

Fig. 5.3. Geographical distribution of postinfective malabsorption (tropical sprue).

which are probably, but not certainly, cases of this syndrome, subacute degeneration of the spinal cord has been recorded. The individual (frequently a young adult) is wasted, anaemic and the tongue may be sore and fissured; although earlier reports stressed aphthous ulceration as being common, this is now rarely a feature of the disease. It is important to differentiate the syndrome from other causes of 'malabsorption in the tropics' (Table 5.9, p. 93).

The cause of PIM was until recently obscure. Genetic factors have been postulated and might be relevant. The disease was for example common in European and Indian soldiers in Asia during World War II, whereas it rarely affected African soldiers serving in the same area. It is now clear that continuing small intestinal luminal colonisation continues after the acute infection and that this is responsible at least in part for the mucosal changes— blunting of villi (but rarely a flat mucosa) and B cell infiltration of the lamina propria. Overgrowth consists of a mixed flora of enterotoxigenic enterobacteriaceae, with *Klebsiella pneumoniae*, *Enterobacter cloacae* and *Escherichia coli* predominant. This is basically different from that in the blind-loop syndrome which in contrast is anaerobic. Claims in south India that coronavirus is aetiologically important there have not been substantiated elsewhere. The cause of the continuing colonisation seems to be associated with delay in small intestinal transit; plasma enteroglucagon concentration is grossly elevated. Immunological abnormalities are not causally involved. Fig. 5.4 summarises the possible pathogenesis of PIM. The role of the colon in this syndrome is unclear. Treatment, which has been in use for over three decades, consists of tetracycline (250 mg t.d.s. for 4 weeks) and folic acid (5 mg t.d.s. for 4 weeks). Recovery is rapid and complete (usually within 2–3 weeks); whereas in the preantibiotic era, death occurred in some 20% of patients, this is now a rare event. Relapse can occur however, especially on removal back to an area where the disease is common.

ORAL REHYDRATION THERAPY (ORT)

Until two decades ago, rehydration in all acute gastrointestinal diseases was carried out by the intravenous route. During the 1970s realisation that it could be accomplished by the oral route became clear. Fig. 5.5 summarises the pathophysiological basis of this form of management. When glucose at a concentration of

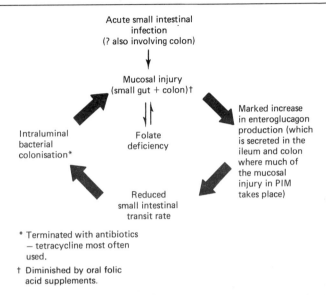

Fig. 5.4. Possible series of events leading to the production of PIM.

approximately 110 mmol/l is introduced into the small intestinal lumen, active transfer across the mucosa is possible even in the presence of bacterial toxin; by 'coupling' with sodium, water transfer follows. Other solutes can also be used. For example sucrose ('refined sugar') is often more readily available in 'Third World' countries, and is an acceptable alternative to glucose unless there is severe morphological damage of the enterocyte, in which case secondary sucrase deficiency may be present. Alternatively, glycine, can be substituted for glucose. Various cereals too, if given at correct concentration, are also effective. Except in severely ill patients and those who are vomiting, the intravenous route is therefore rendered unnecessary. In a world context this is in fact an extremely important contribution to the therapy of acute diarrhoeal disease, especially in children in developing 'Third World' countries. The *Lancet* (1978) concluded that this discovery represented 'potentially the most important medical advance this century'*. It is the duty of every medical practitioner therefore to make certain that this technique is more widely used.

*Editorial. (1978). Water with sugar and salt. *Lancet*; **2**: 300–1.

Gastrointestinal Infections 97

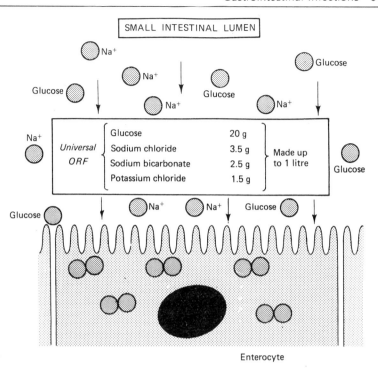

COMPOSITION OF THREE ORAL REHYDRATION FLUIDS (mmol/l)

	Universal ORF (see above)	Adults with severe diarrhoea (e.g. cholera)	Children
Glucose	110	110	110
Na+	90	120	75
K+	20	25	35
Cl−	80	97	70
HCO3−	30	18	40

Fig. 5.5. Principle of oral rehydration.

FURTHER READING

Cook G. C. (1980). *Tropical Gastroenterology*, pp. 225–445. Oxford: Oxford University Press.

Cook G. C. (1983). Travellers' diarrhoea: an insoluble problem. *Gut*; **24**: 1105–8.

Cook G. C. (1984). Aetiology and pathogenesis of postinfective tropical malabsorption (tropical sprue). *Lancet* **1:** 721–3.
Cook G. C. (1984). Hypolactasia: geographical distribution, diagnosis and practical significance. In *Critical Reviews in Tropical Medicine*, Vol. 2, pp. 117–39. (Chandra, R. K., ed). New York, London: Plenum Press.
Cook G. C. (1985). Parasitic infection. In *Disorders of the Small Intestine*, pp. 283–98. (Booth, C. C., Neale G., ed). Oxford: Blackwell Scientific Publications.
Cook G. C. (1986). The clinical significance of gastrointestinal helminths—a review. *Trans. R. Soc. Trop. Med. Hyg*; **80:** 675–85.
Cook G. C. (1986). Colorectal parasitic and mycotic infection. *Ital. J. Gastroent*; **18:** 338–42.
Cook G. C. (1987). Intestinal parasitic infection. *Curr. Opinion Gastroent*; **3:** 130–41.
Cook G. C. (1987). Postinfective malabsorption (including 'tropical sprue'). In *Oxford Textbook of Medicine*, 2nd ed., 12.115–12.120. (Weatherall D. J., Ledingham J. G. G., Warrell D. A., eds.). Oxford: Oxford University Press.
Cook G. C. (1987). *Strongyloides stercoralis* hyperinfection syndrome: how often is it missed? *Q. J. Med*; **64:** 625–9.
Editorial. (1985). Is that amoeba harmful or not? *Lancet*; **1:** 732–4.
Editorial. (1986). Clostridium difficile—a neglected pathogen in chronic-care wards? *Lancet*; **2:** 790–1.
Feldman M. (1984). Traveler's diarrhea. *Am. J. Med. Sci*; **288:** 136–48.
Gorbach S. L., ed. (1986). *Infectious Diarrhea*, p. 328. Boston, Oxford: Blackwell Scientific Publications.
Harries A. D., Myers B., Cook G. C. (1985). Inflammatory bowel disease: a common cause of bloody diarrhoea in visitors to the tropics. *Brit. Med. J*; **291:** 1686–7.
Igra-Siegman Y., Kapila R., Sen P., *et al.* (1981) Syndrome of hyperinfection with *Strongyloides stercoralis. Rev. Infect. Dis;* **3:** 397–407.
Jokipii L., Jokipii A. M. M. (1986). Timing of symptoms and oocyst excretion in human cryptosporidiosis. *N. Engl. J. Med*; **315:** 1643–7.
McNulty C. A. M., Gearty J. C., Crump B., *et al.* (1986). Campylobacter pyloridis and associated gastritis: investigator blind, placebo controlled trial of bismuth salicylate and erythromycin ethylsuccinate. *Brit. Med. J*; **293:** 645–9.
Mahalanabis D. (1984). Oral rehydration therapy. In *Critical Reviews in Tropical Medicine*, Vol. 2, pp. 77–91. (Chandra R. K., ed). New York, London: Plenum Press.
Montgomery R. D., Chesner I. M. (1985). Post-infective malabsorption in the temperate zone. *Trans. R. Soc. Trop. Med. Hyg*; **79:** 322–7.
Sprott V., Selby C. D., Ispahani P., Toghill P. J. (1987). Indigenous strongyloidiasis in Nottingham. *Brit. Med. J*; **294:** 741–2.
Steffen R, Linde F. van der, Gyr K., Schär M. (1983). Epidemiology of diarrhea in travelers. *J. Am. Med. Ass*; **249:** 1176–80.

Chapter Six

Infections Involving the Liver and Biliary System

THE VIRAL HEPATITIDES (A, B, NANB AND D)

The viruses responsible for 'viral hepatitis' occur worldwide. In developing 'Third World' countries they all are extremely important and are associated with substantial morbidity, and in some areas great mortality. In 'Third World' countries, HAV is usually acquired early in life, and HBV is frequently transmitted in the neonatal period. NANB, which consists of several distinct viruses probably varies a good deal locally (*see* p. 102). The HDV (or δ) virus is also more common in some areas than others; it is particularly lethal.

Hepatitis A (HAV)

The faecal–oral route is the usual mode of infection. Therefore, the incidence of this disease depends very largely on the underlying standards of sanitation, etc. The highest incidence in travellers to the tropics occurs in those going to the Indian subcontinent; rates in Africa, the Middle-east and south-east Asia are rather lower. The Mediterranean littoral does not have an especially high rate. The incubation period is short (15–49 days) and the illness—anorexia, nausea, jaundice, dark urine and pale stools—is a self-limiting one. The virus is able to replicate in the intestine, kidneys and other sites, also. After the icteric phase, HAV is complexed with antibody and is no longer infectious. Occasionally, a cholestatic phase with continuing pruritus proves troublesome; other long-term sequelae are very unusual. Fig. 6.1 summarises the serum immunological findings; HAV IgG remains elevated for the remainder of the patient's life. There is no

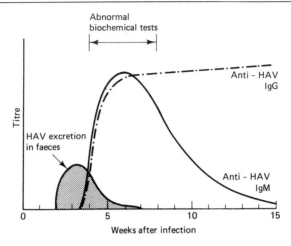

Fig. 6.1. Serum immunological findings in relation to HAV infection.

specific treatment; bed-rest might be of value in the acute phase (although this is unproven); a high calorie intake seems to be beneficial. Dietary fat is not contraindicated. Alcohol should be avoided until the liver function tests return to normal. Prophylaxis with pooled γ-globulin renders temporary protection for several months.

Hepatitis B (HBV)

Fig. 6.2 shows the HBV virus in diagrammatic form; e antigen is a subunit of the core protein. This infection is usually spread by the parenteral route. It is a major problem (and has increased in frequency during the last decade) in drug-addicts; evidence is now available that, in the UK, this is now declining. Male homosexuals also have a high rate of infection. In developing 'Third World' countries, the portal of entry is: neonatal infection, tattooing, scarifications inflicted by local medicine men (witch-doctors), ritual circumcision, etc. Following infection, HBV is integrated into the host's DNA. A rise in IgM and transaminases are synonymous.

Fig. 6.3 summarises the immunological events after an HBV infection. Various subtypes of HBV have different geographical distributions; although of academic interest in helping to locate

Infections Involving the Liver and Biliary System 101

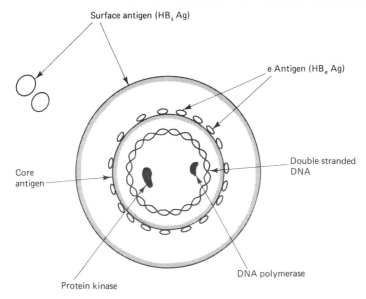

Fig. 6.2. Schematic diagram of the HB virus, showing the various antigenic components.

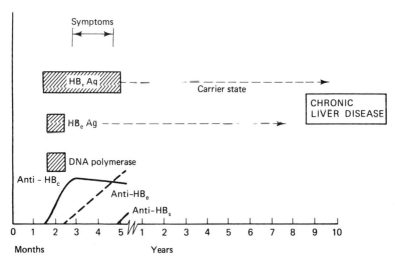

Fig. 6.3. Serum immunological findings in relation to an HBV infection.

the site of infection they have little, if any, clinical importance. The incubation period is a long one (60–180 days). Grades of illness vary from subclinical to a serious complicated disease. An acute glomerulonephritis is an occasional manifestation. Acute hepatic necrosis is associated with a high mortality rate. There are some 200 million HBV carriers worldwide; this state is caused by a failure to clear the virus due to a defect in the production of endogenous α-interferon. When possible, the carrier state should be treated early with interferon or adenine arabinoside. However, interferon is of no value in neonatal infections. When HIV infection is present simultaneously, there is no response to interferon. The incidence of the HB_sAg carrier state varies in different geographical areas; thus in the 'Western World' (including the UK), the rate is approximately 0.1%, in much of tropical Africa the figure is approximately 10%, and much higher rates have been recorded in Pacific populations. More important numerically are the chronic sequelae described below (*see* p. 112). Hepatocytes are destroyed by cytotoxic T cells.

Delta (δ) Agent (HDV)

This incomplete virus, which is homologous with plant viroids, can only replicate in the presence of HBV. It was first described in Italy, but is now known to be widespread geographically, especially in the Middle-east, south America and northern Africa. There are probably several different subtypes of the incomplete virus. Infection with HBV plus δ agent (HDV) produces an acute fulminant hepatitis and severe chronic disease; with progressive disease, death tends to occur after 2–3 months rather than 20–30 years (with HBV infection alone). In northern parts of south America a severe fatal form of hepatitis known for many years as *labrea* hepatitis is caused by this agent. The virus is susceptible to interferon.

Non-A Non-B (NANB)

NANB is a term given to a group of viruses with varying incubation periods and routes of infection. Because there are as yet no serological markers it is impossible to distinguish them positively from HAV and HBV infections. Some are faecal–oral and others parenterally transmitted infections. Large epidemics of water-borne NANB infection with faecal–oral spread have occurred in India and Kashmir; a high incidence of acute hepatic necrosis, especially in pregnancy, has been reported. With parenterally transmitted strains, both the carrier state and nature of the chronic complications are similar to those caused by HBV infection; these are relatively common in Western populations and up to 90% are post-transfusional.

By no means all cases of acute hepatitis, especially in a tropical and subtropical context, are caused by the viruses so far described; Table 6.1 summarises some of the main differential diagnoses.

Table 6.1

SOME CAUSES OF ACUTE HEPATITIS IN A TROPICAL OR SUBTROPICAL SETTING

Viral hepatitis
    HAV, HBV, HDV and NANB

Other viral causes
    Yellow fever
    Viral haemorrhagic fevers
    Others, e.g.
        Epstein-Barr virus (EBV)
        Cytomegalovirus (CMV)

Bacterial causes
    Leptospirosis
    Salmonella typhi

Parasitic causes
    Plasmodium falciparum
    Visceral leishmaniasis

Toxins/therapeutic agents

Alcoholic hepatitis

Jaundice of systemic bacterial infection
    Pneumococcal pneumonia
    Pyomyositis

OTHER VIRAL INFECTIONS

Yellow Fever

Confined to tropical Africa and southern America (Fig. 6.4), this disease affects up to hundreds of thousands of people with many thousands of deaths (case fatality rate is up to 50%) in its epidemic form; recent outbreaks have occurred in Nigeria. It was first recognised as a nosological entity in the 17th century but was for long confused with viral hepatitis. It caused much mortality in sailors and others in affected areas and the designation of west Africa as the 'white man's grave' had much to do with this. Mosquito transmission was established by Reed in 1900; the virus (a member of the *Flavivirus* genus) was isolated in 1927 by inoculation of blood from a Ghanaian man into highly susceptible rhesus monkeys. In the 1930s, an effective vaccine (17D)—live and attenuated—was developed; although effective immunisation campaigns led to a dramatic decline in incidence, reduction in surveillance has resulted in a resurgence of the disease in Africa. The vaccine is mandatory for travellers to the affected countries; a certificate is valid for 10 years. Vaccination is not advised in the first 9 months of life, in other circumstances where live vaccines are contraindicated, and during the first trimester of pregnancy. Newer techniques of vaccine production are anticipated now that the nucleotide sequence of the virus has been unravelled. The reservoir of infection is in susceptible mosquito species (which include *Aedes aegypti*), in which infection continues throughout life and is transmitted transovarially through infected eggs. Entomological and virological aspects of transmission are complex; urban and jungle cycles have been described.

The acute disease (incubation period 3–6 days) which is undoubtedly underdiagnosed in affected areas, is characterised by two clinical stages: a viraemia, and a hepatorenal stage (including acute tubular necrosis) with haemorrhagic manifestations; these are separated by a short remission. Following recovery, hepatic histology returns to normal. Diagnosis is by virus isolation, serology (appropriately timed paired samples), and virus detection in serum or blood by means of an antigen-capture ELISA technique. Needle liver biopsy is absolutely contraindicated; histology is rarely diagnostic. Virus isolation from hepatic tissue, in which Councilman bodies may be demonstrated histologically, at necropsy can give a definitive diagnosis.

Infections Involving the Liver and Biliary System 105

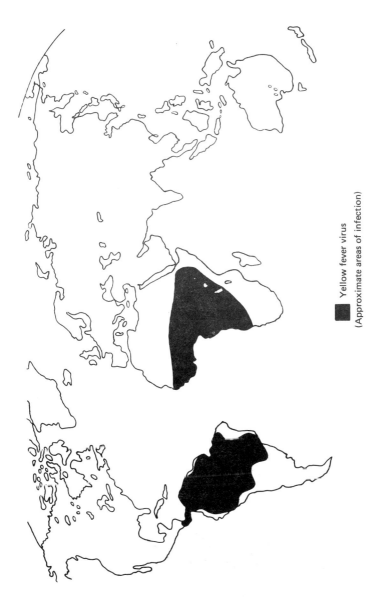

Fig. 6.4. Geographical distribution of yellow fever.

■ Yellow fever virus (Approximate areas of infection)

Clinical management is merely supportive; apart from hepatic (death is rarely attributable to hepatic failure) and renal complications, bleeding, electrolyte disturbances, acidosis, oliguria, delirium, shock and superimposed infections (bacterial and parasitic, including malaria) are potentially amenable to treatment.

Viral Haemorrhagic Fevers and other Viruses

The viral haemorrhagic fevers are discussed in Chapter 15. Jaundice may be an important clinical manifestation in Marburg and Ebola diseases. Epstein–Barr virus and cytomegalovirus hepatitis are also dealt with in Chapter 15. Although jaundice is unusual, derangement of liver function is present in 100% of cases of EBV hepatitis. CMV hepatitis is common throughout the world, especially in immunocompromised individuals. Acute hepatic involvement is common in CMV hepatitis; histological changes are characteristic and cholestatic features are common.

BACTERIAL INFECTIONS

Leptospirosis

Leptospirosis is caused by many different serotypes of leptospires (finely coiled spirochaetes), the best known being *Leptospira icterohaemorrhagiae* and *L. canicola*. Weil's disease was first described in 1887, being associated with working in sewers. The disease occurs worldwide in tropical and temperate countries; it is a major problem in south-east Asia (especially in paddy fields) and central (including the Caribbean) and south America. The range of animal hosts is wide; a carrier state develops and the leptospires are excreted in urine. Infection is either by direct contact with urine from an infected animal or from contaminated water, soil or vegetation; entry is through skin lesions or mucous membranes. Liver, kidneys and muscle are especially affected although all organs may be involved. The incubation period is 2–26 (usually 7–13) days. In the initial (leptospiraemic) phase of the illness, organisms are present in blood and CSF; fever, muscle pains and headache are common, and pulmonary symptoms less so. Examination reveals a febrile patient with a relative bradycardia (as in typhoid) and conjunctivitis; there may be a rash—usually macular or maculopapular. In the second ('immune') phase which occurs after 4–9 days (and coincides with IgM antibody production), fever and meningismus (aseptic meningitis) occur. In severe cases, jaundice, renal failure and haemorrhagic manifestations may ensue. A neutrophil leucocytosis may be marked. Proteinuria, with casts and cells may be present in the first phase, when abnormal liver function tests are often present; the serum creatinine kinase concentration is usually elevated. Diagnosis depends on culture of leptospires from blood or CSF (first phase) or urine (second phase); serological tests are of value in the second phase of the disease.

Prognosis is variable and depends on the age of the patient and the serotype involved. Penicillin, streptomycin, tetracyclines, chloramphenicol and erythromycin have been used therapeutically. Penicillin G 600 mg 4-hourly given intramuscularly, started very early in the disease, probably offers the best results; within 4–6 h a Jarisch–Herxheimer reaction may occur. Jaundice and renal failure should be managed on merit.

Jaundice of Acute Systemic Bacterial Infection

A complex form of hepatic insult is a common accompaniment of acute bacterial infection, especially pneumococcal pneumonia and pyomyositis. This seems especially common in Africa and Papua New Guinea. It is presumably a 'toxic' hepatitis; hepatocellular, cholestatic and haemolytic elements may all be present, the incidence of the latter largely depending on the underlying incidence of glucose-6-phosphate dehydrogenase (G–6–PD) deficiency in the community. It is self-limiting and rapidly resolves as the underlying bacterial infection subsides; no specific treatment is required. It is important, however, to exclude this entity from other causes of acute hepatitis) especially the viral hepatitides (*see* p. 99).

PARASITIC INFECTIONS

The liver can undergo acute involvement in the presence of parasitic infections. Severe acute *Plasmodium falciparum* malaria may produce gross derangement of hepatocellular function; the underlying mechanism is largely a vascular one, but the precise pathogenetic bases are unclear. This is important in the context of pharmacodynamics of antimalarial agents. Other conditions, e.g. visceral leishmaniasis (*see* Chapter 15) can also produce significant functional hepatic derangement.

Hepatic Amoebiasis

The life-cycle and intestinal manifestations of *Entamoeba histolytica* infection have been described in Chapter 5. Invasive hepatic disease is, however, the most important complication of this infection. 'Abscesses' (which are actually areas of necrotic liver tissue in the absence of pus) can form in any part or parts of the liver. However, they tend to be peripheral in distribution and occur in a normal or cirrhotic liver. Presentation is frequently with symptoms and signs in the right lower chest; a tender liver and fever are accompanying features. Confirmation of diagnosis is by serology; the immunofluorescent antibody test (IFAT) is positive in approximately 95% of cases of acute invasive amoebiasis, while in the remainder nearly all become positive as the disease progresses. Ultrasonography is of great value in differentiation from other space-occupying lesions (e.g. pyogenic abscess and hydatid cyst), and also in localisation. Treatment is with metronidazole (800 mg t.d.s. for 10 days), followed by diloxanide furoate ('Furamide') (500 mg t.d.s. for 10 days) to eliminate intestinal luminal cysts. Aspiration should be reserved for:

(i) A large 'abscess', or 'abscesses' in a severely ill patient.
(ii) Cases where the lesion(s) impinges upon a vital structure, e.g. the pericardial cavity.

Amoebic pericarditis is potentially a lethal complication. Rupture of 'abscesses' can pursue many routes, and may involve most viscera in proximity to the liver.

Differentiation from a pyogenic abscess is important because management is entirely different. Pyogenic abscess(es) occurs more commonly in older people and there is frequently an underlying cause (e.g. appendicitis, diverticulitis, Crohn's disease, etc). In this disease serology is negative and ultrasonography is of value in differentiation. The aspirate from the lesion is foul-smelling, in contradistinction to that in invasive amoebic disease. Whereas the only acceptable form of treatment was formerly laparotomy, needle aspiration under antibiotic cover (e.g. cloxacillin + gentamicin) using ultrasound guidance has recently given promising results. However, laparotomy is still sometimes necessary, and this is a serious condition which carries a high mortality rate.

Hepatic Schistosomiasis

One estimate is that 100 million of the world's population suffers from hepatic schistosomiasis. Intestinal schistosomiasis, which is acquired by skin exposure to fresh-water infected with cercariae has been outlined in Chapter 5. Intermediate hosts consist of various species of fresh-water snail (*see* p. 12). Fig. 6.5 shows the geographical distribution of *Schistosoma mansoni* and *S. japonicum* infections. The liver may be involved in the acute invasive phase of the disease (Katayama fever). Hepatic granulomas subsequently form around ova and these slowly fibrose with the production of 'pipe-stem' fibrosis (of Symmers). Hepatocellular function is usually well maintained until late in the disease; while ascites and encephalopathy are usually late manifestations, portal hypertension and bleeding varices occur as in cirrhosis (*see* p. 113). The HB_sAg carrier state is significantly higher in people with advanced hepatic schistosomiasis. An immune-complex mediated glomerulonephritis occurs in individuals with *S. mansoni* infections, especially if accompanied by chronic salmonellosis—a common complication.

Diagnosis has been simplified by serology (the ELISA technique being highly sensitive and specific), but if a parasite diagnosis is required, faecal samples and/or rectal and liver biopsy specimens should be examined. Investigation of portal hypertension and hepatocellular function is identical with that for cirrhosis.

Treatment is either with praziquantel (40–50 mg/kg as a single oral dose) or oxamniquine (20–30 mg/kg orally for 3 days). These agents can be safely given in the presence of portal-systemic shunting. Older agents should now be confined to the therapeutic museum.

Hepatic Hydatidosis

The life-cycle of *Echinococcus granulosus* involves the dog and sheep (although other mammals including the camel may be infected). The disease occurs, therefore, whenever man lives in close rela-

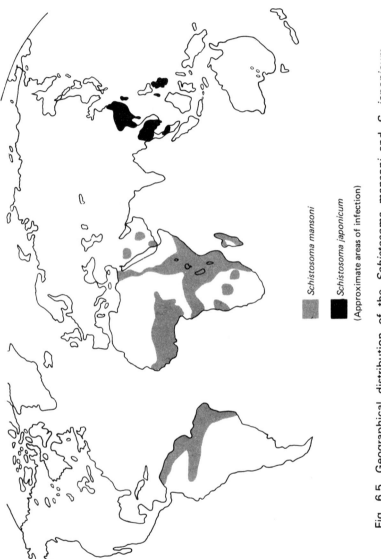

Fig. 6.5. Geographical distribution of the *Schistosoma mansoni* and *S. japonicum* parasites.

tionship to sheep and dogs. Hydatid cysts can form in most organs, but the liver is the most common site.

Diagnosis is assisted by serology; an ELISA test—preferably using factor 5 component of human hydatid fluid—now gives excellent results. Ultrasonography is of value in differentiating this from other lesions and in localisation.

In former days, the only treatment was to enucleate the cyst(s) at laparotomy after prior injection of either formalin or cetrimide (spillage of fluid may produce either an anaphylactic reaction or seeding throughout the peritoneal cavity). This immediate hypersensitivity (type I) reaction is caused by the release of large amounts of hydatid antigen into the circulation and its subsequent reaction with IgE-sensitised mast cells. The benzimidazole compounds are currently being evaluated and are giving promising results; albendazole (which is well absorbed) is given over several weeks, and assuming high plasma and more importantly intracyst concentration can be achieved, death of the protoscolices frequently takes place. Controlled trials are however urgently required to assess accurately this group of compounds in the medical management of this disease.

Biliary Infections

Biliary ascariasis (*see* Chapter 5) is a potential problem throughout the tropics and subtropics, and in people who have travelled to these areas. Cases are also reported in people who have not left a temperate area, e.g. the UK, Canada and Sweden. Large-duct obstruction with an obstructive-type jaundice may be a sequel to infection; it is important to recognise this and not confuse it with other causes of biliary tract obstruction. *Fasciola hepatica* (the liver fluke) occurs sporadically throughout the world and is usually contracted from contaminated vegetables. It is often accompanied by a peripheral eosinophilia. Although praziquantel has been used in treatment, the more toxic agent bithionol (30–50 mg/kg on alternate days for 10 doses) probably gives superior results.

Clonorchiasis and opisthorchiasis are important biliary parasites in south-east Asia. Diagnosis is by demonstration of characteristic ova in faecal samples. When untreated, adenocarcinoma of the hepatic ducts is an important complication with both of these infections. Treatment is with praziquantel (25 mg/kg given 3 times during 1 day) or niclofolan; the latter agent is more toxic.

CHRONIC LIVER DISEASE

The majority of cases of chronic liver disease in a tropical country originate from viral hepatitis (usually HBV or NANB infections). Prevalence of HBV carriers varies greatly geographically (*see* p. 102). Carriers who are also e positive are much more infective; an infant born to an e-positive mother has an approximately 70% chance of becoming a carrier. Between 20 and 30% of infants infected in the postnatal period (during the first 2 years of life) become chronic carriers; however, only 5–10% of infected adults become carriers. Expression of the e-antigen is determined genetically, e.g. most Chinese, but far fewer African mothers who are HB_sAg positive, are also HB_eAg positive. Overall, of children born to Chinese, African, Asian and European mothers, approximately 40–70%, 30%, 6–8% and none, respectively, become carriers. Table 6.2 lists some important differential diagnoses of chronic liver disease.

Table 6.2

DIFFERENTIAL DIAGNOSIS OF CHRONIC LIVER DISEASE IN THE TROPICS AND SUBTROPICS

Post-viral
    CAH → macronodular cirrhosis → HCC (*see* p. 113)

Schistosomiasis
    S. mansoni
    S. japonicum
    S. intercalatum
    S. mekongi
    S. mattheei

Alcoholic
    Chronic hepatitis
    Micronodular cirrhosis

Haemosiderosis

Indian childhood cirrhosis

Veno-occlusive disease

Biliary disease
    Clonorchiasis
    Opisthorchiasis

Chronic Hepatitis

The major forms of chronic hepatitis are chronic persistent hepatitis (CPH) and chronic active hepatitis (CAH); both usually (but not always) result from viral hepatitis. While the former is in most cases benign—periportal infiltration resolves with time and does not progress to serious chronic liver disease—the latter often pursues a relentless course with long-term complications. Indeed, progression from HBV or NANB, to CAH, and thence to macronodular cirrhosis, and ultimately, hepatocellular carcinoma (HCC) is a very common sequence of events in the context of liver disease in the 'Third World'. Other causes of CAH which should be differentiated include: autoimmune type, Wilson's disease, α_1-antitrypsin deficiency, therapeutic agents (methyldopa, isoniazid, oxyphenacetin and nitrofurantoin being examples), and alcohol.

Whereas corticosteroids are of benefit in the 'autoimmune' group, they are positively contraindicated in the 'HBV' group where they are accompanied by progressive viral replication; in this latter group, interferon and adenine arabinoside may be of value, but controlled evidence for this is still lacking. Alternatively high dose 'short burst' corticosteroids occasionally initiate an e antibody response and cessation of HBV antigenaemia; this line of management is, however, not without potential hazard.

Macronodular cirrhosis

Serological indicators of likely progression to chronicity are persistence of HB_sAg especially when combined with HB_eAg (Fig. 6.3). Macronodular cirrhosis may present with the various clinical stigmata of hepatocellular dysfunction: muscle wasting, palmar erythema, white opaque nails, loss of axillary hair, and gynaecomastia (in men), and later fluid retention, dilated anterior abdominal wall veins, etc. Cutaneous stigmata, e.g. spider naevi are, however, extremely difficult to detect in brown and black skins.

Treatment should be directed at the various complications of the disease: fluid retention (diuretics), oesophageal haemorrhage (Sengstaken tube, pitressin and sclerotherapy, when available) and encephalopathy (lactulose and/or neomycin).

Hepatocellular Carcinoma

Development of hepatocellular carcinoma (HCC), perhaps the world's most common malignancy, is the final stage on the fateful pathway. This highly malignant tumour is more common in men than women (7:1); it is highly vascular and produces metastases early in the lungs and other organs. Present evidence that HBV is important aetiologically is summarised in Table 6.3. HBV–DNA stimulates growth factor, which is probably oncogenic. The role of aflatoxin (derived from ground-nuts contaminated with *Aspergillus flavus*) is still unclear; it might be more important in some geographical locations (e.g. India), possibly acting as a cocarcinogen.

There is no satisfactory treatment; cytotoxic agents (including 5-fluorouracil and adriamycin) have been used (both intravenously and directly into the hepatic artery) but with only very limited success; hepatic artery embolisation is also of limited value. Resection is rarely possible because the tumour is usually multifocal and rarely localised to a single lobe or segment. Prophylaxis with HBV vaccine offers the only hope of success. Good evidence now exists that if this vaccine or immune globulin

Table 6.3

EVIDENCE THAT HBV IS IMPORTANT AETIOLOGICALLY IN HEPATOCELLULAR CARCINOMA

(i) Good correlation geographically between HCC and HB$_s$Ag carrier state

(ii) Over a 5-year period, an HB$_s$Ag carrier has an approximately 1000 times greater chance of developing HCC compared with a non-carrier

(iii) HB$_s$Ag carrier state is approximately 100 times higher in patients with HCC compared with controls

(iv) HBV infections precede liver damage (and not vice versa); they progress from chronic hepatitis, via macronodular cirrhosis to HCC (in this order)

(v) HBV–DNA is present in the genome of HCC cells

(vi) HEPADNA (hepatitis DNA) virus infections in woodchucks and Pekin ducks behave in a very similar way to human HBV infections, with progression to chronic hepatitis, cirrhosis and HCC (or preferably both) are given to infants of HB_sAg/HB_eAg positive mothers in the perinatal period, a highly significant protection can be acquired against the continuing antigenaemia. Both passive and active immunisation prevent horizontal transmission. Vaccine prepared from blood antigen gives good protection to infants born of mothers who are carriers, if the first dose is given at birth. Hepatitis B immunoglobulin alone merely delays the appearance of chronic antigenaemia. In some infants, infection is acquired *in utero*: here it is impossible to protect with either vaccine or immunoglobulin. Therefore, there is no chance of protecting every newborn child.

Ideally, worldwide immunisation would solve the problem, but this is impossible to achieve (*see* p. 313). The alternative is to screen all mothers and to immunize babies at birth; it has been suggested in the UK that all mothers of Chinese, African, Asian and west Indian origin should be screened. Table 6.4 summarises other high risk groups who should be considered for HBV vaccination. Regrettably, the cost of vaccination is still far too high for developing 'Third World' country health budgets; interest has now turned to using recombinant DNA technology in vaccine manufacture. Overall, there is no immediate chance of successful eradication of HCC and other forms of chronic liver disease in a world context.

Table 6.4

INDICATIONS FOR HBV VACCINATION

Developing countries
   Infants of HB_sAg/HB_eAg positive mothers in the neonatal period

Developed countries
   Drug addicts
   Active male homosexuals
   Health care workers
   Oncology units
   Renal dialysis units—staff and students
   Institutions for mentally retarded, etc
   Sexual/household contacts of HB_sAg carriers
   Immigrants from areas with a high incidence of HBV infection

Other Causes of Chronic Liver Disease in the Tropics

Alcoholic liver disease

This is increasing rapidly in most 'Third World' countries; WHO figures demonstrate a colossal increase in some. It is likely that moderate alcohol consumption in an HB_sAg carrier leads to a higher incidence of chronic liver disease than when only one of those insults is present. Micronodular cirrhosis is not infrequently complicated by HCC. Alcohol consumption should be considered in the differential diagnosis of chronic liver disease even in countries where alcohol is prohibited; there usually seem to be means of acquiring supplies.

Malnutrition

There is no evidence that severe malnutrition (including Kwashiorkor) results in chronic liver disease. Good evidence points to the fact that after the malnutrition is treated, hepatic histology returns to normal.

Haemosiderosis

Often known as 'Bantu siderosis', this is a major problem in southern Africa; it also occurs in other parts of the continent. Male incidence predominates. A high iron intake from iron cooking pots is undoubtedly important; however, genetic factors which might also be important have not been excluded. Other suggested factors are: alcohol intake *per se*, locally brewed beer, maize diet, chronic malnutrition and folate deficiency.

Indian childhood cirrhosis

This disease, which also has acute and subacute presentations, occurs in parts of India (Punjab, Calcutta, etc), Pakistan, Burma, Malaysia and Sri Lanka. It is especially common in some ethnic groups including Brahmins, Kayasthas, Agrawals, Rajputs and Sikhs, and has a male predominance. Copper has been implicated in the pathogenesis of the disease, and an increased intake from milk stored in copper vessels in childhood has been demonstrated on epidemiological grounds. However, a genetic factor is also likely to be important. Other aetiological theories implicate:

congenital hepatitis, 'autoimmunity', aflatoxins, abnormal tryptophan metabolism, etc. Prophylaxis is by reducing copper intake in infancy and childhood; an increased dietary tryptophan and vitamin B6 content might be of value in treatment.

Veno-occlusive disease

This was first described in the Caribbean, but it is also a significant problem in India, Afghanistan, Jordan and south Africa. The basic pathology consists of central and sublobular hepatic venous occlusion, which results from the ingestion of various pyrrolizidine alkaloids—Crotolaria, Senecio and Heliotropium—components of 'bush' teas. The sex incidence is equal. Various clinical forms of the disease—acute, subacute and chronic are recognised. There is no specific treatment once the disease has occurred.

FURTHER READING

Buitrago B., Popper H., Hadler S. C., *et al.* (1986). Specific histological features of Santa Marta hepatitis: a severe form of hepatitis δ-virus infection in Northern South America. *Hepatology*; **6:** 1285–91.
Cook G. C. (1980). *Tropical Gastroenterology*, pp. 59–190. Oxford: Oxford University Press.
Cook G. C. (1985). Hepatocellular carcinoma: one of the world's most common malignancies. *Quart. J. Med*; **57:** 705–8.
Cook G. C. (1986). Tropical infections and the liver. In: *Advanced Medicine*, Vol. 22, pp. 193–202. (Triger D. R., ed). London, Philadelphia: Baillière Tindall.
Cook G. C. (1986). Schistosomiasis: a major world scourge with few signs of hope! *Ann. Saudi Med*; **6:** 237–41.
Coursaget P., Yvonnet B., Chotard J., *et al.* (1986). Seven-year study of hepatitis B vaccine efficacy in infants from an endemic area (Senegal). *Lancet*; **2:** 1143–5.
Editorial. (1986). Yellow fever in Africa. *Lancet*; **2:** 1315–16.
Editorial. (1987). Man, dogs, and hydatid disease. *Lancet*; **1:** 21–2.
Flewett T. H. (1986). Can we eradicate hepatitis B? *Brit. Med. J*; **293:** 404–5.
Hoofnagle J. H., Mullen K. D., Jones D. B., *et al.* (1986). Treatment of chronic non-A, non-B hepatitis with recombinant human alpha interferon. *New Engl. J. Med*; **315:** 1575–8.
Hyams K. C., El Alamy M. A., Pazzaglia G., *et al.* (1986). Risk of hepatitis B infection among Egyptians infected with *Schistosoma mansoni*. *Am. J. Trop. Med. Hyg*; **35:** 1035–9.
Nash T. E., Cheever A. W., Ottesen E. A., Cook J. A. (1982). Schistosome infections in humans: perspectives and recent findings. *Ann. Intern. Med*; **97:** 740–54.

Sacks S. L., Freeman H. J. (1984). Cytomegalovirus hepatitis: evidence for direct hepatic viral infection using monoclonal antibodies. *Gastroenterology*; **86:** 346–50.

Seeff L. B., Beebe G. W., Hoofnagle J. H., *et al.* (1987). A serologic follow-up of the 1942 epidemic of post-vaccination hepatitis in the United States army. *New Engl. J. Med*; **316:** 965–70.

Yokosuka O., Omata M., Imazeki F., *et al.* (1986). Hepatitis B virus RNA transcripts and DNA in chronic liver disease. *New Engl. J. Med*; **315:** 1187–92.

Wright R., Millward-Sadler G. H., Alberti K. G. M. M., Karran S. (eds). (1985). *Liver and Biliary Disease*: pathophysiology, diagnosis, management, 2nd ed., p. 1608. London, Philadelphia: Baillière Tindall, WB Saunders Co.

Chapter Seven

Respiratory Infections (Excluding Tuberculosis)

Excluding tuberculosis (Chapter 3)—probably the world's most common bacterial infection—respiratory tract infections account for a vast amount of morbidity and mortality in infants, children and adults in both developing and developed countries. In the former, they are placed second only to infective diarrhoea in importance in children, and in the latter, they are responsible for a greater loss of schooling and working hours than any other group of communicable diseases. Viral, rickettsial, bacterial, fungal, protozoal and helminthic causes are all important. In the context of immunosuppression, fungal and protozoal infections dominate the scene. Only a minority have a specific geographical distribution.

Where and when available, radiological techniques are of great value in diagnosis; however, in most 'Third World' countries these are only available at tertiary referral centres and diagnosis has usually to be based on clinical symptoms and signs.

ACUTE UPPER RESPIRATORY TRACT INFECTIONS (URTI)

The upper respiratory tract (which comprises the nose and throat) is normally colonised by a wide range of organisms; Table 7.1 summarises some of them. Mechanisms of host defence include:

(i) Ciliated epithelium (nose and sinuses).
(ii) Salivary lysozyme.
(iii) Immunoglobulins, especially IgA (mucous secretions and serum).

In infants and children, URTIs are extremely common; the

Table 7.1

UPPER RESPIRATORY TRACT BACTERIAL AND FUNGAL FLORA IN THE NORMAL SUBJECT

Normal flora
  Streptococcus viridans
  Neisseria spp.
  Diphtheroids
  Anaerobic cocci, fusiform bacilli and *Bacteroides*

Respiratory 'pathogens' which are sometimes present without symptoms
  Strep. pyogenes
  Strep. pneumoniae
  Haemophilus influenzae
  (Corynebacterium diphtheriae)

Transient flora sometimes associated with antibiotic therapy
  Coliforms—*Klebsiella spp.*, *E. coli*, etc
  Pseudomonas spp.
  Candida albicans

---

majority have a viral aetiology and occur in winter. Spread of these infections to the middle-ear (via the Eustachian tube) is especially common in children. Sinusitis is a common complication in both children and adults.

Acute Coryza (The Common Cold)

This occurs at any age. Incubation period is 2–4 days. The major symptoms are nasal discharge, sneezing, sore throat and occasional fever and headache. Length of illness is up to 1 week. Rhinoviruses, of which there are over 100 serotypes constitute the usual pathogens; other viruses (corona, respiratory syncytial, parainfluenza, Coxsackie, Echo and adenoviruses), subsequently followed by bacteria (as secondary invaders) can also be involved. No specific treatment is indicated unless there is a clear predisposition to bronchitis (*see* p. 123).

Sore Throat/Tonsillitis

These symptoms are often associated with dysphagia and painful cervical lymphadenopathy; in young children, fever and anorexia are also common. Mild pharyngitis may be accompanied by a purulent follicular exudate; diphtheria and EBV infections (both of which are usually accompanied by an exudate) should always be suspected when symptoms and signs are severe. Table 7.2 summarises some causes of sore throat. Investigations should include: throat and nasal swabs, virus isolation (a special transport medium is required), and peripheral blood (blood slide for atypical lymphocytes) and serological (EBV, CMV and toxoplasma) testing; in addition antistreptolysin antibodies should be estimated. Penicillin should be given for a *Streptococcus pyogenes* infection (unless there is penicillin 'allergy'). Ampicillin and amoxycillin should not be given because if EBV is the cause, a generalised rash will result. Metronidazole or penicillin should be given for Vincent's infection. *Strep. pyogenes* throat infections can be complicated by: (i) Peritonsillar abscess ('quinsy'), otitis media, or 'scarlet fever' (*see* Chapter 2), or (ii) Rheumatic fever (*see* Chapter 8), acute glomerulonephritis (*see* Chapter 10), or streptococcal skin rashes.

Table 7.2

SOME CAUSATIVE ORGANISMS OF SORE THROAT/TONSILLITIS

Viruses
  Adenoviruses (33 types)*
  EBV*
  Enteroviruses*
  Common cold viruses (*see* text)*
  Measles (prodromal stage)
  CMV
  Herpes simplex
  Lassa fever† (*see* p. 234)

Bacteria
  Strep. pyogenes (Lancefield group A β-haemolytic streptococcus)*
  Strep. pyogenes (Lancefield groups C and G)
  Corynebacterium diphtheriae†
  Corynebacterium ulcerans†
  Vincent's organisms (*Borrelia vincenti* and anaerobic Gram-negative fusiform bacilli)
  Treponema pallidum†
  Neisseria gonorrhoeae†

* = Common cause of sore throat; † = Rare cause of sore throat.

Oral Candidiasis ('Thrush')

While *Candida albicans* infections can occur in the young and elderly, they are now more commonly opportunistic infections in immunosuppressed individuals, e.g. those with AIDS (*see* Chapter 11) (where infection often spreads to the oesophagus), an underlying malignancy, or in association with corticosteroid or broad-spectrum antibiotic treatment. Treatment is with oral nystatin or amphotericin B lozenges; a systemic antifungal agent (e.g. 5-fluorocytosine, miconazole or ketoconazole) is required in the immunosuppressed state.

ACUTE LOWER RESPIRATORY TRACT INFECTIONS

Mechanisms protecting the lower respiratory tract from infection are similar to those in the upper tract (*see* p. 119):

(i) Upward movement of mucus by the ciliated epithelium.
(ii) Phagocytosis by polymorphs and macrophages.
(iii) Local lysozyme production.
(iv) Interferon and secretory IgA production.

When these mechanisms fail, for example in chronic bronchitis, the bronchial tree becomes intermittently or even persistently colonised by bacteria such as *Strep. pneumoniae* and *Haemophilus influenzae*.

Non-specific Causes

Tracheobronchitis

Most acute infections are caused by viruses—rhino, influenza and para-influenza viruses. Secondary infection by *Strep. pneumoniae*, *Haemophilus influenzae* and less commonly *Staph. aureus* occasionally occurs; in this case, ampicillin (or amoxycillin), co-trimoxazole or erythromycin are appropriate antibiotics, unless penicillinase-producing *Staph. aureus* is suspected (*see* p. 123). In tropical countries it is important to distinguish acute bronchitis from tuberculous bronchitis with or without bronchopneumonia (*see* Chapter 3); absence of cough and a negative tuberculin test do not necessarily exclude this diagnosis. In children in developing countries, acute bronchitis (followed by bronchopneumonia) is a common sequel to measles and carries a high mortality rate.

Exacerbations of chronic bronchitis

Table 7.3 summarises some of the responsible organisms. Viruses are sometimes important (they may be complicated by secondary bacterial involvement) in this disease, but overall bacterial (especially *Haemophilus influenzae*) infections are more common. Because in most cases, frequent antibiotic courses have previously been given, 'resistant' bacteria are common. Investigation rárely provides worthwhile data (except occasionally in advanced cases) and antibiotic treatment should be started immediately the sputum appears infected. The two most likely causative bacteria (*see* Table 7.3) are covered by:

(i) Ampicillin (500 mg q.d.s. orally for 5–7 days) or amoxycillin (250–500 mg t.d.s. orally for 5–7 days).
(ii) Co-trimoxazole (2 tab b.d. orally for 5–7 days).
(iii) Oxytetracycline (250 mg q.d.s. orally for 5–7 days) or doxycycline (100 mg orally daily for 5–7 days).

Tetracycline or co-trimoxazole can be given if a history of penicillin 'allergy' is obtained. In advanced cases which are non-responsive, parenteral cephalosporins (cefuroxime and cefamandole), which are active against penicillinase-producing *Staph. aureus* and also *H. influenzae* should be considered.

Table 7.3

INFECTIVE AGENTS RESPONSIBLE FOR EXACERBATIONS OF CHRONIC BRONCHITIS

Agents	Stage of disease Early	Advanced
Haemophilus influenzae	+ + +	+ + + +
Strep. pneumoniae	+ + +	+ + +
Pseudomonas	–	+
Coliforms (some resistant to ampicillin and other broad spectrum antibiotics)	–	+
Non-sporing anaerobes	–	+
Staph. aureus	–	+
Mycoplasma pneumoniae	+	+
Viruses	+ +	+ +

In prevention, smoking must be stopped completely, exposure to cold and foggy weather avoided, and influenza immunisation recommended. In a tropical country, e.g. the Papua New Guinea highlands, cooking in smoky, enclosed huts may be important. Dust inhalation may also be relevant. In addition, a prophylactic antibiotic, e.g. oxytetracycline (500 g b.d. orally), taken throughout the winter months often reduces frequency of exacerbations; an alternative agent is co-trimoxazole (2 tab b.d.). A polyvalent pneumococcal vaccine for use in patients with known predisposing factors is undergoing investigation.

Transient 'pneumonitis' in the tropics

While passing through the lung parenchyma, the larvae of several parasites can cause a diffuse pneumonitis (Löffler's syndrome); multiple opacities throughout both lung fields are present radiologically and must be differentiated from miliary tuberculosis (*see* Chapter 3); hilar lymphadenopathy is not present however, and the apices are spared. This condition is associated with a peripheral eosinophilia and in *Ascaris lumbricoides* infections bronchospasm is common. This is caused by release of a potent allergen from the migrating helminthic larvae. Similar symptoms can occur in hookworm, *Strongyloides stercoralis*, visceral larval migrans and acute schistosomal infections (*see* p. 109). Larvae are frequently present in sputum even though absent in faecal samples. Clinical and radiological recovery occur within a few weeks.

In acute schistosomiasis (Katayama fever), approximately 3–6 weeks after an initial (primary) infection with *Schistosoma mansoni* or *S. japonicum* and less frequently *S. haematobium*, bronchospasm is often accompanied by mild hepatosplenomegaly and generalised giant urticaria.

Opportunistic pneumonias

As well as being common in immunosuppressed patients (including those with AIDS), these can occur in the presence of previous lower respiratory tract disease, general debilitation, following broad-spectrum antibiotics, and in intensive care units. The numerous organisms involved include:

(i) Gram-negative bacilli (*Klebsiella, Pseudomonas, Serratia*, and other coliforms and *Legionella pneumophila* (*see* p. 130)).
(ii) *M. tuberculosis* and atypical mycobacteria.
(iii) Fungi (including *Aspergillus, Cryptococcus, Mucor* and *Histoplasma*).
(iv) Viruses (including CMV, varicella-zoster, herpes simplex and measles).
(v) Protozoa (e.g. *Pneumocystis carinii*).
(vi) Helminths (e.g. *Strongyloides stercoralis* (*see* Chapter 5).

Viral Causes

Influenza

This common lower respiratory tract infection results from the *myxoviruses* A, B and C. The major disease is caused by type A which shows minor antigenic 'drift' every year, and marked antigenic 'shift' approximately every 10 years; the haemagglutinin (H) and neuraminidase (N) surface antigens are involved. Radically new strains originate every 30 years or so. This virus also causes disease in a wide range of mammals and birds. Between pandemics, small influenza A epidemics usually occur every or in alternate years, mainly during the winter months. Influenza B usually causes small epidemics every 2–3 years and affects children and young people principally; 'drift' and 'shift' of surface antigens are much less common. Influenza C virus causes mild sporadic infections only. Para-influenza viruses I–IV produce a less severe disease, usually but not always restricted to the upper respiratory tract.

Respiratory droplet infection is the main method of transmission, although fomites contaminated by respiratory secretions can also be responsible. After an incubation period of 1–3 days, the virus replicates in the respiratory (both upper and lower) tract epithelium and damages cilia. Defence mechanisms—interferon, local IgA and serum antibody production (active against haemagglutinin and other surface antigens)—are triggered off, but in a small minority of individuals, a rapidly fatal alveolitis is produced before these come into play. Onset is usually abrupt, with fever, headache, malaise and a cough which is usually associated with acute tracheitis or bronchitis; sore throat, anorexia and muscle aches complete the clinical picture. Although the symptoms usually subside within 4 days, mild tiredness and depression may continue for several more days, and even weeks.

The most important complication is secondary bacterial infection with *Staph. aureus*, *Strep. pneumoniae*, *Strep. pyogenes* or *H. influenzae*. *Staph. aureus*, and to a lesser extent *Strep. pyogenes*, can cause a very rapidly progressive disease which does not respond to antibiotics and results in death within a few days; this can be a major problem even in healthy young adults in an influenza A pandemic (the Asian 'flu epidemic of 1957 produced many such cases in the UK). The reason why *Staph. aureus* superinfection is so deadly is that it produces a protease which cleaves and activates haemagglutinin on the surface of viral particles enabling far more of them to affect the cells and multiply; therefore, there is more cellular damage, they become more vulnerable to *Staph. aureus* infection (which in turn produces more protease), and a vicious cycle is set in motion. In infants and the elderly, in particular, this cycle can be difficult to interrupt. Primary influenzal pneumonia is less common than the secondary variety but is even more lethal; the clinical course can be extremely fulminant with respiratory distress and cyanosis proceeding to death within hours. Myocarditis, pericarditis, encephalitis and polyneuropathy rarely follow influenza infection.

Virus isolation can often be made from a throat swab or nasopharyngeal washing (a special transport medium is necessary). Paired serum samples should be collected to detect a rise in antibody titre.

Whereas the average case should be treated with bed-rest and salicylates only, a complicated case demands prompt antibiotic administration; co-trimoxazole, and in a severe case intravenous high-dose cloxacillin + ampicillin are indicated. Prophylaxis is important in the elderly and those with chronic cardiac and respiratory tract disease; the vaccine should include the currently prevalent strain and be given by subcutaneous or intramuscular injection in the preceding September; a second dose should be given after 4–6 weeks. An antiviral agent, amantadine, is active against the influenza A virus (*see* Chapter 16).

Bacterial Causes

Symptoms of bacterial pneumonia are characteristically: cough (initially unproductive), fever and pleuritic chest pain; as the disease progresses, the cough becomes productive (except in atypical pneumonia). Physical findings are: consolidation of a lobe (or lobes) which can be confirmed by radiography; in early cases, evidence of this may be minimal. In *Klebsiella* pneumonia, bowing of the adjacent pleural fissure (e.g. horizontal fissure on the right) is characteristic and of value in differentiating this from pneumococcal disease. Those pneumonias caused by bacteria are usually, but not always, more acute and of greater severity than those resulting from *Mycoplasma* and other organisms (the atypical pneumonias).

Mycobacterium tuberculosis occasionally presents with an acute pneumonia (*see* Chapter 3), usually in elderly men and immigrants to the UK—especially from India. In atypical pneumonia, chest signs are often minimal and cough and fever dominant clinical features; there is usually no leucocytosis and chest radiography merely shows patchy consolidation. Table 7.4 summarises some causative organisms in various groups of individuals (factors involved in group (ii) include: previous respiratory tract disease, impaired defences, influenza, alcoholism, chronic hepatic and renal disease, and old age. In addition, *Staph. aureus* pneumonia is more common in drug addicts and infants with impaired immune responses). This list is largely based on probabilities; all organisms can affect any group, and in addition the following can cause pneumonia: influenza A, respiratory syncytial, para-influenza, adeno, and other viruses including measles and varicella-zoster, *Coxiella burnetii* (Q fever), fungi, protozoa and helminths.

In all groups *Strep. pneumoniae* is the most common causative agent; there are approximately 80 serotypes of this organism— related to the capsular polypeptide antigens. A particularly virulent example is type III. There is no cross immunity between different serotypes. Classical pneumococcal lobar pneumonia is still extremely common in tropical countries and accounts for a vast amount of morbidity and mortality; at presentation patients often do not appear particularly ill. It is frequently accompanied by the jaundice of acute bacterial infection (*see* Chapter 6). Empyema and meningitis are occasional sequelae. In some countries, e.g. South Africa and Papua New Guinea, pneumococci have become resistant to several antibiotics including the penicillins, tetracycline and aminoglycosides.

Multiple lung abscesses, empyema and septicaemia are complications of *Staph. aureus* pneumonia; these can be especially troublesome when associated with influenza (*see* p. 126).

Legionella pneumophila pneumonia (Legionnaire's disease) (*see* p. 130) is also a cause of bacterial pneumonia.

Table 7.4
SOME CAUSATIVE ORGANISMS OF ADULT PNEUMONIA, AND APPROPRIATE INITIAL ANTIBIOTIC THERAPY

		Initial antibiotic
(i)	*Previously healthy individual*	
	Streptococcus pneumoniae*	Benzylpenicillin or amoxycillin†
	Mycoplasma pneumoniae*	Erythromycin or tetracycline
	Chlamydia B (psittacosis)	Tetracycline
(ii)	*Debilitated, elderly or predisposed individual ('secondary' infection)*	
	Strep. pneumoniae*	Amoxycillin or ampicillin
	Staph. aureus	Flucloxacillin + fusidic acid + benzylpenicillin‡
	Haemophilus influenzae	Amoxycillin or ampicillin§
	Legionella pneumophila	Erythromycin (or tetracycline)
	Mycobacterium tuberculosis	Rifampicin + INAH + streptomycin
	Mycoplasma pneumoniae	(as above)
(iii)	*Hospital in-patient ('secondary' infection; partly dependent on hospital flora)*	
	Strep. pneumoniae*	Amoxycillin or ampicillin
	Staph. aureus	(as above)
	Haemophilus influenzae	(as above)
	Coliforms (e.g. *Klebsiella*)	Gentamicin or cefuroxime
	Pseudomonas aeruginosa	Tobramycin + carbenicillin
	Anaerobes (e.g. *Bacteroides*)	Metronidazole

* = Common infecting organism; † = Erythromycin or co-trimoxazole may be used in patients with penicillin 'allergy'; ‡ = Erythromycin + fusidic acid, or cefuroxime may be used in patients with penicillin 'allergy'; § = Co-trimoxazole or cefuroxime may be used in patients with penicillin 'allergy'.

Salmonella typhi infections can result in pulmonary consolidation. Primary tuberculosis should be excluded (*see* Chapter 3). Invasive amoebiasis (*see* p. 88) may cause pulmonary consolidation, especially in the right lower lobe; where diagnostic facilities are unavailable, a trial of metronidazole is often warranted. Pneumonic plague (caused by *Yersinia pestis*) can present with pulmonary consolidation; a febrile illness of sudden onset with productive cough and blood-stained sputum can mimic pneumococcal and *Klebsiella* pneumonia; progression to involve multiple lobes is rapid in the untreated. Acute pneumonia, usually of bronchial distribution, can also occur in anthrax, glanders and acute *Plasmodium falciparum* malaria. In marasmic and immunocompromised children, *Pneumocystis carinii* pneumonia should be considered in the differential diagnoses (*see* p. 134).

Both pleural effusion and dry pleurisy can follow any bacterial, and several of the parasitic pneumonias. The presence of many lymphocytes and a raised protein concentration in the pleural fluid should suggest tuberculosis; acid-fast bacteria are sometimes detected in a pleural biopsy. Invasive amoebiasis (involving the liver), paragonimiasis and strongyloidiasis can give rise to pleural effusion.

When acute pneumonia resolves slowly or incompletely, several possibilities should be considered:

(i) Incorrect or inadequate antibiotic administration.
(ii) Legionnaire's disease; erythromycin (or tetracycline) should be given, there being no response to β-lactam antibiotics and aminoglycosides.
(iii) Tuberculosis has been missed.
(iv) Infection is secondary to an obstructed bronchus (caused by a bronchial carcinoma, tuberculous or malignant hilar lymphadenopathy, or a foreign body).
(v) Primary atypical pneumonia; *Mycoplasma pneumoniae*, psittacosis and *Coxiella burnetii* are examples and they do not respond to penicillin, ampicillin or cephalosporins.

Pneumonia following bronchial obstruction, often caused by tuberculous hilar lymphadenopathy, is common in many parts of the tropics including Africa and Papua New Guinea; a complete 'white-out' of the lung representing complete destruction, on radiography, is a common finding. A chronic 'destructive' pneumonia, probably caused by aspiration of anaerobic flora is also common in African men; this can proceed to bronchiectasis (*see* p. 132).

Investigations in patients with acute pneumonia should include:

(i) Total and differential polymorphonuclear leucocyte count.
(ii) Sputum culture (mucopurulent specimens should reach the laboratory as soon as possible) for diagnosis and antibiotic sensitivity tests.
(iii) Pleural fluid for microscopy, culture and when relevant antibiotic sensitivity tests.
(iv) Pneumococcal antigen immunoelectrophoresis of sputum, blood and urine (this is often positive when *Strep. pneumoniae* cannot be detected in sputum or blood).
(v) Blood cultures (before starting antibiotics).
(vi) Paired serum samples (for primary atypical pneumonia (*see* p. 129), Legionnaire's disease, CMV, influenza and fungal infections).
(vii) Cold agglutinins (in atypical mycoplasma pneumonia).

Table 7.4 (p. 128) summarises initial antibiotic regimens for acute pneumonia while laboratory results of organism and antibiotic sensitivities are awaited. In a severely ill patient, in whom the cause(s) is unknown, a combination of high-dose intravenous erythromycin + benzylpenicillin + gentamicin is of value. In 'secondary' infections (where a mixed flora is considered likely), antibiotic combinations should be given after consultation with a microbiologist.

Legionnaire's disease

This disease which is caused by an unusual Gram-negative bacillus—*Legionella pneumophila*—was first recognised in war veterans who were attending a conference in Philadelphia, USA, in 1976. The organism is, however, present throughout the world; it was previously unrecognised because the causative organism is not readily identified by Gram-staining and therefore a silver stain should be used. It is endemic in the UK, and unlike pneumococcal pneumonia occurs in the summer months. It usually afflicts individuals more than 45 years old (younger individuals usually suffer a mild illness only), and onset of illness is frequently associated with a stay in an hotel; humidifier (air-conditioning) or shower apparatus usually provides the source of infection. There is no evidence of case-to-case transmission. The incubation period is about 5 days. Men are affected twice as frequently as women. Chronic chest disease and smoking are known predisposing factors.

Onset is usually with an 'influenza-like' illness, dry cough and mental confusion; psychiatric or neurological features complicate approximately 50% of cases. Bilateral patchy areas of pulmonary consolidation (occasionally of lobar distribution) which 'migrate' to different zones are characteristic. Deterioration accompanied by respiratory failure is rapidly progressive; unconsciousness may supervene. Pleural and hepatic failure may occur. The mortality rate is at least 15%. Characteristic results of laboratory investigation include: lymphopenia ($<1\cdot0 \times 10^9/l$), low plasma sodium (<130 mmol/l), reduced serum albumin (<20 g/l), and raised plasma aminotransferase and creatine phosphokinase concentrations. Although the causative organisms can often be isolated, serology is the main diagnostic technique; paired serum samples show a rise in immunofluorescent antibody.

Treatment with erythromycin (initially 1·5 g intravenously 6-hourly) is usually satisfactory. Rifampicin (300–600 mg b.d.) should be added to the regimen and continued for at least 3 weeks (to avoid relapse) if the response is poor.

CHRONIC LOWER RESPIRATORY TRACT INFECTIONS

Empyema, Lung Abscess and Bronchiectasis

All acute lower respiratory tract infections can proceed to chronicity, including empyema, lung abscesses and bronchiectasis.

Empyema

Empyema (pus in the pleural cavity) can occur after untreated or inadequately treated pneumonia of almost any cause (*see* p. 128). The causative organism can usually be isolated from aspirated pus. Treatment is with the appropriate antibiotic(s) and drainage (surgical in severe cases). Presentation of an amoebic 'empyema' is sometimes with the coughing up of the 'abscess' content following development of a bronchopleural fistula.

Lung abscess

This complication follows a pulmonary infection usually caused by *Staph. aureus*, or occasionally *Klebsiella spp.* This may follow influenza A, but also occurs in drug addicts (where abscesses are frequently multiple); secondary infection distal to a bronchial obstruction caused by a foreign body, malignancy or hilar lymph-node can cause an abscess (anaerobes (e.g. *Bacteroides necrophorus*) are important). In the tropics, the most common cause of lung abscess is aspiration of anaerobic buccal flora; this often follows unconsciousness resulting from trauma or an alcoholic bout. A swinging pyrexia and respiratory symptoms are present; the clinical diagnosis is confirmed by chest radiography. An anaerobic lung abscess usually causes a relatively thick-walled cavity with local parenchymal reaction. Sputum and blood cultures, and frequently an endoscopy are required for diagnosis. Postural drainage and appropriate antibiotic therapy are essential; surgical drainage or resection of a malignancy, segment or lobe of damaged lung may also be necessary. A further cause of lung abscess (frequently multiple) is melioidosis, resulting from *Pseudomonas pseudomallei* infection. This disease is particularly common in south-east Asia and may mimic tuberculosis; treatment is with tetracycline. *Strongyloides spp.* has occasionally been demonstrated in a lung abscess. Amoebic lung abscess caused by *Entamoeba histolytica* may follow invasive disease involving the liver (*see* Chapter 6); treatment is with metronidazole.

Bronchiectasis

Bronchial dilatation leading to chronic infection, fibrosis and ultimately calcification, may follow numerous acute infections of the lower respiratory tract, e.g. childhood pertussis, tuberculosis, bronchial obstruction caused by a foreign body, cystic fibrosis, hypogammaglobulinaemia with repeated infections, bronchopulmonary aspergillosis or paragonimiasis (*see* p. 136). Kartagener's syndrome is a rare cause. It is a major problem in developing countries, and usually results from inadequate treatment of an acute pneumonia. Clinically, cough, haemoptyses and production of thick purulent sputum (often several cupfuls daily) during acute episodes of infection are characteristic. A chest radiograph may show cystic changes and in an advanced case fluid levels also. Finger clubbing may be gross. Sputum microscopy and culture are important investigations, and blood culture is sometimes useful; many causative organisms for pneumonia may be present (*see* Table 7.4, p. 128), in addition *Aspergillus spp.* may often be found (*see* below) in combination with these. Postural drainage, physiotherapy and appropriate antibiotic treatment (usually for at least 10 days) are essential. When the disease is localised, resection of an affected segment or lobe may be indicated.

Upper respiratory tract disease should be treated adequately; a postnasal 'drip' from a chronic nasal sinusitis can lead to a vicious cycle of infection. When present concurrently, tuberculosis must also be treated. Complications include: recurrent episodes of bronchitis or pneumonia, empyema, lung or cerebral abscess, massive haemoptyses, respiratory failure, cor pulmonale and secondary amyloidosis.

Fungal Causes

Fungi may produce granulomatous pulmonary disease resulting in nodules, solitary tumours or thin-walled cavities with a cystic appearance.

Aspergillosis

This group of fungi, the most common example of which is *Aspergillus fumigatus* (which can be inhaled into the lower respiratory tract), can produce disease presenting as:

(i) *Asthma.* A type I (IgE) hypersensitivity response to the fungus (sputum contains eosinophils).

(ii) *Allergic bronchopulmonary aspergillosis.* This sometimes occurs in malt workers—an extrinsic allergic bronchoalveolitis caused by types I or III hypersensitivity; asthma and a chronic productive cough are common features which can be complicated by bronchial obstruction and bronchiectasis.

(iii) *'Aspergilloma'.* This lesion, demonstrated by chest radiography, occurs in a previously damaged area of lung, e.g. a tuberculous cavity, which may fill with a 'mycetoma'; it may also be the seat of a secondary bacterial infection. Cough, haemoptysis, occasionally massive, may occur. A type III response with fever and constitutional upset may also be present.

(iv) *Disseminated aspergillosis.*

Sputum examination with culture, and aspergillus serology (which is strongly positive in more than 90% of patients with aspergilloma, and 75% with bronchopulmonary disease, but is weakly positive or negative in the other two groups) are of value diagnostically. In those with asthma and bronchopulmonary disease, skin tests are usually positive. In groups (i) and (ii) treatment of the 'allergy' is indicated; corticosteroids are often necessary in group (ii). In groups (iii) and (iv) treatment is with systemic amphotericin B; a 'mycetoma' may have to be resected surgically.

Farmer's Lung

This consists of an extrinsic allergic alveolitis (type III hypersensitivity reaction) following the inhalation of mouldy hay (usually during the winter months). Cough and breathlessness (with bronchospasm) occur several hours after exposure. Scattered nodular shadows, later with resultant fibrosis, can be demonstrated on chest radiography. The responsible organisms are thermophilic actinomyces, e.g. *Micropolyspora faeni* and *Thermoactinomyces vulgaris*. Precipitating antibodies to actinomycete antigens are present in about 80% of infections. The acute symptoms should be treated with corticosteroids and avoidance of further exposure to mouldy hay is important.

Parasitic Causes

Entamoeba histolytica 'abscess' (which is occasionally chronic) is described on p. 132 and in Chapter 6.

Pneumocystis carinii

This is important as an opportunistic pulmonary infection in AIDS sufferers; this is the most common opportunistic parasitic infection in this disease in the UK and USA. It is also important in malnourished children (including those with Kwashiorkor) in tropical countries. The protozoan is usually confined to the lung; whereas most infections are asymptomatic, in the presence of compromised immunity it may cause widespread consolidation (most marked in the mid and lower zones) and diffuse patchy opacities on chest radiography. The organism is sometimes found in sputum samples, but more invasive techniques are often required for a positive identification. Treatment is with co-trimoxazole or pentamidine; in severe disease oxygen is required.

Filarial hypereosinophilia (tropical pulmonary eosinophilia)

This disease is most common in southern India and Sri Lanka. It is associated with filariasis—*Brugia malayi*, *Wuchereria bancrofti* and filarial worms of animal origin (e.g. *Dirofilaria immitis*—the dog heartworm). A severe non-productive cough is associated with nocturnal bronchospasm and sometimes a rash or urticaria; a marked peripheral eosinophilia (usually $>3\cdot0 \times 10^9/l$) is usual except in immunocompromised individuals. Microfilariae are not usually found in peripheral blood, but filarial serology is strongly positive. The pulmonary lesions consist of granulomas containing many eosinophils. Differential diagnoses include: Löffler's syndrome (*see* p. 124), allergic aspergillosis and other helminthic infections including strongyloidiasis. Radiological findings are diffuse fine opacities throughout both lung fields. Treatment is with diethyl-carbamazine (DEC) (2 mg/kg t.d.s. for 21 days); a corticosteroid cover is often advisable at the commencement of DEC treatment.

Hydatid cysts (*see* Chapter 6)

Pulmonary cysts are often discovered incidentally in a chest radiograph; they should be distinguished from tuberculomas, and primary and secondary neoplasia. They are smooth, circular, well-defined lesions which closely mimic 'cannon-ball secondaries'; cysts can be single or multiple, and the diameter ranges from 1-20 cm. Growth is relatively slow and they rarely calcify. When symptomatic (cough, haemoptyses, dyspnoea, chest pain, etc), there is often pressure on surrounding structures. Secondary infection, empyema, leakage and rupture, and pneumothorax are relatively uncommon however; occasionally a cyst ruptures into the pleural space or a bronchus, and the patient complains of coughing up 'grape skins'. Examination of sputum using a Ziehl–Neelsen stain may reveal *Echinococcus* hooks. In approximately one-quarter of individuals with pulmonary disease the liver also contains cysts. Treatment was formerly surgical. Response to oral albendazole is usually excellent (presumably because penetration into the thin-walled cyst is good); results are far better than for those involving the liver.

Schistosomiasis

In chronic infections (usually with *S. mansoni*) ova embolise to the pre-arteriolar pulmonary circulation. This results in an obliterative endarteritis and a diffuse, fine, nodular radiological appearance caused by interarterial and para-arterial granulomas. Pulmonary hypertension and right-sided dilatation results. Cor pulmonale is a further sequel (*see* Chapter 8) which is invariably accompanied by hepatosplenomegaly.

Paragonimiasis

Paragonimus westermani (a lung fluke) produces chronic pulmonary disease closely resembling active chronic tuberculosis (with which it sometimes coexists). The disease is confined to south-east Asia, India and west Africa. Other lung flukes cause disease in southern America. Infection is acquired by ingestion of raw freshwater crayfish or crabs. Chest pain and productive cough, with sticky, rusty sputum may persist for many years; haemoptyses are common especially when bronchiectasis has developed, and may be gross. Most patients are clinically well, afebrile, and chest radiography may be normal; lesions, when present, are often at the periphery of the mid and lower lung unlike those in chronic tuberculosis. The lesions consist of circular or oval nodules or may be cystic (ranging from 0·5 to 4·0 cm in diameter); there may be aggregates of up to 5 lesions. Eggs can sometimes be detected in a sputum sample, especially during an episode of haemoptysis; they are not detected by the Ziehl–Neelsen stain. During treatment the radiological appearances often worsen in the absence of symptoms. Following death of the parasite, a 2–5 cm calcification may remain. Bithionol has been most widely used for treatment; however, praziquantel has recently given promising results.

FURTHER READING

Barrett-Connor E. (1982). Parasitic pulmonary disease. *Am. Rev. Resp. Dis*; **126**: 558–63.

Editorial. (1980). Chronic destructive pneumonia. *Lancet*; **2:** 350–1.
Editorial. (1986). Penicillin prophylaxis for babies with sickle-cell disease. *Lancet*; **2:** 1432–3.
Everett E. D., Nelson R. A. (1975). Pulmonary melioidosis: observations in thirty-nine cases. *Am. Rev. Resp. Dis*; **112:** 331–40.
Igra-Siegman Y., Kapila R., Sen P., *et al.* (1981). Syndrome of hyperinfection with *Strongyloides stercoralis*. *Rev. Infect. Dis*; **3:** 397–407.
Kum P. N., Nchinda T. C. (1982). Pulmonary paragonimiasis in Cameroon. *Trans. R. Soc. Trop. Med. Hyg*; **76:** 768–72.
Ludman H. (1981). ABC of ENT: throat infections. *Brit. Med. J*; **282:** 628–31.
Miller A. C. (1981). Erythromycin in Legionnaire's disease; a re-appraisal. *J. Antimicrob. Chemother*; **7:** 217–22.
Neva F. A., Ottesen E. A. (1978). Tropical (filarial) eosinophilia. *New Engl. J. Med*; **298:** 1129–31.
Riley I. D., Lehmann D., Alpers M. P., *et al.* (1986). Pneumococcal vaccine prevents death from acute lower-respiratory-tract infections in Papua New Guinean children. *Lancet*; **2:** 877–81.
Seeff L. B., Beebe G. W., Hoofnagle J. H., *et al.* (1987). A serologic follow-up of the 1942 epidemic of post-vaccination hepatitis in the United States army. *New Engl. J. Med*; **316:** 965–70.
Simberkoff M. S., Cross A. P., Al-Ibrahim M., *et al.* (1986). Efficacy of pneumococcal vaccine in high-risk patients: results of a veterans administration cooperative study. *New Engl. J. Med*; **315:** 1318–27.
Tashiro M., Ciborowski P., Klenk H-D., *et al.* (1987). Role of *Staphylococcus* protease in the development of influenza pneumonia. *Nature*; **325:** 536–7.
Woodhead M. A., Macfarlane J. T., McCracken J. S., *et al.* (1987). Prospective study of the aetiology and outcome of pneumonia in the community. *Lancet*; **1:** 671–4.

Chapter Eight

Infections of the Cardiovascular System

There are major geographical variations in the incidence rates of infective cardiac and pericardial disease. Acute rheumatic fever and its chronic sequelae are now very unusual events in developed countries; however, in most parts of the 'Third World' they constitute a major problem which accounts for widespread morbidity and mortality. Numerically, acute rheumatic fever and bacterial endocarditis are the most serious manifestations of infective cardiac disease, even in the late 1980s. Constrictive pericarditis, which is usually but by no means always caused by tuberculosis, is a relatively common problem in developing countries, but a rarity in most developed ones. Schistosomal cor pulmonale and south American trypanosomiasis (Chagas' disease) are examples of diseases with serious cardiac complications which have circumscribed areas of distribution. When approached from a clinical viewpoint, cardiac disease with a non-infective aetiology—congenital, hypertensive and atherosclerotic (very unusual in rural communities of Africa)—must however enter the list of differential diagnoses.

ACUTE RHEUMATIC FEVER

Because streptococcal sore throat (pharyngitis) occurs worldwide, so likewise do rheumatic fever and rheumatic heart disease (RHD); in throat swab culture surveys of primary school children, a prevalence rate of β-haemolytic streptococcus isolation of at least 30% is a common finding. RHD, a sequel to acute rheumatic fever, remains the most common form of cardiac disease in childhood even in developed countries; this remains so up to the third decade of life. Certain M types of Group A β-haemolytic streptococcus (e.g. types 5, 14 and 24) are especially likely to cause acute rheumatic fever. Development of cardiac damage might result from a cell-mediated immune reaction rather than streptococcal antibody alone. Whether genetic or ethnic host factors are involved in susceptibility is unclear, but this seems likely. Socioeconomic conditions are undoubtedly important, and there is good evidence that as standards of living improve, the prevalence of acute rheumatic fever declines.

Although the basic lesion is the Aschoff nodule, myocardial fibril fragmentation and lymphocytic interstitial infiltration are the predominant histological features during the acute illness; the pericardium produces a fibrinous exudate often resulting in a small effusion. The mitral and aortic valves are the major sites of endocardial involvement; the tricuspid is occasionally, and the pulmonary valve rarely affected. Stenosis and/or regurgitation result from organisation of the fibrinous deposits.

Clinically, carditis is more likely in those who develop the disease early in life, and a transient arthropathy is more common in those who are older. A history of sore throat, and rarely of scarlet fever is common. Joint involvement is characteristically a 'flitting' migratory polyarthropathy; Sydenham's chorea (which only rarely occurs in association with arthritis) and the presence of subcutaneous rheumatic nodules, erythema marginatum (on the trunk), and erythema nodosum (characteristically over the anterior tibial borders) are occasional accompanying features. There is usually fever and a tachycardia. Atrial fibrillation is a common sequel to cardiac involvement. Cardiac decompensation with right-sided failure, pulmonary hypertension and pericarditis are important complications.

ESR, C-reactive protein (CRP) and antistreptolysin titre are elevated; the total polymorphonuclear leucocyte count is usually raised also. Throat swab culture frequently yields streptococci. A rising streptococcal antibody titre is valuable diagnostically. Electrocardiographic examination may reveal a prolonged PR interval and first-degree AV block. Chest radiography frequently shows evidence of left atrial appendage enlargement at the left upper cardiac border; this exerts a protective effect on the lungs by limiting the development of mitral regurgitation; dyspnoea is thus a late symptom in most cases. In a severe and advanced case the left atrial outline may be visible beyond the right cardiac border.

Benzathine penicillin (458 mg for a child < 30 kg, and 916 mg for an adult) should be given as a single dose intramuscularly; in penicillin-sensitive individuals, erythromycin (250 mg q.d.s. for 10 days) is an appropriate substitute. Treatment of the carditis consists foremost of bed-rest; duration of disease activity ranges from 2–4 months. Salicylates (aspirin has been used since 1876) are the mainstay of medical treatment; 100 mg/kg daily in 5 divided doses is accompanied by rapid response of fever, tachycardia and arthralgias. Although the CRP rapidly falls, the ESR is much slower in responding. In a severe case, prednisolone (2 mg/kg daily, with a maximum of 60 mg daily for an adult) should be given for the first few weeks and then replaced by salicylates. Complications, such as right-sided cardiac failure, are treated on their merits. As a prophylactic against further attacks of acute rheumatic fever, either the penicillin dosage outlined above, or erythromycin 250 mg b.d. should be repeated at monthly intervals, this regimen continuing into adult life.

The ultimate outcome depends on the degree (if any) of valvular damage, and the activity of the rheumatic disease. Cardiac surgery is rarely available in those parts of the world where the disease is still very common although mitral valvotomy (for stenosis) is occasionally carried out. In developing countries, valve replacement is rarely possible; furthermore, anticoagulation is difficult to control and secondary infection of damaged valves extremely common.

BACTERIAL ENDOCARDITIS

Although many different organisms may involve the endocardium, the most common problems result from a *Streptococcus viridans* and the most devastating from a *Staphylococcus aureus* infection. Overall some 1500 cases occur annually in the UK, but a very high prevalence exists in most 'Third World' countries; even where modern antibiotic therapy is available, the overall mortality rate ranges from 15–30%. Previous rheumatic (*see* p. 138), congenital and atherosclerotic cardiac disease, the presence of prosthetic heart valves, and addiction to hard-line drugs are all well established predisposing factors.

Roughened endothelium in proximity to a high pressure gradient (usually around a valve or septal defect) with resultant turbulence, forms an ideal site for platelet and fibrin deposition. Infective organisms reach this site by way of a bacteraemia originating in teeth, gums (*Strep. viridans*) and less frequently, other portals of entry. Microbial vegetations result. The outcome depends largely on (i) the nature and concentration of the invading organism, and (ii) the efficiency (or otherwise) of the host defence mechanisms. This equilibrium is also dependent, however, on the site and nature of the cardiac (usually valvular) defect. Less commonly, the endocardium can be infected in the absence of previous damage; *Staph. aureus* and rarely *Strep. pyogenes* or *Strep. pneumoniae* are then the most likely causative organisms.

Onset, especially in elderly patients, is frequently insidious; tiredness, low grade pyrexia, anaemia, progressive cardiac failure and changing cardiac murmurs may be present. Clinically it is sometimes difficult to distinguish the disease from acute rheumatic fever. Osler's nodes (tender areas in the pulp of the fingers and less commonly toes) and acute glomerulonephritis (which is rarely fatal) result from the deposition of immune complexes originating from the high antibody titres produced against the infecting organism. Tender splenomegaly (typhoid fever and brucellosis may be simulated) and clubbing may be present. Embolic episodes (both sterile and 'septic') originating at the infective cardiac lesion can affect the skin and fingers ('splinter haemorrhages'), and more importantly the central nervous system and also other organs. Death may be a sequel to cardiac decompensation; this usually depends on the magnitude of valvular damage.

A definitive diagnosis is dependent on microbiology and in a minority of cases serology; echocardiography is of value in identifying and localising vegetations. Whenever there is clinical suspicion of endocarditis, three samples of blood for culture (ideally separated by a few hours, but depending on the condition of the patient) must be obtained before any form of treatment is started; a strictly aseptic technique is absolutely essential. In approximately 25% of patients, blood cultures are negative because:

of previous antibiotic therapy;
of the presence of fastidious bacteria;
the cause is non-bacterial;
in a minority of cases the original clinical diagnosis was incorrect.

Serological tests are of great value in diagnosis in culture-negative cases (paired serum samples should always be obtained).

Table 8.1 summarises some of the likely causative organisms in patients who have and have not undergone preceding cardiac

Table 8.1
SOME CAUSATIVE ORGANISMS INVOLVED IN INFECTIVE ENDOCARDITIS

Organism	'Spontaneous' infection	Infection following cardiac surgery
'Streptococcus viridans'	+ + + +	+ + +
Strep. faecalis	+	+
Staphylococcus aureus	+ +	+ + +
Staph. epidermidis	+	+ +
Haemophilus spp.	+	−
Anaerobic streptococci	+	−
Microaerophilic streptococci	+	−
Chlamydia trachomatis and C. psittaci*	+	−
Brucella spp.*	+	−
Diphtheroids	−	+
Gram-negative bacilli	−	+ +
Fungi (e.g. Candida spp. and Aspergillus spp.*)	−	+
Coxiella burnetii* (Q fever)	+	−

*Diagnosis is usually made by serological examination (paired serum samples); blood cultures are frequently negative.

surgery; 'Strep. viridans' consists of a large group of α-haemolytic and non-haemolytic streptococci which are present in the normal buccal flora. Infection frequently, but by no means always, occurs after dental extraction, when a transient bacteraemia lasting up to 20 min is inevitable. Strep. faecalis is a more common organism in elderly men with genitourinary (e.g. prostatic) disease. In contrast to streptococcal infections, those resulting from Staph. aureus usually pursue a more aggressive course; septicaemia with multiple metastatic abscesses and disseminated intravascular coagulation are often present simultaneously. Portals of entry include the skin and less commonly the lungs; drug abusers are especially vulnerable. In this case the endocardium is frequently normal and a previously healthy valve (the aorta is especially vulnerable) may be affected. Staph. epidermidis infections are relatively common after cardiac surgery; the source of infection is usually the skin of either the patient or surgeon.

Table 8.2 summarises some possible therapeutic regimens which should be started before microbiological confirmation

Table 8.2

ANTIBIOTIC PROPHYLAXIS AT DENTAL OPERATIONS AND OTHER INVASIVE PROCEDURES, AND TREATMENT OF SUSPECTED BACTERIAL ENDOCARDITIS (Therapeutic doses given are for adults with normal renal function.)

Prophylaxis (also see text)	Time before surgical procedure
(i) Fortified benzathine penicillin, BPC 1 Vial (i.m.)	15–30 min
(ii) Amoxycillin 3 g (oral)	1 h (repeat 6–8 h after procedure)
(iii) Fortified benzathine penicillin, BPC 1 Vial (i.m.) + Streptomycin 1 g (i.m.)	15–30 min
(iv) Ampicillin 1 g (i.m.) + Gentamicin 80 mg (i.m.)	15–30 min (repeat at 6 and 12 h after procedure)

Treatment	Drugs and dose
'Spontaneous' infection	Benzylpenicillin (3·0 g 6 hourly—i.v. bolus) + Gentamicin (80 mg 8 hourly i.m.)
After open heart surgery	Benzylpenicillin (1·2 g 6 hourly—i.v. bolus)* + Gentamicin (80 mg 6 hourly—i.v. bolus) + Cloxacillin (2 g 4 hourly—i.v. bolus)

*In late cases (presentation > 2 months after surgery) the dose should be doubled because '*Strep. viridans*' is a more likely causative organism.

when there is a strong clinical suspicion of this diagnosis. Among the 'spontaneous' infections, when there is a strong possibility of a staphylococcal infection, cloxacillin should be added to the regimen. Because organisms are often deeply embedded within the vegetations, complete *bactericidal* treatment is essential. When a satisfactory antibiotic concentration is achieved, the mortality rate should be reduced from 100% to approximately 10%. In developing countries, antibiotics are widely and often incompetently used and a definitive laboratory diagnosis is frequently not obtained; therefore satisfactory management cannot be monitored by microbiological criteria. Following identification of the organism(s), a joint consultation between physician and microbiologist is essential; estimates of minimum bactericidal concentration (MBC) and minimum inhibitory concentration (MIC) (*see* Chapter 16) should be carefully taken into account. In the presence of 'penicillin allergy' expert microbiological advice must be sought. Treatment should be continued for 4–6 weeks in the 'spontaneous' group and at least 6 months in the 'prosthetic valve group'. *Coxiella burnetii* (Q fever) endocarditis (*see* Chapter 15) should be treated with tetracycline for many months and excision of the infected valve is sometimes necessary. Rifampicin may also be used. When a fungus is involved, amphotericin B and surgical intervention are usually combined.

Table 8.2 (p. 143) also summarises some regimens which may be used prophylactically in high risk groups. Although regimen (i) is usually recommended before dental procedures, (ii) can be used for operations undertaken outside hospital. However, in patients who have a prosthetic heart valve or have recently received penicillin, regimen (iii) (with the addition of an aminoglycoside) should be followed. After colonic surgery or genitourinary procedures when *Strep. faecalis* is a likely organism, regimen (iv) should be instituted.

SOME CAUSES OF ACUTE INFECTIVE MYOCARDITIS

Myocarditis, often associated with pericarditis, frequently presents as an acute illness with breathlessness, and sometimes chest pain, in young adults. Electrocardiography may be required to differentiate the disease from a myocardial infarction. Table 8.3 summarises some of the causes of acute myocarditis. Whereas the Coxsackie and influenza viruses account for most cases in the UK, arboviruses are important in many tropical countries. Rare viral

Table 8.3
SOME CAUSES OF ACUTE INFECTIVE MYOCARDITIS AND PERICARDITIS

Viruses
Coxsackie B1–B6
Influenza A
Arboviruses
Rubella

Common causes of acute myocarditis and pericarditis in the UK'

Myocarditis in the fetus

Miscellaneous
Mycoplasma pneumoniae
Chlamydia psittaci
Coxiella burnetii (Q fever)

Bacteria
Many of the organisms responsible for acute rheumatic fever and bacterial endocarditis
Strep. pneumoniae
Neisseria meningitidis
Neisseria gonorrhoeae
Corynebacterium diphtheriae toxin (*see* Chapter 2)
Salmonella typhi
Treponema pallidum (?)
Leptospira spp.

Protozoa
Toxoplasma gondii
Trypanosoma cruzi (acute infection)
Entamoeba histolytica (?)

Helminths
Several intestinal and blood nematodes during their migratory cycles
Trichinella spiralis

Fungi
Cryptococcus neoformans

---

causes are EBV, mumps and poliomyelitis; typhus (especially scrub typhus) is an unusual rickettsial cause. Although acute myocarditis has been reported in primary tuberculosis, usually in association with erythema nodosum, this is a most unusual event.

In the investigation of acute myocarditis, isolation from throat swabs of Coxsackie B and influenza viruses should be attempted. Paired serum samples (the first obtained as early as possible and the latter at 10–14 days) should be examined for Coxsackie B, influenza, mycoplasma, coxiella and psittacosis antibodies. Paired serum samples can also be examined for leptospires, toxoplasmosis (dye test) and antistreptolysin concentration. Blood cultures might yield *Neisseria spp.*, *Staphylococcus spp.*, and other possible bacterial causes. If pericardial fluid is present, and a diagnostic aspiration carried out, microscopy, culture and sensitivity testing is sometimes of value. Faecal specimens also should be examined for Coxsackie B.

Treatment obviously depends on the cause. Neisseria and leptospiral infections are responsive to penicillins. Mycoplasma, coxiella and chlamydia infections respond to tetracycline. Toxoplasma myocarditis should be treated with pyrimethamine + sulphadiazine, or spiramycin (*see* Chapter 15).

CHRONIC CARDIAC LESIONS WITH AN INFECTIVE BASIS

Syphilitic Cardiac Disease

Whereas this disease is now rarely encountered in developed countries, it is still common in many 'Third World' countries. In some parts of Africa, at least 10% of cardiovascular deaths still result from this disease. Clinically, it is more common in men. Signs of aneurysmal dilatation of the thoracic aorta (interstitial pulsation and a tracheal tug) may be present; evidence of aortic regurgitation is usual. The presence of aortic regurgitation in a young man suffering from angina (resulting from coronary ostial involvement) makes this diagnosis likely. There may also be partial superior vena caval obstruction, and pressure on other thoracic inlet structures is common. A previous history of a primary chancre (*see* Chapter 12), and neurological sequelae of tertiary disease are most unusual. Serological tests may be positive and chest radiography usually reveals aortic dilatation, often containing calcification. Because the changes are irreversible, treatment is of no avail; although penicillin is frequently administered, the aneurysmal size may increase, often suddenly, after treatment.

Takayasu's Disease

This disease, which is most commonly seen in women in Asia, southern America and rarely Africa, consists of a panarteritis (involving the carotids especially) leading to a widespread diminution in peripheral pulsations. Initial presentation is with fever, night sweats, weight-loss and erythema nodosum. Limited circumstantial evidence suggests a mycobacterial aetiology. The tuberculin test is frequently positive. Corticosteroids are of value if started early; the role of antituberculous therapy is unclear.

South American Trypanosomiasis (Chagas' Disease)

The heart is often involved early in this disease which is common in southern America (*see* Chapter 15); an early result of infection is an acute myocarditis (*see* Table 8.3, p. 145). The heart may be enlarged, and in addition a tachycardia, loud systolic murmur and cardiac failure are sometimes present. Electrocardiography may show T-wave changes; first degree AV block is a common finding. In *chronic* myocarditis, sudden death (resulting from conduction defects and arrhythmias is common; however, congestive cardiac failure is the most common presentation. Examination reveals signs similar to those in the acute disease; however, abnormalities of rhythm and conduction dominate the clinical picture: right bundle-branch, and AV block (with Stokes–Adams attacks), intraventricular block and premature ventricular contractions (often multifocal) may be present. Cardiac aneurysms (often at the apex of the left ventricle) may be present; these can give rise to arterial embolism. In addition, dysphagia and abnormal bowel function (resulting from megaoesophagus and megacolon respectively) may be present (*see* Chapter 15). This disease should be distinguished from RHD which is common in the same areas; presentation is different however, and although atrial fibrillation is common in RHD, other conduction disturbances are unusual.

Schistosomiasis

Schistosomiasis rarely involves the heart directly (granulomatous myocarditis is reported), but it does so by way of pulmonary disease and cor pulmonale. *Schistosoma mansoni* (*see* Chapter 6) is the usual species to be involved; in some 15% of individuals with severe hepatic fibrosis there is evidence of right ventricular hypertrophy at post-mortem examination. Although schistosomal cor pulmonale is commonly recognised in Egypt (young farmers being especially vulnerable) it has also been recorded in young children less than 10 years old.

Breathlessness, cough, wheezing and syncope are common presenting features; haemoptysis is a late symptom, and atrial fibrillation is unusual. Examination reveals evidence of right ventricular hypertrophy and tricuspid regurgitation; portal hypertension with hepatosplenomegaly and portal-systemic collaterals are usually present concurrently. Electrocardiographic and radiological evidence of right ventricular hypertrophy are present; the latter investigation characteristically outlines a dilated pulmonary artery. Cardiac catheterisation is a hazardous undertaking. If treatment is undertaken, dead adult schistosomes can embolise to the lungs and add to the obstructive process; right pulmonary artery thrombosis, aneurysmal dissection, and cardiac arrhythmias may lead to sudden death.

ENDOMYOCARDIAL FIBROSIS (EMF)

While most common in tropical Africa (especially Uganda and Nigeria), EMF has also been documented in southern America, the Indian subcontinent and south-east Asia. Although an infective aetiology has not been established, epidemiological evidence makes this likely; in Uganda it is, for example, far more common in Rwandan people who have migrated there in childhood, making an environmental (probably an infective) factor more likely than a genetic one. Although many infections have been incriminated, none has been proved to be responsible. Streptococcal infection is one possibility. Filariasis (including loaiasis) with resultant eosinophilia has also received attention. Endomyocardial damage can follow a high sustained eosinophilia from any cause; this might be due to eosinophil infiltration of the myocardium, or the direct action of a component of eosinophil granules. By the time EMF has developed, a peripheral eosinophilia is usually absent and evidence of active filariasis is not usually demonstrable. EMF usually presents after cardiac failure has supervened, when it consists of a restrictive cardiomyopathy in which both inflow tracts and the ventricular apices are involved. The myocardium is scarred; acute and chronic inflammatory cells, mast cells and eosinophils are present. Ventricular expansion is impaired by a severe fibrotic process with the production of mitral and tricuspid regurgitation. Differential diagnosis from RHD and constrictive pericarditis may be difficult but nevertheless important because those conditions both require prompt treatment. Cardiac surgery has occasionally been attempted in severely affected individuals but there is no adequate treatment.

Chronic cardiac disease has also been documented in the presence of a very high peripheral eosinophil concentration in the absence of clear evidence of a filarial or other helminthic infection.

PERICARDITIS

Pericardial disease most commonly results from acute rheumatic fever (*see* p. 138), pyogenic infections and tuberculosis (*see* Chapter 3). Viral infections (e.g. Coxsackie) can also be responsible. Amoebic involvement (*see* p. 108) is a rarity but when it occurs is associated with a high mortality rate. Acute pericarditis frequently accompanies acute myocarditis of many varying aetiologies (*see* p. 144 and Table 8.3, p. 145).

Pyogenic pericarditis is most common in infants and children; it is usually secondary to an acute systemic infection, e.g. osteomyelitis or pneumonia. Presentation is frequently delayed until cardiac tamponade is present. A pericardial friction rub, and low voltage electrocardiogram (with ST-segment elevation) are helpful diagnostically; chest radiography usually reveals a 'globular' cardiac outline. Echocardiography, when available, is an important investigative technique. Pericardial aspiration produces purulent fluid which must be cultured; the responsible organism is usually a staphylococcus. Treatment with a penicillinase-resistant penicillin should be started immediately; surgical drainage may also be necessary. Assuming recovery occurs, some cases proceed to constrictive pericarditis which in a tropical setting should not necessarily be assumed to be of tuberculous origin.

Tuberculous pericarditis is usually a secondary manifestation of the disease, and occurs in adult life. Whereas pulmonary disease and pleural effusion(s) are usually present concurrently, this is not always so. Pericardial aspiration yields yellow straw-coloured fluid which clots on standing; lymphocytes are frequently plentiful. *M. tuberculosis* is not often obtained on culture; tuberculin testing is usually positive. Frequently, a therapeutic trial of antituberculous therapy is necessary in the absence of a definitive diagnosis. Constrictive pericarditis (ultimately with calcification visible on a chest radiograph) is a late sequel. Pericardiectomy is often required, especially when constriction has developed.

Histoplasma capsulatum and coccidioidomycosis have rarely been incriminated in the pathogenesis of pericarditis; effusion and constriction have been reported.

Amoebic pericarditis results from rupture of an amoebic 'abscess', usually in the left lobe of the liver (*see* Chapter 6), into the pericardial cavity; it may have escaped detection on clinical grounds. Cardiac tamponade may occur. When a left lobe 'abscess' is detected therefore, either clinically or by ultrasonography or CT scanning (and especially when it impinges on the pericardial sac) it should be aspirated before this catastrophe develops. Urgent pericardial aspiration is essential. It is most unusual for *Entamoeba histolytica* to be detected in the 'necrotic' aspirate; neutrophil leucocytes are usually present in large numbers. Serology for invasive amoebiasis is positive in at least 95% of cases. A metronidazole or tinidazole course should be given; in addition, surgical pericardial drainage should be carried out if suitable facilities exist. Drainage of sub-diaphragmatic fluid may also be necessary.

Hydatid cysts occasionally occur within the pericardium. These are usually discovered incidentally by routine chest radiography and are often calcified; they should be differentiated from other pericardial cysts. Rupture of a cyst into the pericardial sac is a rare event.

FURTHER READING

Bisno A. L. (1987). Acute rheumatic fever: forgotten but not gone. *New Engl. J. Med;* **316:** 476–8.

Davies J., Spry C. J. F., Sapsford R., *et al.* (1983). Cardiovascular features of 11 patients with eosinophilic endomyocardial disease. *Q. J. Med*; **52:** 23–39.

Drug and Therapeutics Bulletin (1987). *Antibiotic Treatment of Bacterial Endocarditis*; **25:** 49–51.

Gray I. R. (1981). Management of infective endocarditis. *J. R. Coll. Physns*; **15:** 173–8.

Morris G. K. (1985). Infective endocarditis: a preventable disease? *Brit. Med. J*; **290**: 1532–33.

Neu H. C., ed. (1985). Emerging perspectives in management and prevention of infectious diseases: Endocarditis. *Am. J. Med*; **78(6B)**: 1–236.

Oakley C. M., Sommerville W. (1981). Prevention of infective endocarditis. *Brit. Heart J*; **45**: 233–5.

Okoroma E. O., Ihenacho H. N. C., Anyanwu C. H. (1981). Rheumatic fever in Nigerian children. *Am. J. Dis. Childh*; **135**: 236–8.

Parry E. H. O., Abrahams D. G. (1965). The natural history of endomyocardial fibrosis. *Q. J. Med*; **34**: 383–408.

Pitcher D. W., Papouchado M., Channer K. S., James M. A. (1986). Endocarditis prophylaxis: do patients remember advice and know what to do? *Brit. Med. J*; **293**: 1539–40.

Shanson D. C. (1981). Prophylaxis and treatment of infective endocarditis. *J. R. Coll. Physns*; **15**: 169–72.

Spry C. J. F., Davies J., Tai P. C., et al. (1983). Clinical features of fifteen patients with the hypereosinophilic syndrome. *Q. J. Med*; **52**: 1–22.

Tai P-C., Ackerman S. J., Spry C. J. F., et al. (1987). Deposits of eosinophil granule proteins in cardiac tissues of patients with eosinophilic endomyocardial disease. *Lancet*; **1**: 643–7.

Chapter Nine

Infections of the Central Nervous System

Bacterial meningitis is a major cause of morbidity and mortality in developing countries. It is dominated by meningococcal, *Haemophilus influenzae* and pneumococcal infections. Although outbreaks (usually affecting children and young adults) occur from time to time this is not however a major problem in developed countries, where viral meningitis (usually followed by spontaneous recovery) is a far more common problem. Poliomyelitis, tetanus and rabies are also more common than in the developed countries; neurological manifestations of diphtheria are covered in Chapter 2. Tuberculous disease (meningitis and tuberculoma) is a major 'Third World' problem. In much of the developing world, cerebral malaria resulting from *Plasmodium falciparum* infection is a common cause of death; in children it frequently presents with febrile convulsions. Some infections have a clear geographical distribution. African trypanosomiasis, for example, causes substantial morbidity and mortality in central and west Africa. Spinal cord compression (paraparesis and tetraparesis are common sequelae) in developing countries is most often caused by vertebral tuberculosis (*see* Chapter 3); transverse myelitis frequently caused by viruses and parasites also occurs (*see* p. 172). Tropical spastic paresis has now been shown to be associated with HTLV-I infection. Leprosy is a frequent cause of peripheral nerve disorders (*see* Chapter 14).

Congenital infections with central nervous defects can be contracted *in utero*: viruses (CMV, rubella and herpes simplex), bacteria (*Treponema pallidum*, Group B haemolytic streptococcus and *Listeria monocytogenes*), protozoa (*Toxoplasma gondii*) and helminths (*Toxocara canis*) can all be involved.

ACUTE MENINGITIS

Acute meningitis can be caused by viruses, bacteria, fungi and protozoa. Table 9.1 summarises the major causative organisms. When it occurs, it is always a serious disease and the patient must be managed as a medical emergency. Whatever the causative agent, clinical features are dominated by headache, irritability, fever, neck stiffness, and Kernig's sign is frequently positive; these events are accompanied or followed by nausea, vomiting and coma. However, at the extremes of life and especially in neonates, specific signs and symptoms may be absent.

Viral Causes

Table 9.1 summarises some of the aetiological factors in viral meningitis, largely a disease of children (*see* Chapter 2). Although the clinical features are similar to those of bacterial meningitis (*see* below), the course is usually more benign and the mortality rate much lower. Enteroviruses (picornaviruses) usually produce an influenza-like illness with headache and sore throat; frequently this subsides for 1-2 weeks and then accounts for a secondary meningitic or encephalitic illness corresponding to a phase of viral replication in the CNS. In a minority with poliomyelitis, and some with Echo and Coxsackie (A and B) infections, anterior horn-cell involvement with lower motor neurone paralysis, or rashes and vesicles may occur, respectively. Mumps is occasionally accompanied by a mild degree of meningeal irritation. A minority of patients with severe genital herpes and varicella-zoster infections also develop *aseptic* meningitis. Differential diagnoses on CSF examination, include: partially treated bacterial meningitis (*see* p. 156), leptospiral meningitis, encephalitis, cerebral abscess, and tuberculous and fungal meningitis. Virus isolation can often be made from CSF, throat swabs and faeces; a rising titre of neutralising antibodies in convalescent compared with acute serum is of value in enterovirus and mumps infections. There is no specific treatment for any of these infections. Prophylaxis with live and attenuated poliomyelitis I, II and III viruses will prevent the paralytic disease (*see* Chapter 2); pregnancy and impaired immunity from whatever cause, are contraindications.

Bacterial Causes

Primary bacterial meningitis (*see* Table 9.1) usually results from a

Table 9.1
AETIOLOGICAL AGENTS IN ACUTE AND CHRONIC MENINGITIS, WITH CORRESPONDING CEREBROSPINAL FLUID CHANGES

Agents	Appearance	Cerebrospinal fluid† Cells	Gram-stain	Protein (g/l)
Viruses				
Enteroviruses — Echo, Coxsackie A and B, Poliomyelitis	Clear or slight opalescence	Lymphocytes	−	0·5–1·0
Paramyxoviruses — Mumps				
Herpes viruses — Herpes simplex, Varicella-zoster				
Adenoviruses				
Arboviruses — Louping-ill (tick borne)				
Bacteria				
'Primary' — *Neisseria meningitidis*, *Haemophilus influenzae*, *Strep. pneumoniae*	Turbid or purulent	Polymorphs	+	0·5–3·0
'Secondary' — Staphylococci and streptococci, *Strep. pneumoniae*, Coliforms, *Pseudomonas aeruginosa*, Anaerobes, *Listeria monocytogenes**				

Infections of the Central Nervous System 155

Neonatal	E. coli other coliforms Group B haemolytic streptococcus Staph. epidermidis Salmonella spp. Pseudomonas spp. Listeria monocytogenes (flavobacteria, Bacillus cereus)	(see p. 156)			
Acid-fast	Mycobacterium tuberculosis	Clear or slightly turbid	Lymphocytes + polymorphs	(Ziehl-Neelsen) +	0·8–5·0
Spirochaetes	Leptospira canicola Leptospira icterohaemorrhagiae Treponema ballidum	Clear or slightly turbid	Lymphocytes	+	0·5–1·0
Fungi Yeasts Filamentous	Cryptococcus neoformans* Candida spp. Aspergillus spp. Mucor	Clear or slightly turbid	Lymphocytes	+	0·5–1·0
Protozoa Free-living amoebae	Naegleria Acanthamoeba spp. Hartmanella	Turbid	Polymorphs, red cells	+	0·5–3·0

* = In adults this is frequently associated with a compromised immune response; † = Glucose concentration is reduced in 'purulent' and tuberculous meningitis (TBM).

bacteraemia and spread of bacteria to the meninges. Secondary disease, which is far less common, results from spread of focal infection in ears, sinuses, traumatic sites, surgery or congenital defects, e.g. spina bifida. In the UK, approximately 2000 cases (two-thirds in children under 5 years old) of bacterial meningitis are reported annually; the most common cause of primary meningitis is *Neisseria meningitidis*, with *Haemophilus influenzae* in second place. The vast majority of cases of *H. influenzae* occur in children. In developing countries, *Strep. pneumoniae* which carries a far worse prognosis is a common cause. Differential diagnoses on CSF examination include cerebral abscess and amoebic meningitis. Treatment must always be started *immediately* and often has to be undertaken 'blind'. Table 9.2 summarises those antimicrobial agents which cross the blood–brain barrier; intrathecal antibiotics are not of proven value.

Meningococcal meningitis

This infection, which has an incubation period of 1–3 days is spread by respiratory droplets and is carried asymptomatically by 2–25% of people (rates are higher in children and where living conditions are overcrowded). There are three main serological types (A, B and C) of this Gram-negative diplococcus. In the UK,

Table 9.2

ANTIMICROBIAL AGENTS AND THE BLOOD–BRAIN BARRIER

Antimicrobial drugs	CSF penetration Normal meninges	Inflamed meninges (meningitis)
Sulphonamides	+	+
Benzylpenicillin	−	+
Ampicillin	−	+
Chloramphenicol	+	+
Trimethoprim	+	+
Gentamicin	−	−
Streptomycin	−	−
Rifampicin	±	+
Isonicotinic acid hydrazide (INAH)	+	+
Pyrazinamide	?	+

most cases, which are caused by the group B serotype are sporadic, and family contacts (usually children) can contract the disease at home. The epidemics, which are associated with very high mortality rates, are common in Africa and Brazil, and now in the Middle East, and are caused by group A and C organisms.

The disease usually starts with a sore throat and/or headache and may progress extremely rapidly, with a dramatic deterioration to drowsiness and coma within several hours. A rash, which is haemorrhagic (petechial, eccymotic and even gangrenous) accompanies the septicaemia (*see* Chapter 15); this probably results from locally formed immune complexes. Gram-negative shock, acute renal failure and disseminated intravascular coagulation (DIC) rapidly supervene. Haemorrhage into many organs including the brain and adrenal glands (producing acute adrenal cortical failure) may accompany a fulminant septicaemia. The overall mortality rate is approximately 10% but this depends on rapidity of diagnosis and treatment. A minority develop 'allergic' manifestations associated with immune complex disease. Blood and CSF cultures should be initiated before antibiotic treatment is commenced. Table 9.1 (p. 154–5) summarises some of the CSF features; a Gram-stain usually shows both intra- and extracellular Gram-negative diplococci. Meningococcal polysaccharide antigen, which can be detected by immunoelectrophoresis, is of value in the rapid diagnosis of types A and C.

N. meningitidis is sensitive to benzylpenicillin; in many areas, resistance to sulphonamides is rapidly emerging. Intravenous benzylpenicillin (30 mg/kg 4-hourly) should be started immediately and continued for 10 days; chloramphenicol may be used in patients 'allergic' to penicillin. If treatment is started early, recovery is usually uneventful. Close contacts of patients should be given immediate chemoprophylaxis; rifampicin orally for 2 days is usually recommended, but nasopharyngeal carriage can also be eliminated with sulphadiazine and minocycline. A meningococcal vaccine against serotype A is being used with some success in parts of Africa and Brazil.

Haemophilus meningitis

This coccobacillus which is a common cause of respiratory tract infection in young children, frequently colonises the respiratory tract of infants. It sporadically causes a bacteraemia, and meningitis is a sequel. Peak incidence is at about 2 years old, and by 12 years most children have developed specific serum antibodies; maternal antibody provides protection during the first few months of life. After an incubation period of about 5 days, meningitis supervenes insidiously; it is altogether far less dramatic than meningococcal disease and is not accompanied by a rash. When there is delay in starting treatment, cerebral and cranial nerve palsies and subdural effusions may complicate the disease. Overall, the mortality rate is around 5%. The responsible organism can be identified in a Gram-stained centrifuged deposit of CSF. Chloramphenicol is the antibiotic of choice; it is bactericidal in CSF and 50–100 mg/kg daily should be administered for 10 days. Although most strains are sensitive to ampicillin, resistance to this antibiotic is developing; furthermore, the relapse rate is higher than with chloramphenicol.

Pneumococcal meningitis

Strep. pneumoniae is a common cause of respiratory tract disease both in children and adults (*see* Chapter 7). Certain capsular serotypes (e.g. type III) can be associated with bacteraemia and meningitic involvement; these events are more common in: infants less than 3 years old and adults more than 60 years old, the malnourished and also alcoholic individuals. Direct spread from an infected nasal sinus or middle ear may occur, especially in young infants; in the presence of a congenital defect or fractured skull, recurrent pneumococcal meningitis may also result from local spread. Onset of disease is rapid and coma can supervene within several hours; there is no rash. The mortality rate is around 30% and higher than in the other two types of 'primary' meningitis, especially when antibiotic treatment is delayed. When survival occurs, cranial nerve damage, intraventricular adhesions and intracranial loculation of pus are common sequelae; this disease is thus a major source of morbidity in 'Third World' countries. Gram-positive diplococci can usually be visualised in a Gram-stained CSF deposit; CSF immunoelectrophoresis usually gives a positive result for pneumococcal antigen. Whereas in the UK, most *Strep. pneumoniae* are sensitive to penicillin, this is frequently not the case in some tropical countries including South Africa, Tanzania and Papua New Guinea. Intravenous benzylpenicillin (60 mg/kg 4-hourly in children, and 1.2 g every 2 h in an adult) should be given without delay, and continued for 10 days. Chloramphenicol may be used in individuals 'allergic' to penicillin. A polyvalent pneumococcal polysaccharide vaccine is of value in prophylaxis and has been widely used in the Papua New Guinea highlands and some other areas.

'Secondary' meningitis

Table 9.1 (p. 154–5) summarises some organisms primarily localised to other sites but which can also produce a bacterial meningitis. Although CSF examination is usually required for a definitive diagnosis, antibiotics should immediately be started when meningitis is diagnosed; for a guide to probable antibiotic sensitivities *see* Chapter 16.

Neonatal meningitis

Table 9.1 (p. 154–5) summarises some causes of this disease which carries a very high morbidity and mortality rate. At least one-third of cases die; long-term complications are also very common. Infection is derived from the umbilical stump, respiratory tract, urinary tract, ear, and less commonly other sites, or from the mother; it may also result from a meningomyelocoele. Classical signs are: a bulging fontanelle, neck stiffness and altered consciousness; however, these are often late and may not occur at all. An urgent Gram-stain of the CSF, and blood cultures are essential; swabs from other sites may also give valuable information. 'Blind' antibiotic treatment is necessary while results of laboratory investigations are awaited; benzylpenicillin + chloramphenicol should be started immediately. To prevent a relapse, courses should be for at least 2 weeks and usually much longer.

Leptospiral meningitis

This disease (*see* Chapter 6) frequently presents with fever and meningitis; jaundice and nephritis are also usually present. Conjunctival injection is often a marked feature of the disease. Leptospira can be detected in the CSF by dark-ground illumination; blood culture and paired serum samples should be examined for a rising antibody titre to *Leptospira spp*. When started early, benzylpenicillin is of value; however, most cases recover spontaneously.

ACUTE ENCEPHALITIS

Table 9.3 summarises some causes of acute encephalitis and encephalomyelitis. Although viruses are usually responsible, es-

Table 9.3

SOME CAUSES OF ACUTE ENCEPHALITIS AND ENCEPHALOMYELITIS

Acute viral encephalitis or meningoencephalitis		*Non-viral causes*	
Epidemic Eastern equine* Western equine* Louping-ill (tick-borne) Japanese B* St Louis* Murray valley*	} arboviruses	*Coxiella burnetii* Rickettsiae *Mycoplasma pneumoniae* *Legionella pneumophila* *Neisseria meningitidis* *Treponema pallidum* *Leptospira spp.* Relapsing fever	} Bacterial causes not associated with cerebral abscess
Echo Coxsackie A and B Poliomyelitis Influenza	} enteroviruses	Streptococci Pneumococci Staphylococci Anaerobes Gram-negative	} Bacterial causes which can proceed to a pyogenic cerebral abscess
Sporadic Herpes simplex Mumps Enteroviruses Varicella-zoster EBV Rabies		*Cryptococcus neoformans* *Aspergillus spp.* *Histoplasma spp.*	} Fungal causes
		Toxoplasma gondii *Plasmodium falciparum* (see Chapter 4) African trypanosomiasis Free-living amoebae	} Protozoal causes

continued

Infections of the Central Nervous System 161

Acute viral encephalitis or meningoencephalitis		*Non-viral causes*
Post-infective encephalomyelitis†		
Measles	*Taenia solium*	⎫
Rubella	Echinococcosis	⎪
	Trichinella spiralis	⎪
Post-vaccination	*Schistosoma*	⎬ Helminthic
Measles	*japonicum*	⎪ causes
Pertussis, etc	*Toxocara canis*	⎪
	Angiostrongylus cantonensis	⎪
	Onchocerciasis	⎭

* = Mosquito-borne infection; † = *See* Chapter 2.

pecially in children and young adults, many other organisms, including bacteria and protozoa may be involved.

Drowsiness (sometimes progressing to coma), confusion, headache, a personality change and fits are common features. Localising signs, e.g. cranial nerve palsies, dysphasia, nystagmus and hemiparesis may also be present in a severe case. However, most infections produce a mild, transient illness only. Complications include: permanent memory loss, emotional disturbances, loss of intellectual ability or impairment of motor functions. Death may occur, especially in herpes simplex, varicella-zoster and measles infections. Virological studies on CSF and brain biopsy are important investigations, especially in differentiating the disease from meningitis. CSF examination may initially be normal, but a moderate lymphocytosis and rise in protein may be present later; evidence of bacterial, fungal or protozoal causes may be demonstrable in either a direct smear or culture. A rising serum antibody titre is of value in the diagnosis of herpes simplex, mumps, coxiella, rickettsia, *Mycoplasma pneumoniae*, *Legionella pneumophila* and *Toxoplasma gondii* infections. Occasionally, viruses can be isolated from blood, throat swabs or faecal samples. An EEG, CT scan, isotopic brain scan and carotid angiography are important investigations in differentiation from cerebral abscess or tumour, subarachnoid haemorrhage, and cerebrovascular disease.

The most common cause of severe encephalitis is a herpes simplex infection; this may occur either in previously normal healthy people, or in the immunosuppressed; only rarely is cutaneous evidence of the disease present. Severe necrotising encephalitis involving the temporal lobes and resulting in epilepsy (and other features of a space-occupying lesion) is a relatively common presentation. In herpes simplex and varicella-zoster encephalitis, acycloguanosine (acyclovir) is of value: hyperimmune zoster immunoglobulin should be given as a matter of urgency in the latter disease. Antiviral agents when started early will reduce the mortality rate, which untreated is of the order of 70%. Some non-viral causes are also summarised in Table 9.3 (p. 160). *Coxiella burnetii*, rickettsial and *Mycoplasma pneumoniae* encephalitis should be treated in the same way as meningitis caused by those organisms.

Individuals who are exposed to chickenpox or herpes zoster infections and who have compromised immunity should immediately receive hyperimmune zoster immunoglobulin.

Table 9.4 summarises some causes of chronic encephalitis resulting from slow virus infection. Subacute sclerosing panencephalitis (SSPE), which is rapidly fatal after progressive intellectual impairment and progressive jerking movements, is a rare complication of measles vaccination. Very high titres of measles antibody are present both in CSF and serum.

Table 9.4

SLOW VIRUS INFECTIONS OF THE CNS (*see also* Chapter 15)

Virus	Resultant disease
Measles	Subacute sclerosing panencephalitis (SSPE)
Kuru	
Creutzfeldt–Jakob	Slow virus diseases
HIV	
JC virus (papovavirus)	Progressive multifocal leucoencephalopathy

RABIES, TETANUS AND THE GUILLAIN–BARRÉ SYNDROME

Some childhood infections which may be complicated by acute CNS involvement, e.g. diphtheria and poliomyelitis, have been covered in Chapter 2.

Rabies

Rabies is present worldwide, with the exception of Britain (since 1921) and Scandinavia; in much of Europe it is endemic and there it is commonly spread by foxes. This lethal viral disease is, however, usually conveyed to man by the bite or scratch of an infected dog; in practice a long list of other mammals, including vampire bats convey the disease. The virus, present in saliva, can penetrate intact mucous membranes, skin abrasions and wounds; therefore, an actual bite from an infected animal is not strictly necessary. Infected animals secrete the virus in saliva for a few days before developing the disease, and die shortly afterwards; if an apparently healthy dog is still healthy 10 days after it bites a man, it is most unlikely that it had rabies on the day of the bite! The incubation period is usually 4–13 weeks but in exceptional cases can be up to 6 months; the nearer the initial lesion is to the brain, the shorter the incubation period. Spread of infection is via peripheral nerves to the CNS where an encephalomyelitis is produced. The virus causes intracytoplasmic inclusions (Negri bodies) within the neurones. The disease is a systemic one and most organs are involved. Following a sore throat, headache, irritability, fever, and discomfort at the site of the wound, CNS symptoms and signs of 'furious' rabies appear; these include: excitement and muscle spasms (affecting the muscles of deglutition when attempting to drink water ('hydrophobia')) which are followed by convulsions progressing to cardiac or respiratory death. Treatment is merely palliative; there is only one well-documented case of survival from this disease. Human diploid cell strain vaccination (HDCSV) is now safe and effective but a course of three injections should probably be restricted to high-risk groups such as veterinary surgeons; post-exposure vaccination is also effective. Therefore, anyone who has been bitten, scratched or licked by a mammal which is possibly infected with rabies should be given: (i) *passive* immunisation with human rabies immunoglobulin immediately, and (ii) *active* vaccination with HDCSV as soon as possible. Diagnosis is by intracerebral inoculation of saliva, urine or brain tissue into rats; a rapid method utilises immunofluorescence of skin biopsy, corneal impression smears, or brain biopsy. Negri bodies can be visualised in the brain of an infected animal.

Tetanus

Although *Clostridium tetani* infection is now unusual in most developed countries, this is still a major problem in the 'Third World'. Muscular spasm is the major clinical manifestation. After an incubation period of 3–21 days (up to several years in very exceptional cases) following accidental inoculation of bacteria into a wound, trismus ('lockjaw') with muscular spasm accounts for the characteristic clinical signs—'risus sardonicus' of the face, and opisthotonos. As the spasms increase in frequency, exhaustion and respiratory failure supervene. Wound swabs sometimes reveal *Clostridium tetani* (a 'drumstick' with a terminal spore which secretes the potent neurotoxin). These bacteria are present in faeces of many mammals including man, but especially horses; they are also present in soil and the environment in general. Any deep wound can become infected following an accident. In developing countries, umbilical sepsis (sometimes resulting from a local custom of placing cowdung on the healing umbilical scar) can be followed by tetanus neonatorum. The toxin reaches the central nervous system (the anterior horn cell is the target) by ascending peripheral nerves to the spinal cord and medulla. Treatment is with human antitetanus immunoglobulin (HAI) (passive immunity) and benzylpenicillin; wound 'debridement' is essential. Sedation and skilled intensive care are essential if the mortality rate is to be kept low; in inexperienced and ill-equipped settings this may approach 100%. All children should be immunised routinely and a booster dose of toxoid given in later life every 5–10 years; if this were carried out efficiently the disease would be extremely rare. All patients with a deep wound should be given toxoid; in the non-immune, HAI should also be given. Hospital dressings and suture materials should always be carefully and adequately sterilised.

Guillain–Barré Syndrome (Infective Polyneuritis)

Paraesthesiae and weakness in the limbs starts acutely; this progresses to involve the respiratory muscles (with respiratory failure), and paraplegia subsequently develops. CSF contains a high protein concentration (up to 1·2 g/l) at the height of the disease; it appears clear and microscopy is normal. Although the cause is frequently unknown, EBV, CMV, *Mycoplasma pneumoniae* and several intestinal infections including *Campylobacter jejuni* sometimes precede this syndrome. Other causes of aseptic meningitis (*see* p. 153) should be eliminated. If an infective cause is detected, appropriate treatment (if available) should be given. The disease is self-limiting provided respiration and other vital functions can be maintained. Careful monitoring of respiratory function is therefore vital, and artificial respiration may be life-saving.

CEREBRAL ABSCESS AND OTHER SPACE-OCCUPYING LESIONS

Cerebral abscess is usually a complication of an acute infection elsewhere; when the infection (usually bacterial) is treated early, abscess rarely occurs. Direct (from ear, sinuses, etc) and haematogenous (from chronic sinusitis, bronchiectasis, osteomyelitis or endocarditis) spread are both possible; the location may be extra- or subdural, or intracerebral. It may occasionally accompany meningitis or meningoencephalitis. Clinically, signs of the systemic diseases dominate the clinical picture, perhaps with a suggestion of neck stiffness and/or a vague personality change; later, fits, coma and localising neurological signs become apparent. Overall mortality rate is around 15–40%. Differentiation from a cerebrovascular accident is important. EEG and urgent CT scan (when available) are important investigations. The causative agent varies and depends on the original site of infection. CSF may be normal (especially with deep-seated abscesses) or consist of thick purulent fluid; pus from the abscess before chemotherapy is started is the most valuable diagnostic material. Blood culture, and culture of pus from any localised infection—otitis media, respiratory tract, etc—are of potential value. Urgent surgical drainage of pus, repeated aspirations and systemic antibiotics (with local instillation) are all vital procedures. Initial antibiotic therapy should be based on probability grounds depending on the likely whereabouts of the initial infection:

(i) *Source unknown:* metronidazole + chloramphenicol + benzylpenicillin.
(ii) *Ear:* metronidazole + chloramphenicol + benzylpenicillin.
(iii) *Nasal sinuses*: benzylpenicillin.

(iv) *Trauma/surgery:* cloxacillin + fusidic acid.

The antibiotic regimen should then be varied in the light of the microbiological results.

Tuberculomas and several parasitic infections (*see* Table 9.3), which must always be considered in the list of differential diagnoses, especially in the developing world, can also produce intracranial space-occupying lesions.

CHRONIC INFECTIONS

Chronic Bacterial Infections

Tuberculous meningitis (*see* Chapter 3)

Although a major problem in developing countries, this disease is now uncommon in most 'westernised' ones in which it is confined largely to immigrants—especially those from the Indian subcontinent—and the elderly and alcoholic. Malaise, low grade fever, intermittent headache and anorexia are prominent early features (in over 50% of cases miliary disease is present concurrently); after several weeks persistent headache, neck stiffness and oculomotor palsies become apparent. Untreated, there may be increasing drowsiness, hemiplegia, multiple cranial nerve palsies and rigidity; death occurs a few weeks later. If antituberculous treatment is not started early, permanent complications, e.g. hydrocephalus, spinal block, epilepsy, deafness, vestibular dysfunction and mental deficiency may ensue. Although choroid tubercles and miliary mottling on a chest radiograph may be present, in association with a positive tuberculin test and raised ESR, CSF examination is required for a definitive diagnosis (*see* Table 9.1, p. 154–5); acid-fast bacilli are usually scanty and a Lowenstein–Jensen culture should be set up. CSF glucose concentration is characteristically low compared with that in a simultaneously obtained peripheral blood sample. Differential diagnoses on CSF examination include: cerebral abscess and cryptococcal meningitis. Table 9.2 (p. 156) summarises the antituberculous agents which cross the blood–brain barrier; rifampicin, INAH and pyrazinamide should all be started immediately; the value of intrathecal streptomycin is controversial. CSF indices should be monitored during treatment. At least three-quarters of affected patients survive when promptly treated, but complications are relatively common.

Tuberculomas, often situated in the cerebellum, are relatively common in parts of the developing world. Presentation is as a space-occupying lesion (*see* p. 165). An increase in size of the lesion commonly occurs after starting antituberculous chemotherapy; this is associated with immunological changes which are as yet poorly understood. Tuberculomas sometimes calcify.

Slow Virus Infections (*see* Chapter 15)

Subacute sclerosing panencephalitis (SSPE) is an example of a latent infection which follows measles and is usually acquired very early in life; in Britain the annual incidence is approximately 1 in 1 million. The best known of the slow virus infections is probably Kuru (first described in 1957); this is a fatal slowly progressive disease which caused an encephalopathy in the Fore tribe in a localised area of the Papua New Guinea eastern highlands. It bears a close resemblance to a transmissible disease of sheep—scrapie. The virus has been successfully transmitted to chimpanzees which develop an illness similar to that in man after at least 18 months. It is similar to other spongiform encephalopathies—including Creutzfeldt–Jakob disease, scrapie in sheep and transmissible (Aleutian) mink encephalopathy. In the 1950s, Kuru accounted for over 50% of deaths in the Fore tribe; children and adult women were mostly affected. Viral transmission was via ritual cannibalism—by self inoculation of infected tissues through skin abrasions and mucosae; oral ingestion was not important. Cannibalistic practices have now been reduced and no new cases are being reported; only a small nucleus still exists. Incubation period can be from 18 months to about 30 years. Onset is gradual with a shivering tremor of the trunk, head and limbs; cerebellar ataxia, dysarthria and dysphagia follow; progressive cachexia and debilitation usually lead to death within 3–9 months, and certainly within 2 years. Dementia is however not a feature of this disease. There is no treatment. The brain at postmortem shows spongiform changes due to vacuolation of astroglial and neuronal processes, diffuse neuronal degeneration, proliferation of glial elements and absence of inflammatory cells; the cerebellum is most severely affected. There is excellent circumstantial evidence that Creutzfeldt–Jakob disease, which is very similar to Kuru, is caused by an infective agent the nature and identity of which is unclear. The term 'prion' has been used for these unknown infective agents.

Fungal Causes

The most common fungal cause of infection of the CNS is *Cryptococcus neoformans*; this occurs sporadically in tropical countries (geographical foci of high prevalence exist, e.g. the Gulf Province of Papua New Guinea), and also in the immunosuppressed (including those with AIDS) where it is an opportunist organism. Headaches, which are recurrent and worsening and sometimes accompanied by pulmonary involvement, may be early presenting features. However, this disease must be included in the list of differential diagnoses of meningitis in vulnerable groups. In some cases, close contact with pigeons (the organism can be found in droppings) has been reported. The simple diagnostic test is negative CSF-staining with Indian ink which reveals the characteristic capsulated yeast; CSF should also be cultured on Sabouraud's agar. Detection of cryptococcal antigen in CSF by a rapid immunological test is also possible. Treatment is with amphotericin B, sometimes combined with 5-fluorocytosine; the disease carries a high mortality rate however.

Parasitic Causes

Protozoa

African trypanosomiasis (sleeping sickness)

This is the most common cause of chronic meningoencephalitis in many parts of Africa. Two morphologically identical parasites are responsible: *Trypanosoma gambiense* (usually transmitted by the tsetse fly *Glossina palpalis*) and *T. rhodesiense* (usually by *G. morsitans*). Fig. 9.1 summarises the geographical distribution, which is confined to sub-Saharan Africa. In an endemic area, less than 1% of tsetse flies are infected. For *T. rhodesiense* a reservoir of infection exists in various members of the antelope species, especially the bushbuck and hartebeest. Widespread involvement

Infections of the Central Nervous System 169

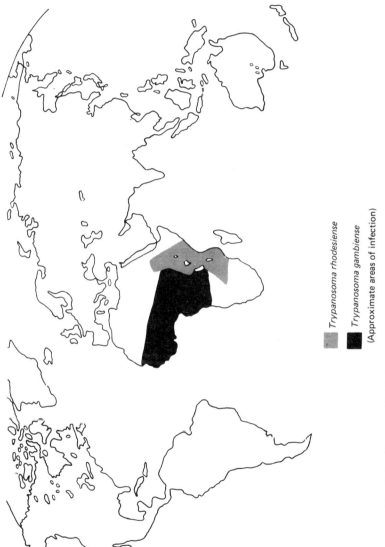

Fig. 9.1 Geographical distribution of *Trypanosoma gambiense* and *T. rhodesiense* (Approximate areas of infection)

of cattle has been a major obstacle to economic development in Africa. The annual incidence of human cases is estimated at 6000 to 10 000; some 35 million people are exposed to the infection. Whereas tourists to game-parks, fishermen and game-wardens are especially vulnerable to *T. rhodesiense* infection, rural populations can be infected with both species. A continuing potential for explosive epidemics exists. Congenital and blood transfusion infections are rare events.

Following a tsetse fly bite a local lesion—the trypanosomal *chancre*—may be present on an exposed part of the body (most frequently in expatriates with a *T. rhodesiense* infection) after an incubation period of 5–15 days. This is followed by fever and often a circinate rash over the trunk, shoulders and thighs. Cervical lymphadenopathy (Winterbottom's sign) sometimes follows in a *T. gambiense* infection. A pancarditis is an important manifestation in *T. rhodesiense* infection; this occasionally proves fatal before central nervous system involvement is present. CNS involvement (meningoencephalomyelitis) supervenes at differing lengths of time after the initial infection, being much earlier (usually 3–4 weeks) in *T. rhodesiense* infections; the degree of parasitaemia and rate of progression is also far more rapid with this infection; CNS involvement and death in the untreated case occurs far more rapidly. Predominant involvement is at the base of the brain. In chronic cases, the meninges are infiltrated with lymphocytes, plasma cells and morular cells of Mott (which are packed with IgM). There is perivascular cuffing around cerebral vessels; severe cerebral damage follows and distortion of the ventricular system is a sequel. Increasing indifference, lassitude, and daytime somnolence with alternating insomnia at night are common features. Extrapyramidal signs frequently occur. Cerebellar ataxia makes walking difficult, and speech becomes slurred. Many other neurological manifestations may also occur. The duration of disease in *T. gambiense* and *T. rhodesiense* infections is of the order of several months to a year or two, and 3–9 months, respectively. Coma and death result either directly from the disease, or from associated malnutrition and intercurrent infection. Diagnosis is by detection of trypanosomes in the 'chancre' or peripheral blood sample in *T. rhodesiense*, and lymph node aspirate in *T. gambiense* infection. In the presence of cerebral involvement they are also to be found in the CSF. Raised CSF IgM is confirmatory evidence of CNS involvement. An increased total protein and total leucocyte count is also common. Serological tests

(IFAT and ELISA) are of value; however, there is cross-reaction with *T. cruzi*.

Treatment in the early stage is with suramin ('Antrypol') given as a slow intravenous infusion (20 mg/kg body weight (maximum dose 1·0 g) on days 1, 3, 7, 14 and 21). Idiosyncratic reactions are rare: collapse and death have rarely been reported. Renal damage is the most important side-effect: urine should be examined prior to each injection. Pentamidine may be used in early *T. gambiense* infections but is inferior to suramine; it also has important toxic effects. When there is evidence of CNS involvement, melarsoprol ('Mel B') (an arsenical preparation) is indicated; some physicians always use this agent in addition to suramine when a *T. rhodesiense* infection seems likely. It is of value at all stages of both diseases, but owing to toxicity should not be the first line of treatment in early disease. Three courses of three daily intravenous injections, with 1 week separating each course constitutes the standard regimen; for an adult weighing more than 60 kg, the doses should be:

(i)   2·5, 3·0 and 3·5 ml.
(ii) 3·5, 4·0 and 4·5 ml.
(iii) 5·0, 5·0 and 5·0 ml.

Toxic effects are: a Herxheimer-type reaction, an encephalopathy (which rarely proves fatal), renal damage and an exfoliative dermatitis. Nitrofurazone has also been used.

Prognosis depends on the point in the disease process when the diagnosis is made and treatment started. Untreated, the disease is invariably fatal. When early infections are adequately treated an almost 100% cure is usual, but with a late infection, especially with *T. rhodesiense*, the outcome is far less satisfactory. Prevention depends on avoidance of heavily infected areas, such as the Luangwa valley in Zambia; exposed parts of the body should be covered. Suramine and pentamidine are effective chemoprophylactics for *T. gambiense* infection, but are not recommended for travellers and those only briefly exposed. Permanent control is aimed at elimination of the tsetse-fly vectors.

Other Protozoa

A meningoencephalitis is rare in south American trypanosomiasis (Chagas' disease) (*see* Chapter 15). Cerebral involvement in

Plasmodium falciparum infection is a serious and often fatal complication (*see* Chapter 4).

Free-living amoebae (*see* Table 9.1, p. 154–5) cause a protozoan meningitis. These organisms multiply in stagnant warm water, often in tropical countries; in England a focus of infection has recently been detected in the Roman baths at Bath. The disease is usually contracted by swimming in contaminated water; children and young adults are most commonly affected. Meningitis and/or encephalitis (usually subacute) is the usual presenting feature. CSF which is purulent and often blood-stained, contains slowly motile amoebic trophozoites which can be detected in a wet, warm preparation; they can also be cultured on special media. Amphotericin B is the agent of choice but the mortality rate is high.

A cerebral abscess caused by *Entamoeba histolytica* is a rare event.

Helminths

Angiostrongylus cantonensis usually produces an eosinophilic meningitis.

Hydatid cyst (*see* Chapter 6) involving the brain often presents as a space-occupying lesion. Cerebral cysticercosis (*see* Chapter 5), presently a major cause of epilepsy in west Iryan, may cause numerous burns as village people fall into their fires during epileptic fits. Treatment is with praziquantel. Several other helminths and/or their eggs can be deposited in the CNS—brain or spinal cord—to produce neurological sequelae (including a transverse myelitis). They include: *Schistosoma mansoni* (which usually produces a cord lesion), *S. japonicum*, paragonimiasis, gnathostomiasis and dracontiasis. Many of these infections present with epilepsy. Diagnosis is frequently difficult, and depends on serology; when there is a strong clinical suspicion, administration of the appropriate anthelmintic is often justified.

FURTHER READING

Ahmadsyah I., Salim A. (1985). Treatment of tetanus: an open study to compare the efficacy of procaine penicillin and metronidazole. *Brit. Med. J*; **291**: 648–50.

Ball A. P. (1987). Cephalosporins in bacterial meningitis: necessity or luxury? *J. Infect*; **15**: 119–23.

Baird D. R., Whittle H. C., Greenwood B, M. (1976). Mortality from pneumococcal meningitis. *Lancet*; **2**: 1344–6.

Behan P. O., Behan W. M. H. (1987). Plasma exchange in neurological disease. *Brit. Med. J*; **295:** 283–4.

Brown F. (1987). Unconventional viruses and the central nervous system. *Brit. Med. J*; **295:** 347–8.

Editorial. (1983). Prevention of neonatal tetanus. *Lancet*; **1:** 1253–4.

Editorial. (1986). Meningococcal infections. *Lancet*; **2:** 551–2.

French G. L., Teoh R., Chan C. Y., *et al.* (1987). Diagnosis of tuberculous meningitis by detection of tuberculostearic acid in cerebrospinal fluid. *Lancet*; **2:** 117–19.

Greenwood B. M., Bradley A. K., Cleland P. G., *et al.* (1979). An epidemic of meningococcal infection at Zaria, Northern Nigeria. 1. General epidemiological features. *Trans. R. Soc. Trop. Med. Hyg*; **73:** 557–62.

Johnson R. T., Griffin D. E., Hirsch R. L., *et al.* (1984). Measles encephalomyelitis—clinical and immunologic studies. *N. Eng. J. Med*; **310:** 137–41.

Montgomery R. D. (1987). Tropical spastic paresis and its relationship to HTLV-I infection. *Q. J. Med*; **64:** in press.

Seale J. R. (1987). Kuru, AIDS and aberrant social behaviour. *J. R. Soc. Med*; **80:** 200–2.

Sotelo J., Escobedo F., Rodriguez-Carbajal J., *et al.* (1984) Therapy of parenchymal brain cysticerosis with praziquantel. *N. Engl. J. Med*; **310:** 1001–7.

Suntharasamai P., Warrell M. J., Warrell D. A., *et al.* (1986). New purified vero-cell vaccine prevents rabies in patients bitten by rabid animals. *Lancet*; **2:** 129–31.

Turner M. (1980). How trypanosomes change coats. *Nature*; **284:** 13–14.

Warrell D. A., Davidson N. M., Pope H. M., *et al.* (1976). Pathophysiologic studies in human rabies. *Am. J. Med*; **60:** 180–90.

Chapter Ten

Renal and Urinary Tract Infections

Urinary tract infections account for significant morbidity and mortality throughout the world. Acute infections, usually bacterial in origin, are especially common in women; this is a result of shorter urethral length, vulnerability to coital trauma, and childbearing. An infection in a young man warrants thorough investigation. They are also common in the elderly. In tropical countries, urinary schistosomiasis accounts for much disease in some parts of Africa and the Middle-east. Renal tuberculosis and the nephropathy resulting from chronic *Plasmodium malariae* infection are other significant diseases in 'Third World' countries.

Urinary tract infections (UTI) can either be primary or associated with underlying congenital abnormalities, stasis, calculi or foreign bodies. Gram-negative bacteria (usually of colonic origin) are the most common organisms. Bacteriuria occasionally occurs in symptomless individuals (*see* p. 175). Acute and chronic pyelonephritis may follow lower urinary tract infections; this can be a consequence of vesicoureteric reflux, obstruction, calculi, congenital abnormalities and other acquired or genetically determined factors.

ACUTE URINARY TRACT INFECTIONS

The entire urinary tract is normally sterile; urinary tract infection can therefore be equated with the presence of micro-organisms, a 'significant bacteriuria' consisting of more than 10^8 bacteria/l (i.e. 10^5 bacteria/ml). However, occasionally in a symptomatic individual, this concentration may be $10^7/l$ or below, in the absence of antibiotics. The clinico-pathological categories are:

(i) *The frequency/dysuria syndrome*. This consists of dysuria and frequency of micturition, and is sometimes accompanied

by suprapubic pain. It is caused by (a) bacterial cystitis—characterised by a 'significant bacteriuria', and often pyuria and haematuria—and (b) abacterial cystitis in which bacteria cannot be demonstrated; the cause of this condition, sometimes known as the 'urethral syndrome', is unknown.
(ii) *Acute bacterial pyelonephritis.* This syndrome consists of loin pain, tenderness and pyrexia, accompanied by bacteriuria and pyuria. Although bacteraemia is usually present, a 'significant bacteriuria' is sometimes absent.
(iii) *Chronic interstitial nephritis.* This syndrome has several causes apart from bacterial infection (which is usually associated with structural abnormalities of the renal tract): analgesic abuse, methicillin nephropathy, and irradiation. The renal interstitium and tubules are chronically inflamed, progressive fibrosis may ultimately produce a 'shrunken' kidney, and tubular function may become progressively impaired.
(iv) *Covert bacteriuria.* In this condition a 'significant bacteriuria' is discovered during screening of an apparently healthy individual; about 5% of pregnant women fall into this category.

Urinary Infection in Special Groups

Urinary tract infections are 2 to 3 times more common in girls compared with boys; approximately 12% of all children with symptomatic urinary tract infections already have renal scarring or reflux at an initial radiological investigation (intravenous pyelography or micturating cystourethrography). Therefore, long-term follow-up and appropriate treatment of urinary tract infection in children is essential in order to prevent hypertension and renal failure in later childhood and adult life. In adults, when there is more than one infection, a structural abnormality on intravenous urography (IVU), indicating the presence of residual urine is a common finding; surgical correction may be possible.

Most acute urinary tract infections are caused by ascending faecal flora, from the perineum and periurethral area. Normal defence mechanisms include: hydrodynamic factors, phagocytosis by polymorphonuclear leucocytes, humoral (IgA) antibody, and non-specific antibacterial compounds in prostatic, urethral and bladder mucosal secretions. When the bladder is incompletely emptied at the end of micturition, e.g. in the presence of a structural abnormality or a neurogenic bladder, infection is more common. Other factors predisposing to infection are: instrumentation and surgery, diabetes mellitus (acute papillary necrosis may be a sequel), and immunosuppression (unusual organisms, e.g. *Salmonella, Serratia, Candida* and *Nocardia* may be present). Most infections are therefore associated with *Escherichia coli* ('O' serotypes) of faecal origin; many of these are adherent organisms, and bacterial fimbriae attach to specific epithelial cell 'receptors'. Following entry to the bladder, a minority of infections ascend to the upper urinary tract; vesicoureteric reflux in infants, and renal calculi in adults often determine this event. The amount and type of polysaccharide 'K' antigen in the capsular surface of an infecting *E. coli* strain may be used to determine the likelihood of subsequent acute bacterial pyelonephritis. Renal infection can also take place by haematogenous spread, e.g. during a *Staphylococcus aureus* bacteraemia; perinephric tissues can thus be infected via this route, with the production of an abscess (which occasionally presents as a pyrexia of undetermined origin) (*see* Chapter 1). Apart from bacteria, fungal agents are less often responsible for a urinary tract infection; in either case their identity depends to some extent on whether they were acquired in or outside hospital. *Staphylococcus albus* (after catheterisation), *Staph. aureus* (following surgery), *Proteus spp., Klebsiella spp., Pseudomonas* and *Serratia spp.* (which are common causes of hospital acquired infection), and *Streptococcus faecalis* are all far less common numerically than *E. coli*. Where there is not a previously demonstrable bacterial cause, *Bacteroides fragilis* should be considered. *Neisseria gonorrhoeae (see* Chapter 12) can cause pyuria but this is a result of urethritis rather than a urinary tract infection. In cases of 'sterile' pyuria, *Mycobacterium tuberculosis* (*see* p. 50) should always be considered. *Candida albicans* is an important cause of urinary tract infection in the presence of diabetes mellitus, in those who have received frequent courses of antibiotics, and in individuals with compromised immune responses.

Site of infection

Clues from the clinical history and examination are often helpful in deciding which part of the urinary tract is infected. In addition, ureteric catheterisation, Fairley's neomycin bladder wash-out test, prostatic massage and culture of renal tissue can provide valuable additional information.

Abacterial cystitis

Approximately 50% of women presenting with frequency and dysuria do *not* have a UTI. The causes, although not usually apparent, include: trauma, and infection with *Chlamydia*, *Mycoplasma* or *Trichomonas*. Gonococcal infection, *Candida albicans*, *Herpes simplex* and *Gardnerella vaginalis* should also be considered.

Investigations

Routine urine specimens are frequently contaminated with normal flora from the perineum and external genitalia, especially in women. A mid-stream specimen after adequate cleansing of the genitalia is a crucial preliminary to accurate microbiological culture. (A microbiology text should be consulted for details of culture techniques, results and their interpretation.)

Treatment

Most cases of UTI consist of bacterial cystitis in women; drinking large quantities of fluids is of value, and in addition, antibiotic therapy is sometimes advisable. *E. coli* infections usually respond to sulphonamides, ampicillin, co-trimoxazole (trimethoprim is probably equally effective and carries a lesser risk of side-effects), nalidixic acid, nitrofurantoin or cephalosporin; however, treatment should when possible be based on sensitivity tests. For children, co-trimoxazole, trimethoprim, ampicillin or cephalexin are usually effective. In hospital practice, a very severe infection might warrant ampicillin + gentamicin until results of sensitivity tests are available. A 3-day course of antibiotic treatment normally gives good results in general practice, but with hospital acquired infections, a 10-day course is usually desirable; such a course is also indicated in cases of acute bacterial pyelonephritis and asymptomatic bacteriuria of pregnancy. Recurrent urinary tract infections can occasionally be cured with surgery if there is an obstructive element or other organic abnormality, but long courses (sometimes months or even years) of antibiotic (e.g. co-trimoxazole, trimethoprim or nitrofurantoin) given at low dosage, are often necessary.

When, in women, there is an association between sexual intercourse and the onset of a UTI, micturition immediately after intercourse is advisable. Rarely, prophylactic nitrofurantoin can be recommended. Regarding hospital acquired infection, catheterisation is often responsible for introduction of the organism(s); techniques used for catheterisation, and techniques for long-term indwelling catheterisation should utilise the strictest aseptic conditions.

Post-streptococcal Glomerulonephritis

This disease follows infection by a specific 'nephritogenic' strain of Group A β-haemolytic streptococcus (usually type 1, 4, 25, 41, 49 or 57). It is the best studied example of transient immune complex-mediated glomerulonephritis; genetic host factors are undoubtedly important. The illness occasionally occurs in children after an outbreak of streptococcal infection, usually of pharyngeal origin but which may also be a skin infection (complicating impetigo or scabies) especially in tropical countries (*see* Chapter 13). A clinically identical illness can occur without evidence of a preceding streptococcal infection: pneumococcal pneumonia, typhoid fever, diphtheria, varicella, adenoviral infection, measles, mumps, enteroviral infections and malaria have been incriminated.

Histologically, diffuse exudative and proliferative lesions involve the glomerular tufts; these result from deposition of specific streptococcal antigen–antibody complexes and activation of the complement cascade. A low concentration of serum C3 is present, and deposits of C3 and IgG can be demonstrated on the epithelial side of the glomerular basement membrane.

Streptococcus pyogenes may be detected in pharyngeal culture; antistreptolysin O (ASO) titres are usually, but not always, elevated, but demonstration of an elevated specific antibody titre to streptococcal M antigen is more helpful. Renal biopsy also may be of value. Daily urine analysis is essential in management; creatinine clearance gives an approximate guide to renal function.

Parenteral or oral penicillin should be given and appropriate management of the renal failure instituted. Most patients recover, but a small minority die of acute renal failure and another small group demonstrates residual abnormalities of renal function, sometimes with the development of a nephrotic syndrome. Prognosis overall is better in children than adults.

Other causes of acute nephritis include: infective endocarditis, systemic lupus erythematosus and other autoimmune connective tissue disorders (including Henoch–Schönlein purpura and Goodpasture's syndrome), and mesangiocapillary and focal glomerulonephritides.

Acute Renal Failure

Many infective conditions can predispose to this medical emergency, e.g. acute *Plasmodium falciparum* malaria (*see* Chapter 4), untreated septic abortion, *E. coli* septicaemia, pyomyositis, typhoid fever, cholera, leptospirosis, yellow fever and the viral haemorrhagic fevers. In addition, the haemolytic-uraemic syndrome occasionally occurs in shigellosis, especially in children. Management should be aimed at control of the hypotension, shock and underlying infection. The oliguric phase may last for a few days to more than 1 month; progressive uraemia (hyperkalaemia, acidosis, and/or overhydration) is potentially life-threatening, and may require peritoneal or haemo-dialysis. Gastrointestinal haemorrhage and intercurrent infection are important complications. The diuretic phase usually begins 10–14 days after onset.

CHRONIC URINARY TRACT INFECTIONS

Chronic Nephritis

Chronic glomerulonephritis and pyelonephritis are usually long-term sequelae of inadequately treated acute disease (*see* p. 174); the latter is also a frequent complication of *Schistosoma haematobium* infection (*see* p. 18).

Renal Tuberculosis

This is one form of extrapulmonary infection (*see* Chapter 3). It results from haematogenous spread, usually with delayed reactivation of lesions in the renal parenchyma. Involvement of the prostate, seminal vesicles and epididymes often accompanies renal involvement in men, and the fallopian tubes and other pelvic organs in women. Presentation is classically with frequency, dysuria and/or haematuria, and sterile pyuria in the presence of low grade chronic fever; positive cultures can usually be obtained from early morning urine specimens.

Salmonellosis

Urinary salmonellosis is a complicating factor in sickle-cell (SS) disease. This infection may also be secondary to a *S. haematobium* infection (*see* p. 181); although urinary stasis is a predisposing factor this does not completely explain the association. Both infections should be treated concurrently.

Plasmodium malariae Nephrosis ('Quartan Malarial Nephropathy')

This chronic form of renal disease (which has not been reported with other forms of malaria) is probably the most common cause of the nephrotic syndrome in tropical Africa. Renal biopsy shows: specific malarial antigen in complex with IgG, IgM and C3. Irregular thickening of the capillary wall which has a twisted, plexiform appearance can be visualised histologically; there is also a non-specific trapping of IgM in the glomerulus. The nephrotic syndrome results from the deposition of immune complexes, rather than from other immunological mechanisms, between the basement membrane and malarial products. The reason for the development of immune complex mediated glomerulonephritis in a small minority of individuals infected with *Plasmodium malariae* (and not *P. falciparum* or other species) is unknown; genetic factors are probably relevant. Treatment is extremely unsatisfactory; neither corticosteroids nor azathioprine are of value.

Intravascular deposition of specific immune complexes (immune complex nephropathy) can be demonstrated in many other communicable diseases, e.g. leprosy, *Treponema pallidum* (syphilis), Kala azar (visceral leishmaniasis), onchocerciasis, loaiasis, trypanosomiasis, toxoplasmosis, and also EBV and HBV infections. In Africa, a further differential diagnosis of the nephrotic syndrome is the nephropathy associated with mercury containing skin-lightening creams. Other causes of the nephrotic syndrome should be excluded: these include diabetic nephropathy, systemic lupus erythematosus, amyloid (*see* p. 181), anaphylactoid purpura, renal vein thrombosis, other toxic and therapeutic agents and Hodgkin's disease. Immune complex glomerulonephritis with associated nephrotic syndrome can also result from *Schistosoma mansoni* and *S. haematobium* infections (*see* below).

Renal amyloidosis accompanied by a nephrotic syndrome is a sequel to several chronic bacterial infections, especially tuberculosis and lepromatous leprosy. This disease should be differentiated from renal involvement (with amyloid deposition) in familial Mediterranean fever (FMF).

Urinary Schistosomiasis

Fig. 10.1 shows the world distribution of the trematode *Schistosoma haematobium*; Africa and the Middle-east are the affected areas. This is the only human schistosome known to produce significant urinary tract disease. The life-cycle of the parasite is similar to that of the intestinal form of the disease (*see* Chapter 6). Acute schistosomiasis (Katayama fever) is less common than with other species. Most infections are mild and asymptomatic. *S. haematobium* (and also *S. mansoni*) granulomas are produced by a cell-mediated response to egg antigen; there is good evidence that as adult life is reached, individuals in endemic areas undergo a reduction in the intensity of this immune reaction with a concurrent improvement in symptoms.

Egg deposition in the bladder wall is accompanied by the development of 'sandy patches', and fibrosis with ureteric stenoses. Bladder calcification, which affects large numbers of people in affected areas results in a small non-contractile organ. Chronic bacteriuria is common; infection with *Salmonella spp.* is also a frequent complication. A Gram-negative septicaemia is common in advanced disease. An obstructive uropathy can be demonstrated by intravenous urography; hydroureter, hydronephrosis, pyelonephritis and latterly renal failure may be present. The frequency with which obstructive uropathy progresses to end-stage renal disease increases with worm load and age of the individual. *S. haematobium* accounts for very many cases of chronic renal failure in areas of high endemicity. Bladder carcinoma (usually of squamous cell type) is a further sequel, especially in Egypt; the mechanism of pathogenesis is unclear:

(i) Ova might initiate an inflammatory reaction which reduces elasticity and bladder-filling capacity; this in turn

182 Communicable and Tropical Diseases

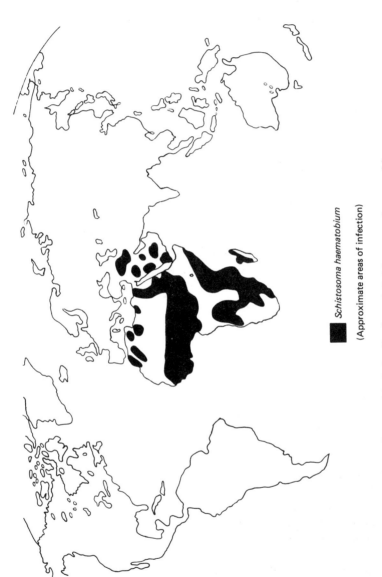

Fig. 10.1 Geographical distribution of *Schistosoma haematobium*

reduces emptying efficiency and a build-up of residual urine occurs which can readily become infected.
(ii) Nitrate-reducing bacteria in the urinary tract then produce nitrites from dietary nitrates which are degraded to carcinogenic nitrosamines.

Nephrotic syndrome can occasionally complicate *S. haematobium* (and less commonly *S. mansoni*) infections. The incidence of these abnormalities correlates with the prevalence of infection in the community.

Presentation of urinary tract schistosomiasis is usually with dysuria, urinary frequency and most characteristically, terminal haematuria. Urinary egg counts have been clearly shown to correlate closely with the degree of haematuria and proteinuria. Diagnosis is by finding ova in a terminal urine specimen (preferably an overnight specimen), by centrifuge sedimentation or a micropore urine-filtration. The eggs, which are characteristically shaped and possess a terminal spine, may also be found in bladder mucosal or rectal biopsies. ELISA serology is almost always positive (*see* Chapter 6).

Renal biopsies may show specific deposits of schistosomal polysaccharide, IgG, IgM and C3; these changes are more likely to occur when there is a heavy worm burden. Slow resolution usually occurs after specific treatment of the schistosomiasis. Renal amyloidosis is an unusual complication of this infection. Although rectal and liver involvement is common (ova are frequently detected in biopsy specimens), progressive changes are very unusual.

Treatment is either with praziquantel (as for *S. mansoni* and *S. japonicum* infections) or the anticholinesterase inhibitor metriphonate (7·5–10 mg/kg body-weight, given on three occasions at biweekly intervals); the latter agent is effective *only* against *S. haematobium* infection; it is considerably cheaper than praziquantel. Bacteriuria should be treated with antibiotics after the appropriate antischistosomal treatment has been given; the same applies to pyelonephritis when present. Surgery may be required for relief of fibrotic lesions causing an obstructive uropathy. Haemodialysis or renal transplant may be required in the presence of advanced renal failure. If bladder carcinoma has already complicated the disease, radical surgery and chemotherapy are of value but only as palliative procedures.

FURTHER READING

Browing M. D., Narooz S. I., Strickland G. T., *et al.* (1984). Clinical characteristics and response to therapy in Egyptian children infected with *Schistosoma haematobium*. *J. Infect. Dis*; **149:** 998–1004.

Cook G. C. (1986). Periodic disease, recurrent polyserositis, Familial Mediterranean Fever, or simply 'FMF'. *Q. J. Med*; **60:** 819–23.

Editorial. (1981). Acute urethral syndrome in women. *Brit. Med. J*; **282:** 3–5.

Hendrickse R. G. (1980). Epidemiology and prevention of kidney disease in Africa. *Trans. R. Soc. Trop. Med. Hyg*; **74:** 8–16.

Hutt M. S. R. (1980). Renal disease in a tropical environment. *Trans. R. Soc. Trop. Med. Hyg*; **74:** 17–21.

Levine M. M. (1986). *Escherichia coli* infections. *N. Engl. J. Med*; **313:** 445–7.

Medical Research Council Bacteriuria Committee. (1979). Recommended terminology of urinary-tract infection. *Brit. Med. J*; **2:** 717–19.

Ngu J. L., Youmbissi T. J. (1987). Special features, pathogenesis and aetiology of glomerular diseases in the tropics. *Clin. Science*; **72:** 519–24.

Chapter Eleven

Acquired Immune Deficiency Syndrome (AIDS)

A pandemic, involving many millions of people, caused by two or more newly recognised lymphotropic viruses currently dominates thought, practice and research in communicable disease throughout the world; it seems likely that with an increasing reservoir of infection, this disease and its complications will continue to be a major world-wide health problem for many years to come. When fully developed (end-stage AIDS), the disease is invariably fatal; no effective vaccine or treatment yet exists. Parallels have been suggested with the syphilis epidemic which swept Europe towards the end of the 15th century; others have referred to it as the modern equivalent of the Black Death. The virus first emerged at the beginning of the 1980s (or possibly as early as 1976), and the first case in the UK was reported in 1981. The number of cases and size of the reservoir of HIV (human immune deficiency virus) infection has grown very rapidly and is perhaps 60 times greater than the disease itself. The origin of the virus is shrouded in mystery (*see* p. 191). Exactly how many infected individuals develop AIDS-related symptoms, and eventually AIDS itself, is so far unclear.

The responsible virus was first isolated in 1983 at the Institut Pasteur in Paris; it was initially named lymphadenopathy-associated virus (LAV). In 1984, a virus present in AIDS sufferers was described at the National Institutes of Health at Bethesda, USA, and was named: human T-cell lymphotrophic virus type III (HTLV III). These two agents were subsequently shown to be virtually identical both on morphological and antigenic grounds. Widespread agreement now exists that the causative agent should be designated HIV-1. It is a retrovirus with an affinity for the T4 antigen site on lymphocytes and other blood-borne cells (including monocytes and macrophages). It replicates within living cells by using its own enzyme *reverse transcriptase*, to convert its RNA into DNA (proviral DNA) which is then integrated into the host DNA. Proviral DNA thus becomes part of the cell's genetic material which on activation, programmes further manufacture of viral components with assembly into the whole virus. The new viruses leave via the cell membrane and thence invade other cells within the same host. In 1986, another virus (LAV II) (now designated HIV–2), which differs by at least 30% in sequence from LAV, was also reported in France in two patients considered on clinical grounds to have AIDS. Whether other closely related viruses remain undiscovered is unknown.

Had this pandemic arisen even a decade ago, there would have been no means of delineating it.

NORTH AMERICAN AND EUROPEAN AIDS

HIV–1 infection has been shown to be largely confined to certain high-risk groups—male homosexuals (especially the very promiscuous), intravenous drug abusers, and haemophiliacs (infected via contaminated Factors VIII and IX). One estimate for the relative HIV–1 carriage rates in these three groups in the UK is: 21, 10 and 31%, respectively; these might however be gross underestimates. Clearly bisexual males (a 'bridging-group') constitute a source of considerable concern, for they could build up a large reservoir of infection in women which could then lead to rapid heterosexual transmission. In northern American and European AIDS the overall importance of female to male transmission is unclear. Genetic, including ethnic factors are probably involved; there is a suggestion that infection is less common in Asians.

One recent estimate is that some 3 million people in the USA are currently infected with HIV–1. In the UK, another estimate is that cases of AIDS will show an annual increase from 144 to 1837 between 1984 and 1988. It has also been suggested that this figure will have risen to at least 10 000 by 1990. A WHO prediction is that by 1991, 100 million people will be infected. However, such predictions are surrounded by a vast amount of uncertainty; they would be made easier if accurate knowledge of the size of the reservoir of HIV–1 infection could be made available, together with the precise numbers of homosexual and bisexual men and of drug abusers involved. While most cases of

AIDS in the UK have been reported in London, a very high incidence of HIV-1 infection exists in Edinburgh in drug abusers.

HIV-1 has been demonstrated in a wide range of body fluids: blood, saliva, tears, breast-milk, semen and cervical and vaginal secretions. There is reasonable evidence that sexual, blood-borne and transplacental routes of transmission explain most of the spread of disease in north America and Europe. Accidental transmission of HIV-1 within households and to health-care workers (including dental practitioners) although documented, is rare. Although infections have been acquired from blood transfusions, this is a rare event in the USA and UK.

Following infection, antibodies to HIV-1 appear in about 8 weeks (seroconversion); however, considerably longer periods of time are sometimes required. These antibodies, although acting as markers of infection, have little or no capacity to neutralise the HIV-1 virus; neither do they reflect either the size of the infecting dose or the likely prognosis. Furthermore, they do not identify an HIV-2 infection.

Acute infection is sometimes accompanied by a transient non-specific illness similar to that of certain other viral infections, EBV in particular, and consisting of: malaise, myalgia, lymphadenopathy, pharyngitis and a rash. However, most acute HIV-1 infections remain subclinical. The ensuing *chronic* phase may also be either asymptomatic or accompanied by an illness of varying degree of severity; the two principal syndromes are: (i) persistent generalised lymphadenopathy (PGL), and (ii) the AIDS-related complex (ARC). Although those with PGL may remain reasonably well, those with ARC experience weight-loss, fever, diarrhoea and mild infections (Table 11.1); furthermore, they have a high risk (a minority may show partial recovery) of progression to end-stage AIDS. Carriers of HIV-1 infection as well as those with AIDS can develop various neurological sequelae (*see* p. 188).

End-stage AIDS represents the most serious sequel of HIV-1 infection; however, the statistical chance of this outcome following an initial infection is so far unclear, estimates ranging from 10 to 100%. Also, the actual course is variable and a wide span of severity undoubtedly exists. Although it was initially considered that most cases had a mean latent period of 3-4 years, this is now considered to be nearer 8-9 years. The disease (AIDS) is diagnosed only at the onset of an opportunistic infection or infections (a somewhat arbitrary dividing line in the progression from ARC). Table 11.2 summarises the opportunistic infections and

Table 11.1

SYMPTOMS, SIGNS AND LABORATORY INVESTIGATIONS ASSOCIATED WITH AIDS-RELATED COMPLEX (ARC)

Symptoms
   Malaise, lethargy
   Weight-loss (>10% body weight)
   Chronic diarrhoea

Signs
   Pyrexia of unknown origin (>2 months)
   Persistent generalised lymphadenopathy
   Hepatosplenomegaly
   Hairy leucoplakia
   Minor infections, e.g. oral candidiasis, herpes zoster

Investigations
   HIV antibodies; HIV isolation
   Leucopenia; lymphopenia
   Anaemia
   Thrombocytopenia
   ESR↑
   Cholesterol↑
   Immunoglobulins↑
   Various immunological abnormalities

other sequelae which are presently known to form an integral part of this disease; many of these infections have undoubtedly been contracted previously by the host but so far held in abeyance. Overt infection results from depletion of T4 lymphocytes, or the fact that they are rendered ineffective; there is a selective effect on these cells. In north American and European AIDS, approximately 70% of sufferers develop one or more of these opportunistic infections, 20% Kaposi's sarcoma, and the remaining 10%, both of them. The infections themselves are in many cases treatable early in the disease, but as time progresses they become increasingly refractory to chemotherapeutic agents. The disease is ultimately fatal in 100% of cases; mean prognosis is approximately 1 year. Individuals initially presenting with Kaposi's sarcoma tend to have a better prognosis (in months) than those presenting with *Pneumocystis carinii*; however, a combination of the two conditions forebodes an especially bad outlook. A further complicating factor in AIDS is neurological involvement; HIV-1 sometimes has a disastrous influence on neurological

Table 11.2

SOME OPPORTUNISTIC INFECTIONS, AND ASSOCIATED DISEASES WHICH ARE IMPORTANT IN AIDS

	Organ involvement
(i) Infective agents	
Viral	
Cytomegalovirus	Lungs, gut, CNS
Herpes simplex	Mucocutaneous, lungs, gut
	Disseminated
?	Progressive multifocal leucoencephalopathy
Bacterial	
Mycobacterium tuberculosis	Disseminated
Atypical mycobacteria (e.g. *M. avium intracellulare*)	Disseminated
Salmonellosis	Gut
Fungal	
Aspergillosis	CNS, disseminated
Candidiasis	Oesophageal, bronchopulmonary
Cryptococcosis	Lungs, CNS, disseminated
Histoplasmosis	Disseminated
Protozoan	
Cryptosporidiosis	Gut, biliary system
Isosporiasis	Gut
Sarcocystis	Gut
Pneumocystis carinii	Lungs
Toxoplasmosis	Lungs, CNS
Helminths	
Strongyloidiasis (?)	Lungs, CNS, disseminated
(ii) Non-infective disease	
Malignancies	
Kaposi's sarcoma	
Cerebral lymphoma	
Non-Hodgkin's lymphoma (diffuse, undifferentiated, B-cell or unknown phenotype)	
Lymphoreticular malignancy	
Burkitt's lymphoma	
Squamous cell carcinomas	
Other	
Chronic lymphoid interstitial pneumonitis	

function as well as on the immune system. Acute, subacute and chronic neurological syndromes—including a subacute encephalitis—have been clearly delineated. One-quarter to one-third of AIDS sufferers develop: headaches, depression, fits, progressive dementia and/or peripheral neuropathy. HIV–1 carriers can also develop these sequelae; it is possible, therefore, that individuals who do not develop end-stage AIDS will, with the passage of time, undergo severe neurological deterioration.

Clearly an enormous preventive medicine ('disease prevention') campaign is required—aimed both at homosexual and to a lesser extent, heterosexual promiscuity. It is essential that publicity campaigns do not produce an impression that this is entirely a 'homosexual disease'. A decrease in numbers of drug abusers, and purer blood products for haemophiliacs must also be sought. It is essential also that individuals from these 'high risk' groups do not donate blood; HIV–1 screening of blood donors is only of limited value, because weeks or months may elapse between infection and positivity of the test. Prevalence of HIV–1 antibody among those not in high risk groups is probably still extremely low in the UK. However, routine screening is not taking place (except with the individual's express permission), and screening of donor blood, or that of individuals with minor illnesses (with a view to establishing the size of the reservoir) is not presently acceptable on ethical grounds. Therefore, the actual size of the problem is unknown. The advisability of screening individuals from Africa before they enter the UK has been suggested; HIV–1 infection in Zaire, Zambia, Uganda and Tanzania is very common (*see* p. 192) and students in particular should perhaps be screened for HIV–1 antibody. However, such a policy would inevitably 'miss' those who had only recently been infected. It would also miss those infected with HIV–2 and other human retroviruses so far unidentified. Government and other prevention campaigns have in some cases recommended the provision of free condoms, and free needles and syringes for drug abusers.

HIV–1 carriers have in some cases been barred from dental treatment, dismissed from employment and refused life insurance cover; very many problems therefore remain to be ironed out.

The cost of dealing with AIDS in the USA and UK, as well as other European countries, etc, will soon be enormous; involvement ranges from counselling of the HIV-positive individual, to funding of hospice and intensive care of terminally ill patients with multiple opportunistic infections. Current research costs are also substantial. If satisfactory treatment regimens are to be forthcoming they might involve very expensive chemotherapeutic agents.

Several agents with a potential for interfering with, or halting viral replication—suramin, ribavirin, azidothymidine (AZT), HPA-23 and phosphonoformate—have now been identified. Of these AZT which can penetrate the blood-brain barrier, has proved most promising. This is not however a cure for AIDS, but merely gives a limited extension of survival. An effective HIV-1 vaccine seems a very long way off. Other research initiatives are examining the possibility of reconstructing the damaged immune system; interleukin-2 and isoprinosine have been tested but results are so far not encouraging. In the treatment of the associated opportunistic infections (*see* p. 189), 9-(1,3-dihydroxy-2-propoxymethyl)-guanine has been used for cytomegalovirus (CMV) infections. In the management of Kaposi's sarcoma, α-interferon, chemotherapy and radiotherapy have been tested. Meanwhile preventive measures must concentrate on halting the spread of infection via blood and blood products. It seems most unlikely, from historical precedents with syphilis, that legal methods would have any impact; unlike the situation with a disease such as smallpox, two consenting sexual partners are usually required to spread this infection; the days of sex without responsibility should be over!

The possibility of a subunit vaccine is at present a remote prospect.

AFRICAN AIDS

Cases of HIV-1 infection in central Africa, of which there are now estimated to be several millions, were first recorded in Zaire in the early 1980s, However, early cases recorded in Haiti, USA, probably originated from Africa; there were also early reports in Europe of infection in Africans who had formerly lived in central Africa. Although a good deal of evidence suggests that the virus originated in Africa, some writers have considered that it was 'man-made', either in the USA or USSR, during efforts to engineer new biological warfare weapons. Infectious disease surveillance in Africa is strictly limited. If in fact it did originate in tropical Africa, the exact site and timing of the event must be the subject of much conjecture; it could even have been present in the population of that continent for many decades. Analysis of the nucleotide sequences of HIV-1 and HIV-2 suggests that these viruses are only distantly related in evolutionary terms, and existed long before the current AIDS epidemic. Retrospective tests on serum samples indicate that HIV-1 infections were present at Kinshasa, Zaire as early as 1959; evidence of infection in the 1960s and 1970s has also been produced from west and east Africa. However, the accuracy of some of these tests has been disputed. Immunodeficiency in the Asian macaque monkey can be caused by an agent designated STLV III MAC. Also, a virus (STLV III AGM) closely related to HIV-1 has been isolated from healthy African vervet (green) monkeys; antibodies to this virus actually cross-react with HIV-1. A similar virus, HIV-2, has more recently been isolated from prostitutes in west Africa; this virus is very similar to STLV III AGM. However, not all workers agree that Africa was the 'cradle' of the human disease.

Because sophisticated methods for recording data and for diagnosis of AIDS in Africa are considerably less advanced than in north America and Europe, it is difficult to assess the true size of the problem there. Urban areas of Zaire, Zambia, Kenya and Rwanda are undoubtedly in the midst of a massive epidemic of HIV-1 infection, and end-stage AIDS. Sex incidence is approximately 1:1; this is *consistent* with heterosexual transmission. The disease is most common in women (of less than 30) and men (more than 40) years old. Up to 88% of female prostitutes have been shown to be infected with HIV-1 in east and central Africa. Highest HIV prevalence rates are thus in the most sexually active groups and up to 5–10% of adults in some cities have HIV antibodies. The infection is also spreading to rural populations and to children. Huge numbers of new AIDS cases are therefore expected within the next few years. The role of needles—used for scarification, tattooing, ritual circumcision, etc in transmission is unclear. Arthropod transmission seems unlikely but has not been completely excluded.

The disease was initially reported on clinical grounds from Uganda and Tanzania as 'Slim disease' (a diarrhoea-wasting syndrome); it is now clear that this is the same as AIDS in the UK and USA. Presentation is usually, therefore, with chronic diarrhoea, weight-loss and oral candidiasis. A generalised pruritic maculopapular eruption, often referred to as 'prurigo', and generalised lymphadenopathy are common clinical features. In children, malnutrition, pneumonia and anaemia are often present. The acute seroconversion syndrome is similar to that in the UK and USA: encephalitis, asymptomatic immunodepression (low T helper cell numbers, with an inverted T lymphocyte-helper/suppressor ratio), PGL, oral candidiasis, herpes zoster, other diverse opportunistic infections and Kaposi's sarcoma.

The range of opportunistic infections probably differs from that in the USA and Europe. Pneumonia caused by *Pneumocystis carinii* is probably less common, and toxoplasmosis more so. Disseminated histoplasmosis has been reported. Cryptococcosis (with meningitis) is also commonly seen. Of viral infections, CMV is probably the most serious. Tuberculosis caused by *Mycobacterium tuberculosis*, is more common than in the western world; HIV-1 infections may complicate strategies for tuberculosis control in Africa. Salmonellosis is common. Although helminthic infections do not seem to be a major problem, limited evidence suggests that *Strongyloides stercoralis* is a frequent opportunistic infection, sometimes in disseminated form. Malaria, leishmaniasis, filariasis and leprosy are, perhaps surprisingly, neither more severe nor more common. Malabsorption with diarrhoea is a major problem; although this is sometimes the result of an opportunistic intestinal infection, the mechanism of villous 'blunting' is unknown—HIV-1 or CMV infections might be important.

Kaposi's sarcoma which seems especially aggressive in Zambia and Uganda, occurs in less than 10% of cases, although regional differences have been demonstrated. It has been recognised for several decades to be common in Africa, especially in young men; however, the AIDS associated tumour (which cannot be differentiated on histological grounds) is markedly more aggressive clinically than that seen hitherto. There is so far no evidence for an increase in incidence rate of B cell non-Hodgkin's lymphoma or Burkitt-like lymphoma as reported in the USA.

Even if an effective treatment for HIV-1 and HIV-2 infections is ultimately forthcoming (*see* p. 191), application of this measure to thousands of infected individuals in Africa would produce impossible logistical problems. Only prevention is likely to have any impact on this major tragedy: educational programmes must be stepped-up. Local traditions however form a major obstacle; thus in rural Zambia it is normal practice when a man dies for one of his male relations to have sexual intercourse with his widow. Methods for eliminating parenteral infection from infected blood, blood transfusions and contaminated needles must be perfected. Travellers to Africa should only receive injections, blood transfusions or surgery when absolutely vital, and all forms of sexual contact with indigenous people must be avoided.

FURTHER READING

Acheson E. D. (1986). AIDS: a challenge for the public health. *Lancet*; **1:** 662–6.
Biggar R. J. (1986). The AIDS problem in Africa. *Lancet*; **1:** 79–83.
Biggar R. J. (1986). The clinical features of HIV infection in Africa. *Brit. Med. J*; **293:** 1453–4.
Colebunders R., Mann J. M., Francis H., *et al.* (1987). Evaluation of a clinical case-definition of acquired immunodeficiency syndrome in Africa. *Lancet*; **1:** 492–4.
Curran J. W., Morgan W. M., Hardy A. M., *et al.* (1985). The epidemiology of AIDS: current status and future prospects. *Science*; **229:** 1352–7.
De Cock K. M. (1984). AIDS: an old disease from Africa? *Brit. Med. J*; **289:** 306–8.
Editorial. (1987). Zidovudine (AZT). *Lancet*; **1:** 957–8.
Farthing C. F., Brown S. E., Staughton R. C. D. (1986). *A Colour Atlas of AIDS: Acquired Immunodeficiency Syndrome*, p. 80. London: Wolfe Medical Publications.
Gillin J. S., Shike M., Alcock N., *et al.* (1985). Malabsorption and mucosal abnormalities of the small intestine in the acquired immunodeficiency syndrome. *Ann. Intern. Med*; **102:** 619–22.
Glasgow B. J., Anders K., Layfield L. J., *et al.* (1985). Clinical and pathologic findings of the liver in the acquired immune deficiency syndrome (AIDS). *Am. J. Clin. Path*; **83:** 582–8.
Guyader M., Emerman M., Sonigo P., *et al.* (1987). Genome organisation and transactivation of the human immunodeficiency virus type 2. *Nature*; **326:** 662–9.
Melbye M. (1986). The natural history of human T lymphotropic virus-III infection: the cause of AIDS. *Brit. Med. J*; **292:** 5–12.
Neequaye A. R., Neequaye J., Mingle J. A., Adjei D. O. (1986). Preponderance of females with AIDS in Ghana. *Lancet* **2:** 978.
Porter R. (1986). History says no to the policeman's response to AIDS. *Brit. Med. J*; **293:** 1589–90.
Quinn T. C., Mann J. M., Curran J. W., Piot P. (1986). AIDS in Africa: an epidemiological paradigm. *Science*; **234:** 955–63.
Vittecoq D., May T., Roue R. T., *et al.* (1987). Acquired immunodeficiency syndrome after travelling in Africa: an epidemiological study in seventeen Caucasian patients. *Lancet*; **1:** 612–15.
Wells N. (1986). *The AIDS Virus: Forecasting its Impact*, p. 60. London: Office of Health Economics.
Wendler I., Schneider J., Gras B., *et al.* (1986). Seroepidemiology of human immunodeficiency virus in Africa. *Brit. Med. J*; **293:** 782–5.
World Health Organization. (1986). Acquired immunodeficiency syndrome (AIDS). WHO/CDC case definition for AIDS. *Wkly. Epidem. Rec*; **61:** 69–73.

Chapter Twelve

Sexually Transmitted Diseases (Excluding AIDS)

This chapter deals with a diverse group of communicable diseases caused by viruses, bacteria, chlamydia, mycoplasma, fungi, protozoa and arthropods. The common feature is that they are all predominantly spread by sexual practices of one form or another. AIDS has been covered in Chapter 11. Some of these diseases are localised largely to tropical countries and are rare in indigenous residents of temperate ones; granuloma inguinale, lymphogranuloma venereum and chancroid are examples. Sexual partners should always be considered infected until laboratory results are shown to be negative.

Historically most emphasis has been placed on syphilis and gonorrhoea; to this list must be added chancroid, lymphogranuloma venereum, and granuloma inguinale, and there are others also. In many countries in the Western World, the incidence of gonorrhoea and non-specific urethritis (NSU) has increased dramatically during the last two decades; this probably also applies to Africa and Asia. Annual notification rates for new cases of those diseases in England and Wales are of the order of 70 000 and over 80 000, respectively. Syphilis is now uncommon in heterosexuals in the UK but remains a major problem in male homosexuals, especially those who are highly promiscuous; about 3000 cases are diagnosed annually. In a world context, WHO estimates indicate that about 50 million new cases of syphilis and 250 million of gonorrhoea occur annually. Unfortunately, however, surveillance methods in most developing countries are often hopelessly inadequate. Genital herpes is common in England and Wales, where several thousand new cases are now diagnosed annually. Overall, the outcome of this group of infections can be extremely serious. Morbidity and diminished productivity are common among men, while infertility, fetal wastage, morbidity and mortality are major problems in women; there is also much neonatal morbidity and mortality.

Table 12.1 summarises some of the organisms which are transmitted during sexual activity. Others, especially in the context of male homosexuality (the 'gay bowel' syndrome), include: CMV and EBV, *Shigella spp.*, *Salmonella spp.*, *Listeria monocytogenes*, *Giardia lamblia*, *Entamoeba histolytica*, *Enterobius vermicularis* and *Strongyloides stercoralis*. This list could be extended to encompass all of the opportunistic infections associated with end-stage AIDS (*see* Chapter 11).

Table 12.2 summarises the distinctive features of some classical sexually transmitted diseases; these manifestations occur at the site of inoculation of the responsible pathogen. Microscopy is essential for a definitive diagnosis: dark-ground microscopy (for *Treponema pallidum*), Gram-smears (for *Haemophilus ducreyi* and *Chlamydia trachomatis*) and scrapings or biopsy material (for *Calymmatobacterium granulomatis*). Genital ulceration may, however, be caused by other agents, including herpes zoster, diphtheria, anthrax, tuberculosis, the eschars of tick and mite-borne typhus, systemic mycoses, amoebiasis and cutaneous leishmaniasis. Behçet's syndrome and various other dermatological conditions should also be considered as differential diagnoses. Aetiological agents involved in NSU include: *Chlamydia trachomatis* and *Trichomonas vaginalis*; Reiter's syndrome should be considered. Causes of vaginal discharge include: *Gardnerella vaginalis*, *Neisseria gonorrhoeae*, *Chlamydia trachomatis*, *Candida albicans* and *Trichomonas vaginalis*. *C. albicans* infections, which are extremely common, especially in warm climates, may be associated with: diabetes mellitus, pregnancy, broad-spectrum antibiotic administration, immunosuppression, oral contraceptive use and hypoparathyroidism. Nystatin, clotrimazole, miconazole and econazole are of value in treatment but long periods of administration may be required. For *Trichomonas vaginalis* infections, metronidazole (400 mg b.d. for 5 days), which should be given simultaneously to both partners, is usually effective.

To date there are few preventive measures apart from the use of a mechanical barrier: the sheath or condom. Male homosexuals constitute one of the high-risk groups for HBV infection (*see* Chapter 6), and should be offered vaccination which gives good protection. Instillation of 1% silver nitrate into the eyes of a newborn infant is essential in the prevention of gonococcal ophthalmia neonatorum (*see* p. 20).

Table 12.1

SOME ORGANISMS WHICH CAN BE TRANSMITTED BY THE SEXUAL ROUTE, AND THE RESULTANT DISEASE

Viruses	
Herpes simplex (type II and type I)	Genital herpes, cervical cancer
Papova	Genital warts
Pox virus (Molluscum contagiosum)	Molluscum contagiosum
HBV*	HB_sAg hepatitis, hepatoma
HIV–1 and HIV–2†	AIDS
Bacteria	
Treponema pallidum	Syphilis
Neisseria gonorrhoeae	Gonorrhoea, ophthalmia neonatorum
Calymmatobacterium granulomatis	Granuloma inguinale
Haemophilus ducreyi	Chancroid
Gardnerella vaginalis	'Non-specific' vaginitis
Chlamydia	
Chlamydia trachomatis	Non-specific urethritis (NSU)
Chlamydia A (L 1, 2, 3 serotypes)	Lymphogranuloma venereum (LGV)
Mycoplasma	
Mycoplasma urealyticum (T-strains)	? Non-specific urethritis
Fungi	
Candida albicans	Vaginal 'thrush', balanitis
Protozoa	
Trichomonas vaginalis	Trichomonal vaginitis, urethritis, balanoposthitis
Arthropods‡	
Sarcoptes scabei	Genital scabies
Phthirus pubis	Pediculosis pubis

* = *See* Chapter 6; † = *See* Chapter 11; ‡ = *See* Chapter 13.

Table 12.2

PRIMARY CUTANEOUS LESIONS OF SOME 'CLASSICAL' SEXUALLY TRANSMITTED DISEASES

Disease	Location of lesion	Description	Associated signs
Syphilis	Genital, anal, lips, tongue, fingers, nipple	Chancre (painless, indurated, rolled margin) (10–90 days after exposure)	Regional lymphadenopathy (non-tender)
Chancroid	Genital	Painful, ragged, undermined margins	Painful lymphadenitis (often suppurative)
Lymphogranuloma venereum	Genital, oral	Inconspicuous, vesicular, evanescent (7–12 days after exposure)	Non-suppurative lymphadenopathy (progressive) (2–6 weeks after infection). Lymphoedema of genitalia, ano-rectal stricture
Granuloma inguinale	Genital, crural, perineal	Elevated, nodular, often extensive ulceration	—

GONORRHOEA

Infection with *Neisseria gonorrhoeae* (an intracellular Gram-negative diplococcus) causes a mucopurulent urethritis in men and endocervicitis in women, and is usually localised to the urogenital tract; asymptomatic infections are common however, and can last for many months. In male homosexuals, proctitis and pharyngitis are common manifestations. Complications include: epididymo-orchitis (often followed by sterility), prostatitis, urethral stricture, bartholinitis, salpingitis, pelvic inflammatory disease (*see* p. 201), perihepatitis (Fitz–Hugh–Curtis syndrome), bacteraemia, an arthritic-dermatitis syndrome, chorioamnionitis, endocarditis and meningitis. When acquired at birth, gonococcal ophthalmia neonatorum and septicaemia are important. Although repeated exposure does not protect against reinfection, recurrences of pelvic inflammatory disease seem less common (*see* p. 202).

Gonorrhoea is extremely common in developing countries; very high infection rates have been recorded in prostitutes in Africa. β-lactamase producing strains, which degrade penicillin (penicillinase-producing *Neisseria gonorrhoeae*, PPNG), are common in Africa and Asia.

Urethritis, which is usually symptomatic, develops within 14 (usually 1–10) days; untreated it usually resolves within 6 months. Table 12.3 summarises some of the differences between the urethral discharge caused by this organism compared with non-gonococcal agents. In women, dysuria rather than a discharge is the usual manifestation; it is thus a cause of 'sterile' pyuria (the 'urethral syndrome') (*see* Chapter 10). In male homosexuals, and occasionally in women, in whom vaginal secretions can infect the anus, a mucopurulent anal discharge, anorectal pruritus, and tenesmus result from infection of the anal crypts. Using a direct

Table 12.3

DIFFERENTIAL FEATURES OF MALE URETHRAL DISCHARGE

Features	Gonococcal	Non-gonococcal
Incubation period (days)	2–7	7–21
Onset	Abrupt	Insidious
Pain	Dysuria	Mild discomfort only
Constancy	Continuous flow	Intermittent drip
Quantity	Copious	Scanty
Consistency	Creamy (purulent)	Thin, mucous
Colour	White, yellow	Clear, green-grey
Gram-smear	Gram-negative diplococci (within leucocytes), many leucocytes	Many leucocytes, normal flora
Other features	May be asymptomatic	Mixed bacterial flora may be present
Complications	Common	Rare

Note: Both gonococcal and non-gonococcal disease may be present concurrently.

Gram-stain on a urethral discharge or early morning urine specimen in men (Gram-negative intracellular diplococci can be visualised in pus cells), or culture of endocervical specimens in women, most cases give positive results. Rectal swabs should be examined in male homosexuals.

Gonococcal bacteraemia can present as fever, tenosynovitis or polyarthritis; painful pustular, haemorrhagic or necrotic skin lesions may develop on the distal extremities. In approximately half, a Gram-stain of the initial lesion, or culture and direct fluorescent antibody reveals the presence of gonococci; blood culture or culture from joint-fluid produces roughly the same yield of positive results.

Treatment of an uncomplicated case (urethritis and cervicitis) should be based on a knowledge of antibiotic sensitivity of the local strains of *N. gonorrhoeae*. The following regimens are usually effective, but in complicated cases should be prolonged:

(i)   Procaine penicillin 2.4 g intramuscularly into each buttock) + 1 g probenecid orally.
(ii) Ampicillin (3·5 g) or amoxycillin (3·0 g) + 1 g probenecid orally.
(iii) Tetracycline (500 mg orally q.d.s. for 5 days).

Where there is a high possibility of *C. trachomatis* being present also, regimen (iii) is preferred. In those areas where PPNG are common, spectinomycin (4 g intramuscularly) and kanamycin are effective, but neither is active against *C. trachomatis* or *Treponema pallidum*. Longer courses using tetracycline + metronidazole, chloramphenicol + tetracycline, or chloramphenicol + sulphafurazole are advisable in the presence of pelvic inflammatory disease (PID); co-trimoxazole and aminoglycosides have been used where PPNG are common.

NON-SPECIFIC URETHRITIS (NSU)

This disease (also known as non-gonococcal urethritis (NGU)) is probably now the most common sexually transmitted disease in the UK. It is less prevalent in some tropical countries, perhaps because *C. trachomatis* is less common; however, in areas where trachoma is endemic, there might be some cross-immunity between the two diseases.

Some clinical differences between NSU and gonorrhoea in men

are summarised in Table 12.3 (p. 199). In women, presentation is usually with an acute 'urethral syndrome' (*see* Chapter 10), or a non-gonococcal mucopurulent cervicitis. The incidence of non-gonococcal cervicitis is probably similar to that of NGU in most parts of the world. Whereas *C. trachomatis* (immunotypes D to K) accounts for the majority of cases, *Ureaplasma urealyticum, Trichomonas vaginalis, Gardnerella vaginalis, Candida albicans,* herpes simplex and mycoplasma can be responsible for others; in approximately one-quarter a cause cannot be found. (Non-infectious NGU can be caused by: excessive ethanol intake, physical stress, 'allergy', frequent changes of sexual partners and local spermicidal agents.) Postgonococcal urethritis is symptomatically and aetiologically similar to NGU; it may begin 2–3 weeks after treatment of gonococcal urethritis with an agent other than tetracycline. This represents, therefore, a urethritis of dual aetiology—*N. gonorrhoeae* and the agent responsible for the NGU. Ascending infection can cause prostatitis, epididymitis and orchitis; sterility and urethral stricture may follow. NGU caused by *C. trachomatis* can produce Reiter's syndrome (especially in those with HLA–B27). Conjunctivitis is a further complication. Diagnosis is by exclusion being dependent on the firm exclusion of a *N. gonorrhoeae* infection. Techniques for the isolation of *C. trachomatis, U. urealyticum* and other causative agents of NGU are not usually available routinely.

Tetracycline (500 mg q.d.s. for 7 days) is highly effective and inexpensive; erythromycin, doxycycline and minocycline have also been used successfully. For a *Gardnerella vaginalis* infection, metronidazole (400 mg b.d. for 7 days) to both partners is usually effective. Approximately 80% are cured by these regimens; the remainder either have persistent symptoms or relapse within 6 weeks of treatment. In this latter group the possibility of a herpes simplex, yeast or *T. vaginalis* infection should be considered. The patient and his or her sexual partner should be treated simultaneously and should abstain from sexual intercourse until the treatment course is completed. Many NGU sufferers with chronic symptoms have a psychogenic overlay.

PELVIC INFLAMMATORY DISEASE (PID)

This disease complex embraces combinations of: salpingitis, oophoritis, pelvic peritonitis and distant intra-abdominal inflam-

Table 12.4

SOME AETIOLOGICAL AGENTS INVOLVED IN PELVIC INFLAMMATORY DISEASE (PID)

	Organism
Sexually transmitted pathogen	*Neisseria gonorrhoeae, Chlamydia trachomatis*
Post-partum, post-abortion sepsis, post-surgery	Coliform bacteria; other enteric or genitourinary flora
Anaerobic infections	*Bacteroides spp., Peptococcus spp., Streptococcus spp.*
Other infective agent	*Haemophilus influenzae* (B), *Streptococcus spp.* (B, D), *Campylobacter spp., Mycoplasma hominis, Ureaplasma urealyticum*
Mycobacterial infections	*Mycobacterium tuberculosis*, atypical mycobacteria
Helminthic infection	*Enterobius vermicularis, Wuchereria bancrofti, Schistosoma haematobium*

mation (most notably, perihepatic adhesions) (*see* p. 202). Table 12.4 summarises some of the aetiological agents. The usual causes are *N. gonorrhoeae* and *C. trachomatis*; anaerobic organisms are present in 20–30% of cases. Clinically, there may be: evidence of genital infection, lower abdominal pain, pelvic tenderness, a palpable adnexal mass, pain on cervical movement and a raised rectal temperature. Infertility, ectopic pregnancy and chronic pelvic pain are long-standing sequelae. Parasitic infections, e.g. schistosomiasis and filariasis, and intrauterine contraceptives may predispose to infection by other organisms. The causative organism should be isolated from the cervix or lower genital tract. As well as examining local swabs, blood should be cultured.

In approximately one-sixth of cases of PID caused by *N. gonorrhoeae* or *C. trachomatis*, the liver capsule becomes inflamed and adhesions form between it and the surrounding peritoneum (the Fitz–Hugh–Curtis syndrome). Signs and symptoms include: fever, right upper quadrant tenderness (especially on percussion) and a friction rub. Although jaundice is rare, serum transaminases are often mildly elevated. As soon as cultures have been obtained, antibiotic treatment should be initiated—ampicillin or metronidazole (a 7–10 day course) is usually effective. Where there is good evidence that *C. trachomatis* is the responsible pathogen, erythromycin should be added.

SYPHILIS

This disease is caused by a spirochaete, *Treponema pallidum* which is about the length of an erythrocyte and cannot be cultured *in vitro*; it requires special staining (silver or immunofluorescent) or dark-ground illumination for it to become visible. The population of Europe was probably first exposed to this disease (the 'great pox') in the late 15th century; contemporary accounts suggest that it was significantly more virulent than it is today. Whether it was introduced to Europe by Columbus' crew after their explorations of south America, or whether it resulted from a new mutation will remain forever conjectural. Since the introduction of penicillin the incidence of the disease has steadily declined in temperate areas of the world; however, it is still very common in many countries of the 'Third World', especially in urban areas. At the *primary* infection, the spirochaete *Treponema pallidum* penetrates either intact mucous membranes or traumatised skin; systemic dissemination results after its entry to subcutaneous blood vessels and lymphatics. After an incubation period of 10–90 days a *chancre* appears at the site of infection; this consists of a small papule which erodes with the production of a shallow, painless punched-out ulcer (up to 3 cm diameter) with indurated margins (the 'hard chancre')—the serous exudate from the granulomatous base contains many spirochaetes. The regional lymph glands are enlarged, firm and painless. Healing takes place within 3–6 weeks. Multiple chancres may result from autoinoculation. Extragenital ones, which are rare, are painful in contrast to those involving the external genitalia.

The *secondary* disease begins from 3 weeks to 4 months after the primary chancre heals. Most commonly, a generalised painless, non-pruritic skin rash appears which may be macular, papular (often maculopapular), follicular, papulosquamous, or pustular; in most it is prominent on the face and thorax, often involving the palms and soles. Most rashes heal within a few weeks without scar formation, but many relapse. As part of a systemic illness, fever with constitutional symptoms, non-tender lymphadenopathy, splenomegaly, hepatitis, meningitis, arthritis, nephrosis, periostitis, iridocyclitis and anterior uveitis may be present.

Tertiary syphilis is a term used to embrace the chronic manifestations which occur after a latent period (3 to 30 years or more) following the secondary disease. Manifestations at this stage may be: cardiovascular (aortic aneurysmal dilatation, aortic insufficiency or coronary ostial stenosis), meningovascular (an obliterative endarteritis), parenchymatous (tabes dorsalis—posterior spinal cord involvement) or gummatous (lesions resembling tuberculomas that can affect any organ). Charcot's joints, Argyll–Robertson pupils and 'general paralysis of the insane' (GPI) are some of the other neurological consequences; the order of frequency of cardiovascular and gummatous lesions, and neurosyphilis is about 80, 10 and 10%, respectively. All of these forms of the disease are much less common than before the antibiotic era.

Congenital syphilis, which can occur at any time during gestation can result in still-birth; alternatively the fetus may subsequently develop a wide variety of anatomical defects, including interstitial keratitis, dental abnormalities and eighth-nerve deafness.

Diagnostically, syphilis can mimic many diseases; frequently another sexually transmitted disease is present concurrently. *T. pallidum* can be visualised by dark-ground microscopy in lesions at all stages of the disease; other spirochaetes must always be excluded. Serological tests are of value in supporting the diagnosis. The Venereal Disease Research Laboratory (VDRL) cardiolipin antigen test, which does not use *T. pallidum* antigen, is of value in screening for syphilis and for assessing activity, but false positive results can occur in many unrelated diseases, including pneumonia, malaria and leprosy. Treponemal antigen tests are more sensitive and specific. In the *T. pallidum* immobilisation (TPI) test (now rarely used except in reference centres), motile *T. pallidum* is immobilised by antibody *in vitro*. The *T. pallidum* haemagglutination assay (TPHA) utilises antigen absorbed to erythrocytes. The fluorescent treponemal antibody (FTA) test uses lyophilised antigen in an indirect fluorescent antibody technique. Yaws and pinta give similar serological results to those of syphilis. A mild polymorphonuclear leucocytosis, raised ESR, serum globulin and transaminases, and a positive test for rheumatoid factor are common findings. Cerebrospinal fluid abnormalities include: increased total protein, mild mononuclear cell pleocytosis and positive serological tests.

Provided there is no evidence of penicillin 'allergy', this (preferably one of the longer-acting preparations) is the antibiotic of choice. For early, latent, and tertiary disease, intramuscular regimens of 10 mg/kg body-weight procaine penicillin for 10, 15 and 20 days, respectively, are usually adequate. Following the initial injection, a *Jarisch–Herxheimer* reaction beginning 6–12 h after the penicillin injection is common; this febrile episode is a result of release of endotoxin from *T. pallidum*. Cutaneous lesions heal rapidly; spirochaetes disappear from them within 48 h. However, in neurovascular and congenital syphilis, prolonged or repeated courses may be necessary to eliminate all viable spirochaetes. Most seropositive individuals with primary and secondary disease become seronegative by 6–12 months after treatment; those with latent or tertiary disease may still be seropositive after 2 years, but this does not usually indicate treatment failure. Because the standard treatment regimens for syphilis do not produce adequate serum penicillin concentrations to cure gonorrhoea, appropriate chemotherapy for this disease should also be given.

Other spirochaetal diseases include yaws, endemic syphilis and pinta; in the main these are not spread by sexual intercourse and are covered in Chapter 15.

GENITAL HERPES

Genital herpes is usually caused by *Herpes simplex* type II virus, although the type I virus (which is usually responsible for herpes labialis) is occasionally responsible. The virus probably lies dormant in peripheral nerve fibres supplying the affected mucocutaneous site. Herpetic lesions consist of vesicles which break down to form shallow painful ulcers, often becoming secondarily infected; they occur after an incubation period of 3–7 days. The primary infection may be accompanied by a mild febrile illness with malaise, and is usually more severe in women than men. Recurrent crops of vesicles, often preceded by local irritation for a day or two, may appear on any part of the penis or vulva; if the urethra is affected, dysuria can be troublesome. Recurrent cervicitis may be present, as a symptomless infection, but severe ulcers may be present on the cervix. The disease must be differentiated from primary syphilis (which may occur concurrently). Complications include:

(i) Aseptic meningitis or encephalitis.
(ii) Hepatitis.
(iii) Neonatal herpes encephalitis or disseminated herpes, which carries a high mortality rate; when the mother is infected near the time of delivery, caesarian section should be carried out.
(iv) Cervical carcinoma.

The *Herpes simplex* virus can be isolated from vesicular fluid; dark-ground microscopy and syphilis serology (which should be repeated 3 months later) is advisable. Provided secondary infection does not occur the lesions heal spontaneously in 8–15 days. In severe cases antiviral therapy is advisable: idoxuridine in 5% dimethyl-sulphoxide. In the presence of systemic symptoms, a parenteral anti-herpes agent, e.g. acycloguanosine, is indicated.

OTHER CAUSES OF SEXUALLY TRANSMITTED DISEASE (STD)

Chancroid

Sometimes designated 'soft chancre', this is an acute, painful, ulcerative disease usually localised to the anogenital region (extragenital lesions can occur by autoinoculation), which is caused by the bacterium *Haemophilus ducreyi*; it may be accompanied by local necrosis and destruction of anogenital tissues, and inguinal buboes. *H. ducreyi* is a short, non-motile, Gram-negative rod with a characteristic strepto-bacillary 'chaining' appearance; it is a facultative anaerobe. Using special culture techniques, 20 to 60% of cases give positive results. The bacillus is autoinoculable and can penetrate the intact dermis. Contaminants and opportunistic pathogens readily invade chancroid ulcers. It is very common in Africa and Asia but occurs worldwide. The florid disease is more common in men than women; asymptomatic prostitutes probably constitute an important reservoir of infection. Other STD infections are often present simultaneously. The incubation period is 2–14 days; an inflammatory papule rapidly erodes with the formation of a painful, non-indurated irregular ulcer(s) with slightly undermined edges; the base is granular and covered with a yellow-grey purulent exudate which bleeds easily (it is unlike the 'hard chancre' of syphilis). Inguinal lymphadenitis develops in about 50% of cases, and is occasionally the initial clinical manifestation. Bacteraemia and systemic complications are rare events. A systemic febrile illness often accompanies infected buboes. Extreme forms of genital mutilation, including penile amputation can result in the untreated disease. There is no immunity to reinfection. Diagnosis depends on identification or isolation of *H. ducreyi* (*see* p. 196). Differentiation from genital herpes, primary and secondary syphilis, lymphogranuloma venereum, and granuloma inguinale (*see* p. 208) is important. Treatment is with co-trimoxazole (ii tab b.d. for 7–10 days) or erythromycin (500 mg q.d.s. for 10 days). Tetracycline also is usually effective. If fluctuant, buboes should be aspirated.

Lymphogranuloma Venereum (LGV)

LGV (tropical bubo, lymphopathia venereum, Nicolas–Favre disease, lymphogranuloma inguinale) is widespread in many tropical countries as well as being sporadic in north America and Europe. Women serve as the reservoir of infection for periods up to several months; they often develop an asymptomatic endocervicitis. It can coexist with other sexually transmitted diseases; extragenital transmission is rare. This is a disease of lymphatic and anogenital tissues and is caused by *Chlamydia trachomatis*—types 1, 2 and 3. An initial (primary) stage, which follows an incubation period of 7–21 days, in which a papule, herpetiform lesion, erosion or endocervicitis appears at the site of infection, often goes unnoticed. After 2–6 weeks, an acute inguinal lymphadenitis, leading to bubo formation or a haemorrhagic proctocolitis, constitutes the secondary stage. If the disease is not treated, tertiary lesions (locally destructive chronic ulcerations, fistulae, abscesses, genital elephantiasis, and stricture) may appear over several years. The disease is now usually treated in the early stages, and the 'tertiary' lesions are unusual. In the 19th century, these three stages of the disease were considered to represent variants of the lesions of syphilis.

Clinical presentation usually occurs in the secondary stage (inguinal buboes in men, and a haemorrhagic proctocolitis in women and male homosexuals); therefore, late complications (rectal stricture, rectovaginal fistula and genital elephantiasis) are more common in women. This stage is often accompanied by systemic symptoms: fever, headache, myalgia and anorexia. A follicular conjunctivitis can occur at any stage by autoinoculation of infected secretions into the conjunctivae. Other diagnoses which should be considered include: other sexually transmitted diseases, Hodgkin's disease, an incarcerated inguinal hernia, acute amoebic dysentery, ulcerative proctocolitis and Crohn's disease. Because culture techniques are often not readily available, diagnosis is frequently based on the clinical presentation in the presence of positive serological (complement fixation) tests. A definitive diagnosis can only be made however by isolating LGV chlamydia from infected tissues or buboes. The CF test is usually strongly positive in the acute phase of the disease; a more specific serological test (IFAT) is not performed routinely. The Frei test lacks sensitivity and is now rarely used. Biopsy histology is non-specific; however, smears from infected secretions or tissue may reveal intracytoplasmic inclusion bodies when stained with fluorescein-labelled chlamydial antibody.

Treatment is with antibiotics: tetracyclines (500 mg q.d.s. for 2–4 weeks), sulphonamides (1 g q.d.s. for 4 weeks), erythromycin (500 mg q.d.s. for 2–4 weeks), chloramphenicol and rifampicin have all been used. Because the disease frequently heals spontaneously, it is difficult to evaluate accurately a response; antibiotics certainly diminish secondary infection. When buboes are fluctuant they should be aspirated. Late complications require plastic surgery after prolonged antibiotic therapy.

Granuloma Inguinale

Granuloma inguinale (donovanosis, lymphogranuloma inguinale) is a chronic granulomatous disease which primarily affects the anogenital region, and is caused by the Gram-negative, non-motile, pleomorphic bacillus *Calymmatobacterium granulomatis* present within the cytoplasm of large mononuclear phagocytes; it is antigenically related to certain species of *Klebsiella*. Limited to the skin and subcutaneous tissues it is autoinoculable. Although it occurs worldwide, peak incidence rates are mostly in tropical areas—especially Africa, Asia, central and southern America, and Papua New Guinea; there might be an ethnic and/or genetic predisposition. The organism is inoculated into skin lesions during sexual intercourse; it can also be isolated from faecal samples.

Incubation period is from a few days to 3 months. The initial lesion is a small painless papule which erodes to form an indurated, slightly elevated ulcer; as it enlarges, the ulcer base becomes granular, red and bleeds easily. Ulcers extend to several centimetres in diameter, spreading subcutaneously into the groin and/or perineum. Secondary infection is common. Because patients often wait for months or years before seeking treatment, secondary infection and destruction of genital tissue has frequently occurred before presentation. Differential diagnoses include: squamous cell carcinoma, syphilis, cutaneous amoebiasis, lymphogranuloma venereum and chancroid.

Complications are: local lymphatic obstruction (with genital elephantiasis in a severe case), fistula formation, bacteraemia and genital destruction; a causative association with squamous cell carcinoma also seems likely. Diagnosis depends on detection of organisms in a biopsy specimen or scraping from the margin of an active lesion; tissue sections should be stained by silver impregnation. In a chronic lesion, repeated examinations may be necessary. Streptomycin, tetracycline, rifampicin, chloramphenicol and co-trimoxazole can all be effective in treatment; however, in Papua New Guinea, where the disease is common, the first two of those agents seem relatively ineffective. Co-trimoxazole (ii tab b.d. for 14 days), and chloramphenicol (500 mg q.d.s. for 10–14 days) are probably most reliable. Surgery may be necessary to close fistulae.

FURTHER READING

Britigan B. E., Cohen M. S., Sparling P. F. (1985). Gonococcal infection: a model of molecular pathogenesis. *N. Engl. J. Med*; **312**: 1683–94.

Editorial. (1980). Genital herpes. *Brit. Med. J*; **280**: 1335–6.

Editorial. (1981). Recalcitrant gonococci, plasmids, and antibiotics. *Lancet*; **1**: 816–17.

Nsanze H., Fast M. V., D'Costa L. J., et al. (1981). Genital ulcers in Kenya: clinical and laboratory study. *Brit. J. Vener. Dis*; **57**: 378–81.

Ridgway G. L. (1986). Human chlamydial infection. In *Advanced Medicine*, Vol. 22, pp. 187–92. (Triger D. R., ed.). London: Baillière Tindall.

Sobel J. D. (1986). Recurrent vulvovaginal candidiasis: A prospective study of the efficacy of maintenance ketoconazole therapy. *N. Engl. J. Med*; **315**: 1455–8.

Thornton J. G. (1984). Fitz–Hugh–Curtis syndrome in Kenya. *Brit. Med. J*; **289**: 470.

Weller I. V. D. (1985). The gay bowel. *Gut*; **26**: 869–75.

Wisdom A. (1973). *A Colour Atlas of Venereology*, p. 352. London: Wolfe Medical Publications.

World Health Organization. (1982). *Treponemal Infections*, p. 75. Technical Report Series No. 674. Geneva: WHO.

Chapter Thirteen

Skin Infections

The skin shares, with the gastrointestinal and respiratory tracts, the role of a major portal of entry for infective organisms present in the environment. Also, very many communicable diseases are accompanied by dermatological manifestations; in a developing country, where sophisticated methods of investigation are sparse, diagnostic clues are frequently obtainable from an adequate dermatological examination—however, skin colour, and the presence of underlying malnutrition and humidity can account for marked differences compared with those in a temperate setting. A careful history with regard to travel and tropical exposure is potentially of great importance. An accurate description of the earliest lesion(s) and the precise distribution of the rash is also essential; associated symptoms should be sought. Good daylight is necessary for an adequate clinical examination, and the use of a magnifying glass is frequently rewarding. In this chapter, therefore, many of the diseases covered are basically generalised or systemic, but a major feature is the skin manifestation.

Human skin harbours two types of flora—(a) resident (*Staphylococcus epidermidis*, micrococci and diphtheroids predominate), and (b) transient. The latter group, the presence of which is determined by several factors, e.g. (i) cleaning and washing, (ii) abrasions, cuts, and bites, (iii) ambient humidity, (iv) skin fatty acids, and (v) antimicrobial substances produced by the resident flora, accounts for many of the diseases mentioned in this chapter. *Staphylococcus aureus* is carried in the anterior nares especially by a minority of individuals; the carrier state is considerably higher in hospital staff than others. Repeated use of antiseptics (e.g. hexachlorophane and chlorhexidine) on affected skin, and hair shampoos, together with frequent laundering of bed clothes and underwear are necessary in carriers possessing an 'epidemic' strain. Occasionally affected hospital staff have to cease work temporarily until they are cleared of infection.

Table 13.1 summarises the dominant lesions in some rashes. A *macule* is a circumscribed area of abnormal skin which is not raised above the surface of its surroundings. A *papule* consists of a small nodular elevation, a *vesicle* a small 'blister' containing clear fluid, and a *pustule* a small elevation containing pus. *Erythema* (which blanches on pressure) may be localised or generalised; an erythematous patch with a pale centre and an intensely red margin is described as *circinate*. *Erythema nodosum* consists of tender and raised circular or oval areas, usually on the anterior tibial borders of the legs; they undergo a colour change from red to bluish-purple over the course of a few days. Acute rheumatic fever, β-haemolytic streptococcal infection, tuberculosis and sarcoidosis are common causes, although this condition may also result from drug sensitivity. Petechiae and ecchymoses are haemorrhagic manifestations, the former much smaller than the latter. Many causes of ulcer with an infective origin exist. In sickle cell (SS) disease, ulcers usually occur around the ankles; they should be differentiated from tropical phagedenic and Buruli ulcers. Pyogenic ulceration can follow pyoderma gangrenosum, a complication of non-specific ulcerative colitis.

Postinflammatory hyper- or hypopigmentation results from many acute communicable diseases; in developing countries, depigmentation associated with malnutrition, especially Kwashiorkor, should be differentiated. In pellagra, the fully developed lesions are hyperpigmented, scaly and localised to the exposed parts; there may be a characteristic 'Casal's necklace'.

VIRAL INFECTIONS

Dermatological manifestations of the viral diseases of childhood are described in Chapter 2; measles, rubella and chickenpox all have their characteristic rashes. A primary herpes simplex infection may occur in childhood presenting with painful vesicular stomatitis, fever and lymphadenopathy which usually resolves spontaneously within 7–14 days. The virus then lies latent, often for many years, and reactivation produces a transient vesicular (sometimes pustular) rash usually around the lips (herpes labialis); this often occurs in the presence of pneumococcal lobar pneumonia, acute *Plasmodium falciparum* malaria, and other infections where there is relative immunosuppression. Herpetic infections may also involve the genitalia (*see* Chapter 12). Viral

Table 13.1

SOME DERMATOLOGICAL MANIFESTATIONS OF INFECTIOUS
DISEASE—CLASSIFIED BY THE BASIC LESION

Macular
  Several rickettsial infections
  Leprosy
  Pinta
  Tinea versicolor
  Onchocerciasis

Papular
  Chickenpox
  Secondary syphilis
  Leprosy
  Cutaneous larva migrans
  Larva currens
  Onchocerciasis
  Scabies
  Flea bites
  Tungiasis
  Myiasis
  Kaposi's sarcoma (AIDS)

Maculopapular
  Measles
  Many rickettsial infections

Vesicular
  Chickenpox
  Monkeypox
  Herpes simplex
  Herpes zoster

Pustules
  Herpes simplex
  Herpes zoster
  Pyoderma
  Paracoccidioidomycosis

Crust (scab)
  Impetigo
  Tick typhus
  African trypanosomiasis (late chancre)

continued

Nodules
  Yaws
  Leprosy
  Chromomycosis
  Sporotrichosis
  Maduromycosis
  Paracoccidioidomycosis
  Myiasis
  Kaposi's sarcoma (AIDS)

Circinate erythema
  Erythema multiforme
  African trypanosomiasis

Ulcers
  Tropical ulcer
  Cancrum oris
  Primary syphilis
  Leprosy
  Buruli ulcer
  Sporotrichosis
  Leishmaniasis

Urticaria/wheal
  'Allergies'
  Acute schistosomiasis (Katayama fever)

Petechiae/ecchymosis
  Viral haemorrhagic fevers
  Meningococcal bacteraemia

culture, a rise in anti-herpes simplex antibodies, or demonstration of balloon and giant cells in the base of a vesicle can be confirmatory. Acyclovir and vidarabine are of value, especially in disseminated disease. Some cases of erythema multiforme are associated with herpes simplex infection; however, sulphonamides can also be incriminated and the aetiology is often unclear. Diagnosis is confirmed by skin biopsy. *Herpes zoster* causes a painful eruption, which later becomes pustular, along the distribution of a sensory nerve; this may be a branch of the fifth cranial nerve or a nerve supplying one of the thoracic dermatomes. The lesions are usually unilateral and cross the midline by only 1–2 cm; they resolve in 7–14 days, but pain after healing may be severe. The same virus as that causing varicella is responsible; it remains latent in ganglia following this disease. Diagnosis is similar to that for *Herpes simplex* infection. Analgesics are usually required in addition to local treatment.

A generalised maculopapular rash is a frequent feature of an EBV infection; the incidence rate increases to about 60% if such patients are given ampicillin. Generalised maculopapular rashes occur in many other systemic viral infections, e.g. Echo and Coxsackie infections, West Nile, Chikungunya and O'nyong nyong fever, etc. In the viral haemorrhagic fevers (*see* Chapter 15), petechiae and ecchymoses of varying size, together with diffuse oozing, are classical manifestations. Dengue haemorrhagic fever may also be complicated by petechiae and ecchymoses, and other spontaneous haemorrhages are common, especially in children. In monkeypox (which is confined to central and west Africa) a generalised vesicular rash (identical with that formerly caused by smallpox) is accompanied by lymphadenopathy (*see* Chapter 15). In tanapox (which is confined to Kenya and Zaire), papulovesicular lesions are characteristic.

A maculopapular rash is present in about 5% of patients with an acute HBV infection; in chronic infection, cutaneous stigmata of chronic hepatocellular disease, including spider naevi (only rarely apparent in brown and black skins) and palmar erythema, are valuable diagnostic signs. In the acquired immune deficiency syndrome (AIDS) (*see* Chapter 11), the major dermatological manifestation is Kaposi's sarcoma. The lesions consist of multiple vascular papules, nodules or plaques which vary in colour from purple to dark blue; there is usually associated oedema of the affected extremity. Diagnosis is confirmed by skin biopsy.

RICKETTSIAL INFECTIONS

This large group of infections includes: murine, and epidemic typhus, Brill–Zinsser disease, Rocky Mountain spotted fever, tick typhus and rickettsialpox, scrub typhus, *Coxiella burnetii* (Q fever), and trench fever (*see* Chapter 15). African tick typhus (especially common in east and southern Africa) is perhaps the best known example and is caused by *Rickettsia conorii*. It is characterised by an *eschar* at the site of infection. This lesion starts as a papule which breaks down with the formation of an ulcer with a black base approximately 2–5 mm in diameter. Regional lymphadenopathy is usual. A generalised maculopapular rash later becoming haemorrhagic, is common. This appears on about the fourth day and rapidly becomes generalised. In the clinical differential diagnosis, measles and meningococcal infections should be considered. An eschar is frequently also present in scrub typhus (Tsutsugamushi fever) and rickettsialpox. In most of the rickettsial diseases a generalised macular or maculopapular rash is a prominent feature; in some there is a petechial or more florid haemorrhagic rash, and in rickettsialpox a vesicular element also. These rashes if untreated last for up to 2 weeks, and rarely longer.

BACTERIAL INFECTIONS

Pyoderma consists of a skin infection caused by *Streptococcus pyogenes* (Group A β-haemolytic streptococci), *Staphylococcus aureus*, or a mixed flora of micro-organisms, together with additional pathogens. Malnutrition and inadequate hygienic standards are important predisposing factors. Impetigo is a term used for the presence of small pustules or vesicles evolving into yellow crusts which heal without scar formation; in young children there may be a bullous component—'bullous impetigo'. A deep skin infection presenting as ulceration and a brown haemorrhagic covering, usually on the legs, is called *ecthyma*; as healing takes place scarring occurs. Pustule formation within hair follicles is termed a *folliculitis*; when an abscess forms this is called a *furuncle* and an aggregation of these lesions is referred to as a *carbuncle*. Erysipelas consists of a skin infection (often on the face or leg) caused by the sudden appearance of an erythematous 'plaque' which enlarges peripherally, and which often has small vesicle formation at the advancing edges; this is accompanied by a systemic febrile illness. Recurrent attacks of erysipelas can produce lymphatic obstruction and lymphoedema. All forms of pyoderma should be treated by local cleansing of the skin with soap, removal of crusts, and systemic antibiotics; either penicillin or a semisynthetic penicillin in full dose should be given for 10–14 days.

A mixed bacterial infection with *Bacillus fusiformis* and *Treponema vincenti* causes tropical (phagedenic) ulcers. These are painful, rapidly enlarging ulcers, usually situated on the legs; they are especially common in malnourished children. After an initial trauma the ulcer, which is well-defined with elevated borders, rapidly expands during some 1–2 weeks. Fibrosis occurs later, and healing takes several years; squamous cell carcinoma is a late complication. Local treatment, nutritional supplements, and systemic antibiotics are all important; plastic surgery may be necessary later. A condition with a similar aetiology—*cancrum oris*—occurs on the face of malnourished children; they frequently have other infections in addition; gross tissue destruction can occur. Cutaneous signs of bacteraemia, especially that caused by the meningococcus (a haemorrhagic rash preceded by macules or papules) and septicaemia, are covered in Chapters 9 and 15. In typhoid and paratyphoid fevers, septicaemic ('rose') spots may be present over the trunk. Signs associated with rheumatic fever (erythema nodosum and erythema marginatum) and bacterial endocarditis (splinter haemorrhages) are summarised in Chapter 8.

Dermatological manifestations of bacterial childhood infections—the cutaneous form of diphtheria and 'scarlet fever' are covered in Chapter 2. Pustules may be a feature of plague; petechial haemorrhages also occur. Localised suppurating granulomatous lesions with sinus formation, especially in the cervicofacial region, are a feature of actinomycosis; pus contains sulphur granules. In cutaneous anthrax ('malignant pustule'), irregular epidermal ulceration and coagulation necrosis is present; there may be a fibrinopurulent membrane) and haemorrhage into the dermis may occur. Penicillin and tetracycline are effective chemotherapeutic agents.

The dermatological lesions of primary and secondary syphilis are summarised in Chapter 12. A chancre is an indurated, painless, oval or circular ulcer with a well-defined border and a clean base; regional lymphadenopathy is present. The basic lesion in the secondary disease is a firm, slightly elevated papule which varies in colour from pink to reddish-brown or copper. Macular lesions, hair loss, erythematous patches on the mucus membranes, fever and generalised lymphadenopathy are common. Skin lesions in other bacterial sexually-transmitted diseases are also summarised in Chapter 12.

Endemic, non-venereal treponematosis (pinta) which is caused by *Treponema carateum*, produces depigmented patches (up to 20 cm or more) at a late stage; these evolve from small scaly papules. Organisms in these spirochaetal diseases can be demonstrated by dark-ground microscopy; serological tests are also positive. In yaws, one of several skin lesions may be present. The initial papule gives rise to the 'mother yaw', a raised raspberry-like lesion (which marks the portal of entry); this is usually acquired by direct contact with a similar lesion at the site of a recent abrasion or laceration. Secondary papillomas follow. In the tertiary disease, chronic ulceration of the extremities and face produces gross mutilation. *T. pertenue* is demonstrated by dark-ground microscopy. Treatment is with benzylpenicillin.

The skin manifestations of tuberculosis (both *M. tuberculosis* and atypical mycobacteria) are summarised in Chapter 3. *M. ulcerans* causes Buruli ulcers in Uganda and Zaire; these usually occur on the legs, and begin as nodules which break down to form large necrotic ulcers; these lesions are painless and there is no regional lymphadenopathy. The causative organisms can be demonstrated in a skin biopsy or culture.

Leprosy (Chapter 14) which is caused by *Mycobacterium leprae* produces depigmented lesions in addition to peripheral nerve involvement. The initial lesions may occur at any site, but are especially common on the buttocks, neck, trunk and extremities; they consist of well-defined, hypopigmented macules which may be mildly erythematous. Loss of pain and temperature sensation, and anhydrosis are usual. Skin biopsy reveals a perineural infiltrate with lymphocytes and mononuclear cells, and a peripheral nerve biopsy often shows *M. leprae* (especially in lepromatous disease); several examinations may be required for a positive diagnosis. Papular lesions can develop in all except the indeterminate stage, and may evolve into hypopigmented, dry, anaesthetic well-defined plaques, or in tuberculoid disease an annular lesion. In lepromatous disease, papules, plaques and nodules (containing histiocytes laden with numerous bacteria) may all be present; these are less well-defined and symmetrical. A generalised febrile reaction with iritis, hepatitis, arthritis and orchitis, and accompanied by tender erythematous nodules (*erythema nodosum leprosum*), may occur in patients at the lepromatous end of the disease spectrum. Later, trophic ulcers resulting from local trauma are common; these are usually on the hands and feet and are often secondarily infected.

FUNGAL INFECTIONS

There are many dermatophytic fungi; ringworm and tinea are two examples and they are caused by *Microsporum spp.* and *Trichophyton spp.* respectively.

Tinea imbricata (caused by *T. concentricum*) is an extreme example of a generalised superficial mycosis. Tinea versicolor (caused by *Pityrosporum orbiculare*) is characterised by asymptomatic, well-defined, scaly macules of variable colour, most being depigmented, and especially marked in a brown or black skin; in some parts of the humid tropics, the majority of the population is affected. These lesions may coalesce to form extensive depigmented areas, especially on the trunk, axillae and groins. Skin 'scrapes' reveal spores and hyphae. Treatment is with antifungal cream: Whitfield's ointment, selenium sulphide, clotrimazole or tolnaftate. The lesions are often very resistant to treatment, but pigmentation ultimately recovers. *Tinea unguium* is the usual cause of ringworm of the nails. *T. pedis* causes athlete's foot, and *T. capitis* scalp ringworm. *Trichophyton rubrum* and *Epidermophyton floccosum* cause tinea in the intertriginous regions in men.

Chromomycosis, a fungal infection acquired by agricultural workers, usually affects the legs and causes chronic granulomatous disease of the skin and mucous membranes. Spores usually enter open wounds; an erythematous nodule develops, subsequently ulcerates, and is followed by scaling and crusting. The affected extremity may become swollen and elephantoid. Diagnosis is by detection of spores or fungi in a skin biopsy specimen. Surgical removal and/or systemic antifungal agents are necessary.

A chronic granulomatous fungal disease which also involves the lymphatics and which is present worldwide affecting agricultural workers and gardeners, is caused by *Sporotrichum schenckii*. An erythematous nodule, which subsequently ulcerates occurs usually on the limbs but sometimes the face or trunk; further lesions appear along the course of the regional lymphatics. Bones and lungs are rarely affected. Skin biopsy or fungal culture reveals characteristic spores. Potassium iodide given orally is the standard treatment.

Maduromycosis or mycetoma (Madura foot) is caused by *Madurella*, *Allescheria* and *Cephalosporium*, and is a further chronic granulomatous fungal disease of skin; however, underlying bone is also involved. It is common in the Indian subcontinent and also in other tropical countries. The foot is most commonly affected.

Nodules, abscesses, sinuses, scarring and other deformities result; secondary infection may produce a periostitis and/or osteomyelitis. The responsible organism can be demonstrated in the pustular exudate, skin biopsy or fungal culture; radiography reveals bone destruction. Chemotherapeutic agents are of only very limited value; the only successful treatment is amputation.

Paracoccidioidomycosis consists of skin, mucous membrane and other organ infection by *Paracoccidioides brasiliensis*; it is endemic in southern America. The mouth is the probable portal of entry. Skin lesions are usually on the face and scalp, consisting of papules, nodules, ulcers, crusts and abscesses with multiple haemorrhagic puncta. Diagnosis is by skin biopsy or culture; chest radiography is abnormal. Long-acting sulphonamides and amphotericin B are effective. Some other deep mycoses (*see* Chapter 15), e.g. blastomycosis, can also produce dermatological lesions.

PROTOZOAN INFECTIONS

Various protozoa of the genus *Leishmania* cause chronic granulomatous skin disease. Cutaneous leishmaniasis ('Oriental sore') is predominantly a disease of Africa, the Middle-east and the Mediterranean littoral; the mucocutaneous variety ('Espundia') occurs in south and central America. Lesions are most commonly on the exposed surfaces—face, arms and legs, and follow sandfly bites. They evolve from a papule to an ulcerated nodule. Most 'Old World' lesions heal spontaneously in about 1 year; however, in the 'New World' varieties, mucous membranes are also affected and extensive destruction of the nose and mouth may result.

'Old World' disease is caused by *Leishmania tropica*, *L. major* and *L. aethiopia*; the reservoir of infection consists of desert rodents and the disease is transmitted by *Phlebotomus* sandflies. Fig. 13.1 shows the approximate distribution of the disease. The incubation period is 2–8 weeks, but may be longer. The lesions have raised edges, and the centre is mildly sunken. The spectrum of disease is comparable to that of leprosy; it varies from a non-healing infection, to a form with an exaggerated hypersensitivity reaction. A chronic form (*leishmaniasis recidivans*) occasionally occurs in Iran and Iraq, while an uncommon manifestation in Ethiopia and Kenya is *diffuse cutaneous leishmaniasis*. Organisms can usually be detected in the margins of the lesions. Serological tests often

220 *Communicable and Tropical Diseases*

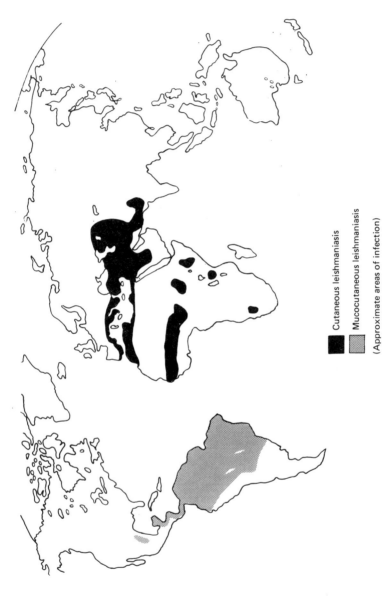

Fig. 13.1. Approximate world distribution of cutaneous and mucocutaneous leishmaniasis.

give negative results; however, a leishmanin skin test is usually positive some 3 months after infection and remains positive for life. The disease is self-limiting in 12 to 18 months but can be severely disfiguring especially when lesions occur on the face. Treatment is with pentavalent antimony compounds. Paromomycin cream is of value. Immunotherapy using BCG has also proved successful in limited studies. Vaccination, using cultured live virulent promastigotes has been used successfully.

In the 'New World' variety, there is also a wide spectrum of disease; the responsible organisms are *L. brasiliensis* and *L. mexicana* but there is considerable conjecture concerning species differentiation. Lesions occur at mucocutaneous junctions. Diagnosis is by demonstrating organisms in the skin lesions. Serological tests are often negative; a leishmanin skin test is usually positive by several months after infection. Treatment is with pentavalent antimony compounds, but relapse is common; amphotericin B has been used successfully.

A form of cutaneous leishmaniasis can be produced by *L. donovani*, the causative organism in Kala-azar (*see* Chapter 15), and the closely related species *L. infantum* (around the Mediterranean littoral); lesions tend to ulcerate rapidly. Cutaneous leishmaniasis sometimes has a very long latent period; the longest the author has experienced is 39 years in a 71-year-old man with compromised immunity who had a newly developed lesion presumed to have resulted from infection in Malta. Post Kala-azar, and disseminated anergic leishmaniasis are other dermatological forms of this disease (*see* Chapter 15); the organisms can be demonstrated in smears, skin biopsy or culture.

African trypanosomiasis usually presents as a febrile illness, sometimes with neurological complications (*see* Chapter 9); careful examination frequently reveals a trypanosomal 'chancre', a painful reddish indurated papule at the site of the tsetse fly bite; this breaks down to a small ulcer during the course of 5–15 days.

Entamoeba histolytica occasionally produces extensive cutaneous ulceration, usually around the anal region and buttocks.

HELMINTHIC INFECTIONS

Intestinal nematodes occasionally produce dermatological lesions. *Larva migrans* ('creeping eruption'), caused by dog hookworms

(*Ankylostoma caninum, A. braziliense* and *Ucinaria stenocephala*) usually produces lesions on the feet. The infection is acquired by walking barefoot on ground (frequently beaches) contaminated by dog faeces; it seems especially common in the Caribbean. Following skin penetration, a pruritic, serpiginous, slightly elevated subcutaneous cord (several centimetres in length) appears; this later becomes erythematous and advances at a rate of up to 5 cm daily. Oral thiabendazole is the most effective chemotherapeutic agent, although topical application of either this agent, piperazine ointment, or ethyl chloride spray meet with some success. *Larva currens*, which usually involves the lower abdomen and buttocks occurs during the migratory phase of a *Strongyloides stercoralis* infection; the lesions, which are raised and linear or serpiginous with an urticarial element, can recur intermittently for many years. Autoinfection produces a typical type I sensitivity reaction. Some former prisoners-of-war in south-east Asia during World War II (1939–1945) are still infected.

Onchocerciasis (*see* Chapter 15), which is caused by the nematode *Onchocerca volvulus* affects the skin, subcutaneous tissue and eyes. After an incubation of about 1 year following the bite of the black-fly, *Simulium*, cutaneous lesions (usually involving the upper part of the body in south America, and the lower in Africa) which start as itchy oedematous papules or nodules, slowly resolve leaving depigmented areas on the shins, groin or abdomen. Later, lichenified papules and secondary bacterial infection result from scratching. In the early stage skin-snips, and in the latter biopsy also reveals the causative organism.

In loaiasis, localised subcutaneous ('Calabar') swellings usually situated over bony prominences, are a transient event. In dracunculiasis (guinea-worm infection), localised abscesses form around a 'blister' caused by the adult female guinea-worm penetrating subcutaneous tissues or joints, usually in the lower limbs; a portion of the female worm may be extruded through the resultant ulcer.

In the acute stage of schistosomiasis (Katayama fever), a generalised urticarial rash may accompany other systemic involvement (*see* Chapter 6).

Multiple subcutaneous nodules may be present in cysticercosis (*see* Chapters 5 and 9).

ARTHROPOD-BORNE INFECTIONS

Some of these infections can be spread by sexual contact (*see* Chapter 12). Scabies, which is exceedingly common in 'Third World' countries, is caused by infection and sensitisation to the bite of the mite *Sarcoptes scabei* var *hominis*; it is characterised by intense itching (especially at night), and burrows. The flexor surfaces of the wrists, finger webs, elbows, nipples, genitalia and anterior axillary folds are common sites of infection, while the hands are usually spared. The burrows are 1–3 mm, whitish and thread-like, with a greyish speck at one end indicating the site of the female mite. Urticarial papules, excoriations and nodule formation result from sensitisation to the mite and also vigorous scratching. They are often secondarily infected (impetigo). The burrow is pathognomonic and the mite can be teased from it with a needle; it can then be placed on to a glass slide and examined microscopically. After a thorough shower, hexachlorobenzene (benzyl benzoate, crotonotoluide and sulphur ointment can also be used) is applied to the entire body-surface and left for 24 h; this should be repeated after 1 week. Secondary bacterial infection may require a systemic antibiotic. Underclothes and bed clothes should be washed thoroughly in hot water.

Flea bites, which result from *Pulex irritans* are common in developing countries; animal fleas also may infect man. The exposed surfaces are usually involved, but with heavy infections other areas also. Small, discrete papules may evolve into vesicles and pustules; they are surrounded by an erythematous ring or wheal. Excoriations and secondary infections are common. Management consists of killing the fleas with an insecticide, and treating secondary infection with an antibiotic.

Tungiasis, characterised by a pruritic papular eruption at the site of penetration of the burrowing female flea *Tunga penetrans* (the 'jigger flea') tends to occur beneath the toenails, sides of the feet and soles, and sometimes on the genitalia, buttocks and hands. Small papules containing a central black dot gradually enlarge and become inflamed and painful; secondary bacterial infection is common. The flea can be teased out with a needle and examined; they are most easily removed by applying chloroform or turpentine; secondary infection requires treatment with an antibiotic.

Myiasis is a term used for the cutaneous lesions produced by several species of fly, usually in tropical countries; mucous membranes, gastrointestinal and urinary tracts can also be involved. The larvae are deposited on to skin, usually by infected clothing which has been left to dry on the ground or under trees where the flies are common. An oedematous, pruritic papule enlarges gradually into a nodule, and a sensation of movement within the lesion is a common symptom. The larvae often protrude through the apex of the lesion; they can then be extracted with forceps. This operation is made much easier after a layer of 'Vaseline' has been spread over the lesion causing suffocation and death of the larvae.

FURTHER READING

Canizares O. (1982). *A Manual of Dermatology for Developing Countries*, p. 355. Oxford, New York, Delhi: Oxford University Press.

Chopra A., Probert A. J., Beer W. E. (1985). Myiasis due to Tumbu fly. *Lancet*; **1:** 1165.

Convit J., Castellanos P. L., Rondon A., *et al.* (1987). Immunotherapy versus chemotherapy in localised cutaneous leishmaniasis. *Lancet*; **1:** 401–5.

Levene G. M., Calnan C. D. (1974). *A Colour Atlas of Dermatology*, p. 368. London: Wolfe Medical Publications.

Pettit J. H. S. (1983). *Manual of Practical Dermatology*, p. 219. Edinburgh, London: Churchill Livingstone.

Pettit J. H. S., Parish L. C. (1984). *Manual of Tropical Dermatology*, p. 260. New York, Berlin, Heidelberg, Tokyo: Springer-Verlag.

Ratnam A. V., Jayaraju K. (1979). Skin diseases in Zambia. *Brit. J. Dermatol*; **101:** 449–53.

Staughton R. (1987). *A Colour Atlas of the Skin as an Indicator of Internal Disorders*, p. 100. London: Wolfe Medical Publications.

Chapter Fourteen

Leprosy

This chronic disease, caused by the bacterium *Mycobacterium leprae*, is currently estimated to affect 15 million people worldwide; approximately 50% of those are in Africa and Asia. The organs principally affected are the skin, upper respiratory tract, eyes (anterior segments), peripheral nerves, and testes, i.e. those parts of the body with a relatively low temperature. Although recognised in ancient writings, including the Old and New Testaments, where it is regarded as a divine punishment, it is impossible to discern at this stage which descriptions truly referred to leprosy. This ancient disease was widespread in Europe, including the UK, in the Middle Ages; some of the Crusaders (11th century) certainly returned with the disease having been infected in the Middle-east. Danish graveyards from the Middle Ages have yielded skulls showing unmistakable evidence of lepromatous leprosy.

BACTERIOLOGY, IMMUNOLOGY AND CLASSIFICATION

The bacillus (acid-fast and $0.3–0.5$ μm $\times$ $4–7$ μm in size) was first visualised in 1873 by Hansen in Norway. The bacillus exhibits the following features:

(i) It does not grow on routine mycobacteriological media.
(ii) It infects footpads of laboratory mice.
(iii) It has acid-fastness which is extractable with pyridine.
(iv) It oxidises DOPA in suspension.
(v) It invades host nerves.
(vi) It produces characteristic dermal responses in tuberculoid leprosy patients in killed suspension.

The only known animal to be highly susceptible to the infection is the nine-banded armadillo, which has a body temperature of 32–35°C. The mode of infection in man is unclear; nasal secretions are in most cases the probable source. Open ulcers also discharge a high concentration of bacilli. In addition, breast milk from lepromatous women contains *M. leprae*. Limited evidence suggests that the disease might be a zoonosis, with a reservoir in armadillos and other animals. Men are more often infected than women by a ratio of 2–3:1. The importance of malnutrition as a predisposing factor is unclear. There is no doubt that underlying socioeconomic conditions are relevant to spread of the disease. Ethnic factors are clearly important in infectivity; whereas the lepromatous form of the disease occurs in 5–10% of Africans, it can exist in up to 50% of those infected in some Asian populations.

The clinical spectrum of disease is governed by the ability of *M. leprae* to survive in macrophages, and to elicit a delayed-type hypersensitivity reaction.

Immunity can be assessed by the *Lepromin* reaction: following an intradermal suspension of killed *M. leprae*, early and late reactions are assessed at 48 h and 3–4 weeks respectively. The late reaction is strongly positive (>5 mm diameter) in tuberculoid, moderately positive (3–5 mm) in borderline, and weak or negative (0–2 mm) in lepromatous cases. These reactions are granulomatous and are a direct reflection of delayed-type hypersensitivity, or cell mediated immunity (CMI) to the *M. leprae* antigen. Cell mediated immunity is therefore markedly suppressed in lepromatous compared with tuberculoid patients; macrophages cannot in this condition clear *M. leprae* from the skin. Also, total T-lymphocyte numbers are decreased in lepromatous patients. The immunological defect in lepromatous disease might therefore reside in lymphocyte–macrophage interaction. A secondary mechanism for depression of CMI in lepromatous disease is that thymus-dependent areas in the lymph-nodes and spleen are largely replaced by infiltrations of bacilli-laden macrophages; this impedes the interaction of antigen with subpopulations of lymphocytes and macrophages, and circulation of T-lymphocytes through these areas. In lepromatous disease, peripheral B-lymphocytes are increased in number, and serum IgG, IgA and IgM concentrations are elevated; many elevated protein fractions are therefore present and a number of diagnostic tests are significantly affected. Raised C-reactive and amyloid-related protein may be present, together with autoantibodies for rheumatoid factor, elevated thyroglobulin antibody, ANF and cryoglobulin, and false-positive tests for syphilis.

Many organs show histological evidence of cellular infiltration; lymph-nodes, liver and spleen are largely replaced by bacillus-laden macrophages and the upper respiratory tract, eye and testes may also be involved. Affected peripheral nerves are also heavily invaded.

In tuberculoid leprosy, a strong cell-mediated (type IV) immune reaction ensures bacteriological recovery in most affected individuals.

CLINICAL ASPECTS

Incubation period for leprosy is from 2 to 20, and usually between 2 and 5 years. Focal paraesthesiae and pruritus often precede the clinical lesions. Indeterminate (I) leprosy is usually the earliest manifestation; this may either heal spontaneously, remain unchanged for months or years, or progress to tuberculoid or lepromatous forms (Table 14.1). It consists either of a single skin macule, or several poorly defined ones; they are mildly hypopigmented or erythematous. Skin smears are negative or contain a few bacilli. Table 14.1 summarises the clinical manifestations of fully developed disease. At the tuberculoid (TT) end of the spectrum, either single or several randomly placed hypopigmented or erythematous skin lesions are present; sensation is impaired, sweating diminished, and there is hair loss. Enlarged cutaneous nerves (especially the ulna, posterior tibial and greater auricular) may be easily palpated. At the lepromatous (LL) end of the spectrum, striking cutaneous manifestations occur, which may be macular and/or nodular. The lateral parts of the eyebrows become thin, and pubic and axillary hair diminishes; testicular atrophy and gynaecomastia are late manifestations of the disease. Laryngeal and ophthalmic (keratitis, conjunctival and scleral changes) lesions may also occur.

Two major types of clinical 'reaction' or inflammatory episode may occur—(i) *reversal*, and (ii) *erythema nodosum leprosum* (ENL). In reversal reactions, the lesions of borderline (BB) (and never LL) disease become erythematous and oedematous, and are often accompanied by an acute neuritis; the disease then moves towards the TT end of the spectrum (with enhanced cell mediated (type IV) immunity), and self-healing or burnt-out disease (accompanied by the characteristic deformities, e.g. claw hand, drop foot) results. ENL is a local immune complex (type III allergic) reaction which occurs in LL and BL patients. A rapid onset of tender

Table 14.1

THE CLINICAL SPECTRUM OF LEPROSY

	Tuberculoid TT	Borderline tuberculoid BT	Borderline (dimorphous, intermediate) BB	Borderline lepromatous BL	Lepromatous LL
Clinical	Single or several well-defined anaesthetic areas; peripheral nerves +	Similar to TT but lesions more numerous and less distinct	Similar to BT but lesions more numerous, with satellites (unstable disease)	Similar to BB. Some nerve damage	Multiple, symmetrical macular or papular non-anaesthetic lesions. No neural lesions until late. Leonine facies, testicular atrophy, etc (late)
Histology	Epithelioid-lymphocyte granulomas in nerves and skin; bacilli rare in nerves	Granulomas as in TT; nerves—infiltrated, bacilli +	Epithelioid cells and histiocytic infiltrations; nerves as in BT	Histiocytic infiltrations; lymphocytes +; nerves less infiltrated	Foamy histiocytes containing bacilli +. Few lymphocytes. Bacilli in nerves and perineurium ++
Lepromin reaction	+++	+	±	−	−
Density of bacteria in skin	−	±	+	++	+++

subcutaneous nodules which become erythematous, and often ulcerate, is accompanied by fever, and often arthritis, iridocyclitis and synovitis. Glomerulonephritis (caused by circulating immune complexes) and subsequently secondary amyloidosis are other sequelae of this form of the disease. An ENL reaction frequently occurs after a few months of chemotherapy. Table 14.2 summarises some of the differential diagnoses of leprosy on clinical grounds.

Diagnosis of leprosy is basically a *clinical* one; however, histology and examination of a skin smear (from the edge of a macule, plaque or nodule, an ear lobe or nasal mucosa) are valuable in confirmation. The lepromin test has no value in diagnosis. The bacterial index (BI) represents the density of bacteria in smears or tissues. The morphologic index (MI), which can also be assessed on a skin smear, expresses the percentage of *solidly* stained acid-fast bacilli (which are presumably therefore viable) by a standardised procedure; non-viable organisms appear irregular, granular or fragmented.

Table 14.2

SOME CLINICAL DIFFERENTIAL DIAGNOSES OF LEPROSY

Dermatological manifestations
 Scars
 Birthmarks
 Actinic dermatitis
 Dermatophytosis
 Filariasis (especially onchocerciasis)
 Leishmaniasis
 Granuloma annulare
 Granuloma multiforme
 Lupus erythematosus
 Psoriasis
 Pityriasis rosea
 Sarcoidosis
 Neurofibromatosis

Peripheral neuropathy
 Carpal tunnel syndrome
 Syringomyelia
 Lead toxicity
 Diabetes mellitus
 Primary amyloidosis of nerves
 Familial hypertrophic neuropathy
 Congenital pain insensitivity

TREATMENT OF LEPROSY

Management of this chronic disease can be divided into:

(i) Specific chemotherapy for the active disease (Table 14.3).
(ii) Prevention and correction of deformities and resultant disabilities.

Treatment is usually on an outpatient basis; patients should not be segregated but managed with those suffering from other medical conditions.

Dapsone (which was the first successful chemotherapeutic agent to be used in this disease, and which is relatively cheap) is *bacteriostatic* and not bactericidal; a major problem is that 'resistant' strains of *M. leprae* are now increasingly encountered. Rifampicin is bactericidal. Clofazimine has anti-inflammatory properties and is of value in ENL reactions; resistance is rarely encountered. Long-term follow-up is extremely important; serial evaluations of MI are of value in monitoring progress. During the reactions (*see* p. 227) additional therapeutic agents are usually required:

(i) *Reversal reactions.* When there is severe nerve involvement, analgesics together with corticosteroids at high dosage (e.g. prednisolone 40–60 mg daily), should be accompanied by physiotherapy.
(ii) *ENL reactions.* Analgesics are often required. In addition, thalidomide (100–400 mg daily) or corticosteroids (as for reversal reactions) are usually necessary. Thalidomide which is potentially teratogenic should not be given to women who are, or who might become pregnant. Iridocyclitis often requires topical corticosteroids.

Management of the neurotropic complications is an extensive and complex problem. Care, with the help of protective devices will minimise further trauma and prevent new lesions especially to limbs and eyes. Careful evaluation by a surgeon with special expertise in correcting the deformities of leprosy is important. If treatment is started early, the prognosis is excellent and mutilations minimised or even prevented. No specific preventive measures are available. However BCG vaccination has been shown to render significant protection. A vaccine is not yet available.

Table 14.3

SINGLE AND MULTIPLE CHEMOTHERAPEUTIC REGIMENS FOR LEPROSY

Therapeutic agent*	Adult dose—when used alone	Duration	Toxic effects
Single chemotherapeutic regimens			
(A) Dapsone (4-4'-diamino-diphenyl-sulphone, DDS)	100 mg daily or 200 mg × 3 weekly	Continue for 18 months after activity is no longer detectable ↓ for life	Allergy Desquamating dermatitis Anaemia Hepatitis Peripheral neuropathy Psychosis
(B) Rifampicin	Not recommended for use alone		
(C) Clofazimine ('Lamprene')	100–300 mg daily		Hyperpigmentation Gastrointestinal disturbances Paralytic ileus

Multiple chemotherapeutic regimens
BB, BL and LL: (A) = 100 mg daily; (B) = 600 mg monthly (at least 2 years);

(C) = 50 mg daily together with 300 mg monthly

BT and TT: (A) = 100 mg daily; (B) = 600 mg monthly (6 months)

* = Prothionamide and ethionamide are alternative agents which are occasionally used.

FURTHER READING

Browne S. G. (1986). Leprosy in the Bible. In *Medicine and the Bible*, pp. 101–25. Exeter: Paternoster Press.
Case 49–1985. (1985). Erythema nodosum leprosum reaction in a patient with lepromatous leprosy. *N. Engl. J. Med*; **313:** 1464–72.
Editorial. (1982). Chemotherapy of leprosy. *Lancet*; **2:** 77–8.
Editorial. (1986). Serological tests for leprosy. *Lancet*; **1:** 533–5.
Fine P. E. M., Ponnighaus J. M., Maine N., et al. (1986). Protective efficacy of BCG against leprosy in northern Malawi. *Lancet*; **2:** 499–502.
Hastings R. C., ed. (1985). *Leprosy*, p. 331. Edinburgh, London, Melbourne, New York: Churchill Livingstone.
Meyers W. M. (1984). Leprosy. In *Hunter's Tropical Medicine*, 6th ed. (Strickland G. T., ed.) pp. 409–22. Philadelphia, London: WB Saunders Co.

Chapter Fifteen

Systemic Infections

In this chapter those infections—viral, rickettsial, bacterial, fungal, protozoal and helminthic—which are associated with multiorgan involvement and widespread systemic manifestations are considered. Clearly there is an overlap with other infections which have a more specific impact on one or another system, most of which have been dealt with in previous chapters.

VIRAL INFECTIONS

Although some viruses replicate and produce cell damage at the site of entry, others disseminate widely with the production of systemic sequelae. Some, e.g. EBV, CMV and the hepatitis viruses can be transmitted via blood transfusions. Others, e.g. yellow fever, rabies, measles and dengue can be prevented by live attenuated or inactivated vaccines. Progress in treatment has been slow; however, interferon and adenine arabinoside are clearly of value in herpes and HBV infections (*see* Chapter 16). Acute coryza and influenza (predominantly respiratory tract infections) are covered in Chapter 7 and herpes simplex and zoster, and rabies in Chapter 9; these infections may also produce systemic manifestations. Those viruses which cause childhood disease in which cutaneous lesions predominate are dealt with in Chapter 2. Viral causes of diarrhoea are summarised in Chapter 5; rotaviruses, which are of special importance in children and neonates, the Norwalk agent and entero, adeno, astro and coronaviruses are all important and their true roles are presently being unravelled. The viral hepatitides are covered in Chapter 6.

Epstein–Barr Virus (EBV)

Maternal antibody protection is often present at birth but is short-lived. Primary infection may be: (i) silent, or associated with (ii) acute infectious mononucleosis (IM), (iii) fatal IM (especially in the X-linked lymphoproliferative syndrome), or (iv) chronic IM. There are three major complications: (a) lymphomas (in organ graft recipients, AIDS sufferers and individuals with the Chédiak–Higashi syndrome), (b) Burkitt's lymphoma (which is a rare tumour even in Uganda where it was first recorded by Sir Albert Cook in 1904); EBV is responsible for 98% of endemic, and 20% of spontaneous cases, and (c) nasopharyngeal carcinoma in which EBV is detectable in 100% of cases. This latter tumour is especially common in China, north Africa (e.g. Libya, Sudan and the Kenya highlands) and in Eskimos.

Infectious mononucleosis (glandular fever) is a common disease, usually affecting young adults. Presentation is with sore throat and associated regional lymphadenopathy; PUO (*see* Chapter 1) may be a further presentation. Differential diagnoses include: CMV, toxoplasmosis and lymphomas. Atypical mononuclear cells are present in a blood film. The Paul–Bunnell test (usually preceded by a positive 'monospot' test, is subsequently positive; this measures heterophile antibodies and can take up to 3 months to become positive.Following infection, a life-long carrier state ensues. Although a vaccine is not yet available, work is currently proceeding using tamorins, the only experimental animal in which the virus will replicate.

Cytomegalovirus (CMV)

Like EBV, this is a DNA virus which can produce congenital or acquired infection. In the latter, presentation is with a systemic illness and lymphadenopathy; a specific hepatitis with cholestatic features may be severe. Pneumonia is a further complication, especially in immunosuppressed individuals; CMV can exist as an opportunistic infection in end-stage AIDS in which colitis is common. Disseminated CMV inclusion disease is a further complication. Viral culture from throat swab, urine and liver biopsy should be attempted. The Paul–Bunnell test is negative; cytomegalovirus CFT should be estimated. An IgM-specific CMV fluorescent antibody test can be carried out; this can be performed on infant serum when congenital infection is suspected. Adenine arabinoside is occasionally effective in CMV pneumonia and disseminated infection.

Viral Febrile Illnesses

Dengue fever and dengue haemorrhagic fever

Classical dengue fever (Table 15.1) is an acute self-limiting illness with biphasic ('saddle-back') fever, associated with severe headache, arthralgias, myalgia, a rash (which may be generalised and erythematous), lymphadenopathy and leucopenia. There are four distinct but closely related serotypes of the dengue virus (genus *Flavivirus*). When various immunological mechanisms (which are poorly understood) come about, *dengue haemorrhagic fever* (DHF), sometimes accompanied by *dengue shock syndrome* may be a sequel; although caused by the same serotypes as classical dengue, the disease then joins the viral haemorrhagic fevers (Table 15.2). Immune complex formation of viral antigen and host antibody origin, with subsequent activation of complement,

Table 15.1

VIRAL FEBRILE ILLNESSES WHICH ARE NOT USUALLY ASSOCIATED WITH HAEMORRHAGIC FEATURES

Disease	Virus	Transmission
Classical dengue	Dengue (serotypes 1–4)	Mosquito
West Nile fever	West Nile	Mosquito
Chikungunya fever	Chikungunya	Mosquito
O'nyong nyong fever	Member of the Semliki Forest complex	Mosquito
Sindbis fever	Member of the Western equine encephalitis complex	Mosquito
Epidemic polyarthritis	Ross River	Mosquito
Mayaro fever	Mayaro	Mosquito
Group C virus fevers	Murutucu, etc	Mosquito
Oropouche virus disease	Oropouche	Mosquito; also midges
Rift Valley fever	Rift Valley	Mosquito
Sandfly fevers	Naples, Sicilian, Chagres, Candiru, Punta Toro, Rift Valley	Sandflies
Other arboviruses	Orungo, Tataguine, etc	Mosquito

Table 15.2
VIRAL HAEMORRAGHIC FEVERS AND THEIR MODES OF TRANSMISSION TO MAN

Disease*	Virus	Transmission
Yellow fever (Chapter 6)	Yellow fever	Mosquito-borne
Dengue HF	Dengue (types 1–4)	Mosquito-borne
Chikungunya HF	Chikungunya	Mosquito-borne
Rift Valley fever	Rift Valley fever	Mosquito-borne
Congo–Crimean HF	Congo-Crimean HF	Tick-borne‡
Kyasanur Forest disease	Kyasanur Forest disease	Tick-borne
Omsk HF†	Omsk HF	Tick-borne
Argentine HF	Junin	Zoonotic‡
Bolivian HF	Machupo	Zoonotic‡
Korean HF†	Hantaan	Zoonotic
Lassa fever	Lassa	Zoonotic
Marburg virus disease	Marburg	?
Ebola virus disease	Ebola	?

*HF = Haemorrhagic fever; † = Occurs in temperate areas only; ‡ = Also spread by person-to-person transmission.

kinin and coagulation pathways has been implicated in this shock/haemorrhagic syndrome.

Dengue was described by Rush at Philadelphia, USA in 1780. Worldwide, epidemics have been documented ever since, especially in south-east Asia. In 1905, *Aedes aegypti* was identified as the principal vector. The causative viruses were isolated in the 1940s and 50s. Epidemics affect large numbers (up to 80%) of exposed individuals; immunity probably continues throughout life, but cross-protection to the different viruses is incomplete and short-lived. Following the mosquito bite, the virus replicates in the regional lymph glands and then becomes widely disseminated. The incubation period is 5–8 days. After the initial illness, the fever falls on the 3rd to 5th day and a morbilliform rash on the trunk spreads centripetally; there is often a brief recrudescence of fever. Leucopenia, neutropenia, and thrombocytopenia are usual. If DHF supervenes, spontaneous haemorrhages, a positive tourniquet test, and evidence of haemoconcentration are present. A 'shock-like' state which has a bad prognosis (mortality rate

>50%) may supervene, especially in children. Myocarditis and encephalopathy may be present. Virus may be isolated from serum during the acute phase of the disease. Serological diagnosis is made from paired serum samples. Treatment of classical dengue is symptomatic, but DHF often necessitates more sophisticated measures. Apart from treatment for shock and disseminated intravascular coagulation (DIC) (which is frequently present), corticosteroids are usually administered although their actual value is unclear. Prophylactically, live attenuated vaccines have received limited tests. Control of the vector should be attempted where possible. Table 15.1 (p. 234) summarises some other causes of viral febrile illnesses not usually associated with haemorrhagic features. Many others have localised areas of distribution; these are usually mosquito-borne and are caused by arboviruses.

Viral Haemorrhagic Fevers

This term refers to a group of at least 13 diseases with a worldwide distribution and which are clinically characterised by: fever, a bleeding diathesis, shock, and in most, abnormal hepatic structure and function. Table 15.2 (p. 235) summarises the diseases and causative agents.

Yellow fever

See Chapter 6.

Lassa fever

This disease is caused by an arenavirus (a single-stranded DNA virus); it has been recognised in west Africa as a disease entity since 1969. The disease is endemic in much of west, and probably central Africa. The virus possesses a reservoir in the rodent *Mastomys natalensis* which contaminates the environment via its secretions, especially urine. The disease is usually mild, especially in children, but carries a mortality rate of 15–20% in patients admitted to hospital. Hospital acquired infection occurs in west Africa via exposure to blood and blood-stained secretions. Outside Africa, person-to-person transmission has not so far occurred. Outbreaks have been recorded in Nigeria, Liberia and Sierra Leone (Fig. 15.1); overall, 17 outbreaks and over 100 deaths have

Systemic Infections 237

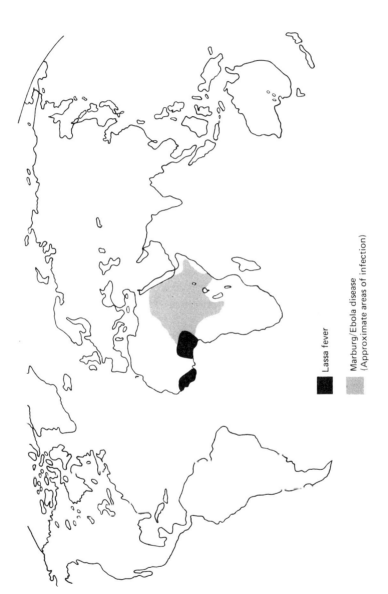

Fig. 15 1. Geographical distribution of Lassa fever, and Marburg/Ebola disease.

been reported but this does not reflect the true incidence of the disease. Since 1971, 10 confirmed cases have been imported to the UK; no secondary cases have so far occurred although some 1500 people have been placed under surveillance. A febrile illness originating in west Africa is far more likely statistically to be caused by malaria or typhoid fever. (To date, none of the other African viral haemorrhagic fevers—Congo/Crimean, Marburg and Ebola—have been imported to the UK). Incubation period is 3–21 days. Early clinical features are non-specific. The virus rapidly becomes generalised throughout the body and replicates in most tissues; generalised pathology is therefore a feature of the disease. Between the 3rd and 6th day symptoms worsen, and an important physical sign is a pharyngitis, with small vesicles and ulcers. The virus is excreted in urine for up to 8 weeks after onset of illness. If death occurs this is usually in the second week and is heralded by haemorrhages, anuria, shock, anoxia, respiratory insufficiency and cardiac arrest.

Febrile patients who have recently been to a rural area where Lassa fever is endemic or have lived or worked in country hospitals in those parts should be admitted to a DHSS designated high security unit. Close contacts of diagnosed patients, i.e. those in direct contact with the patient's blood, secretions, clothing, bedding and fomites should be placed under surveillance; others who have handled laboratory specimens, etc should also be included. Evidence for hospital acquired infection by the airborne route is extremely limited.

Diagnosis is by detection of viral antigen in peripheral blood samples; antibodies are present in the second week of illness. Virus isolation can be carried out from blood, pharyngeal secretions and urine; positive results can usually be obtained in 72 h. Ribavirin administered during the first week of illness reduces the mortality rate substantially; in patients with severe viraemia and/or raised plasma aspartate transaminase (a sign of bad prognosis), mortality is reduced from 55 to 5%. Ribavirin should also be given prophylactically (orally) for 10 days to those who have been exposed to the virus percutaneously. Administration of Lassa immune plasma has no place in management. Supportive measures: fluid balance, blood pressure maintenance, tracheostomy, etc are frequently necessary.

Marburg virus disease

This disease, which is caused by a single-stranded RNA virus, was first recognised in laboratory workers at Marburg and Frankfurt, West Germany and Belgrade, Yugoslavia in 1967. They had become infected by vervet monkeys (*Cercopithecus aethiops*) imported from Uganda; 7 of 25 primary infections were fatal, and 6 secondary cases survived. In Africa, the first recognised case was in a hitch-hiker who had travelled to South Africa via Zimbabwe; a further case was reported in Kenya in 1980. Overall 36 cases with 9 deaths have to date been reported. The disease is probably zoonotic but this has not been confirmed; it seems likely that the natural reservoir is in a subhuman primate population. The mode of human infection is unclear. The incubation period is 3–9 days, and virus can persist in the body for at least 80 days. The illness is heralded by a severe headache, pyrexia and generalised pain, most marked in the lumbar region. Abdominal pain and diarrhoea are also prominent clinical features. Conjunctivitis and a characteristic maculopapular rash is often present between days 5 and 7. Severe bleeding is a prominent feature. Necroses have been demonstrated in all organs. Diagnosis is by virus culture from blood or serum during the acute phase of the disease. The virus can also be directly visualised by electron microscopy of affected tissue. An indirect immunofluorescent antibody test (IFAT) is of value in the recovery phase. Treatment is symptomatic and supportive. Heparin may be of value in the prevention of DIC.

Ebola virus disease

This disease is caused by a virus which is morphologically very similar, if not identical, to the Marburg virus; however, there are antigenic differences. The disease was first recognised in 1976 during two severe outbreaks of haemorrhagic fever in Sudan and Zaire (*see* Fig. 15.1, p. 237); some 600 cases were reported and mortality rates of 53–88% recorded. A further outbreak occurred in southern Sudan in 1979. The reservoir is also unknown. Like Marburg disease, virus transmission seems to be of a low order and direct contact with infected blood, inoculation, or prolonged contact with an infected patient seem important. The incubation period is 4–16 days. The clinical illness and pathological findings are similar and probably identical to those of Marburg disease; respiratory and CNS symptoms, and pharyngitis were prominent features in the Zaire outbreak. Haemorrhagic manifestations are very common. Death occurs between 7 and 16 days after onset.

Diagnostic techniques and management are the same as those for Marburg disease; although Ebola immune serum and interferon have been used with a seeming degree of success this form of treatment is of unproven efficacy.

Other viral haemorrhagic fevers

These are summarised in Table 15.2 (p. 235). Bolivian haemorrhagic fever (BHF), first recognised in 1959 in rural areas of north eastern Bolivia, is caused by the Machupo virus which is rodent (*Calomys callosus*) associated. Two major epidemics occurred in 1962 and 1964, and small localised outbreaks occur more or less annually. The incubation period is 7–14 days and the onset insidious. Multiple organ involvement with interstitial haemorrhage into various organs is characteristic. A case fatality rate of from 5–30% has been recorded. Argentine haemorrhagic fever (AHF), which is caused by the Junin virus, was first recognised in 1958; it occurs annually in rural areas of Buenos Aires. Reservoirs for this virus are *Calomys laucha* and *C. musculinus* and other rodent species. The incubation period is 8–12 days. The diseases are similar but lymphadenopathy is more common in AHF. With both diseases, control measures are based on attempts to reduce the rodent population.

Congo–Crimean haemorrhagic fever was first recognised in western Crimea in Russian soldiers in 1944; however, it had undoubtedly occurred for many years in central Asian areas of the USSR. The virus is identical to the Congo virus first isolated in Zaire in 1956. Small outbreaks have occurred in the Middle-east, eastern Europe and other parts of Africa. It is a rural disease, and is transmitted to man either by infected ticks (in which transovarian transmission occurs), or by direct contact with severely infected patients or domestic animals. The incubation period is 7–21 days. Fever and generalised symptoms are present, and generalised (sometimes massive) haemorrhage into several organs constitutes an important feature of the disease; hepatocellular necrosis is common. Diagnosis is by viral isolation, IFAT, agar gel diffusion precipitation, complement fixation, or indirect haemagglutination tests. Treatment is symptomatic; control of dehydration and haemorrhage are important. The efficacy of a USSR vaccine is unproven. Prevention is by tick control of domestic animals; tick repellents in humans are probably also of value.

Kyasanur Forest disease is confined to Mysore State, southern India; Langur and Macacca monkeys form the reservoir of infection. It is spread to man by *Haemaphysalis* ticks. Human cases occur in the pre-monsoon season. Incubation period is 3–8 days. Fever, severe headache, lymphadenopathy, meningoencephalitis, albuminuria and a haemorrhagic tendency are prominent features. The majority of patients completely recover although there is a significant mortality rate. Diagnosis, management and control are similar to those for the other viral haemorrhagic fevers.

The muroid nephropathies

Haemorrhagic fever with a renal syndrome is a disease of rural communities exposed to the urine of infected rodents (e.g. voles and field mice). Korean haemorrhagic fever which is caused by the Hantaan virus occurs in Asia and eastern USSR (Table 15.2, p. 235). A less severe form, *nephropathia epidemica* has been reported from Scandinavia and eastern Europe.

Monkeypox

This disease bears a very close resemblance to smallpox (variola), a systemic illness with a very long history and which last appeared in 1977; the last recorded case was in Somalia. The only clinical difference is that it is usually accompanied by lymphadenopathy. The virus belongs to the genus *Orthopoxvirus* which also includes: camelpox, cowpox, ectromelia and vaccinia. The disease is confined to small forest villages in central and west Africa (Fig. 15.2) and was first recognised in Zaire in 1970. Because it is prevented by smallpox (variola) vaccination, the incidence rate was probably masked and it was previously misdiagnosed as smallpox. The reservoir is unknown (several mammalian species are known to be infected) although it has been isolated from monkeys of both African and Asian origin; person-to-person transmission is low. The incubation period is probably between 10 and 14 days. It is more common in children than in adults and the fatality rate is of the order of 10–20%.

242 *Communicable and Tropical Diseases*

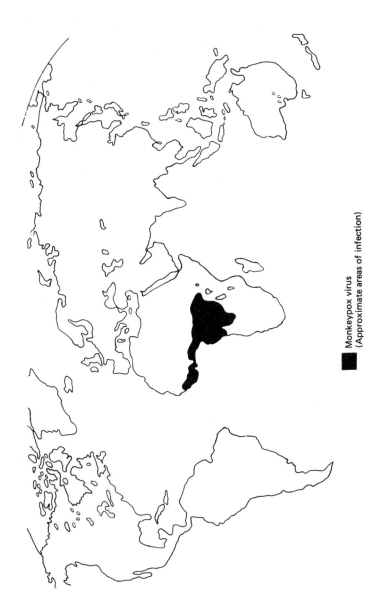

Fig. 15.2. Geographical distribution of monkeypox infection.

Persistent Virus Infections

Table 15.3 summarises some viruses which can persist or lie clinically dormant for long periods of time (*see also* Chapter 9), producing overt disease at a later date. The term 'slow virus infection' has several uses, including—persistent infection, latent infection, and infection following a long incubation period. The most impressive and well documented of these is Kuru (*see* Chapter 9).

EBV and CMV infections can also continue for long periods of time; however, in the event of immunosuppression, e.g. AIDS, overt disease becomes manifest. Table 15.4 summarises some diseases of unknown aetiology but in which a persistent virus infection might be relevant.

Table 15.3

VIRUSES WHICH CAN PRODUCE PERSISTENT INFECTIONS IN MAN

Rubella
Measles
Retroviruses
   HTLV–I
   HTLV–II
   HIV–1 and HIV–2
Unconventional viruses
   Kuru agent
   Creutzfeld–Jakob disease agent
   Gerstmann–Sträussler syndrome
Herpes virus
   Cytomegalovirus (CMV)
   Epstein–Barr virus (EBV)
   Herpes simplex 1 and 2
   Herpes zoster
Papovaviruses
   Polyomaviruses
   Papillomaviruses
   Progressive multifocal leucoencephalopathy (PML)
Adenoviruses
Hepatitis B (HBV) (*see* Chapter 6)

Table 15.4

DISEASES WHICH MIGHT RESULT FROM PERSISTENT VIRAL INFECTIONS

Neurological	Multiple sclerosis
	Amyotrophic lateral sclerosis
	Parkinson's disease
	Presenile dementia
	Schizophrenia
	Depressive illness
Neoplasms	
Birth defects	
Autoimmune	Systemic lupus erythematosus
	Rheumatoid arthritis
	Dermatomyositis
	Periarteritis nodosa
Crohn's disease	
Diabetes mellitus (type I)	
Miscellaneous endocrine deficiencies	
Paget's disease	

CHLAMYDIA INFECTION

The most important organisms in this group are *Chlamydia trachomatis* (*see also* Chapter 12) and *Chlamydia psittaci* (*see* Chapter 7). Trachoma has been recognised since antiquity although the causative organism was not isolated until 1950. It consists of a chronic follicular conjunctivitis which results in corneal scarring, distortion of the upper eyelids, and subsequent blindness. It is common throughout most developing countries.

RICKETTSIAL INFECTION (INCLUDING TYPHUS)

Table 15.5 summarises the distribution and life-cycles of some major rickettsial diseases. While some, e.g. tick typhus have a limited geographical distribution, others, e.g. murine typhus and Q fever, exist throughout the world and are associated with widespread morbidity and occasional mortality. With the exception of louse-borne typhus and trench fever, all are zoonoses (*see* Chapter 1); man is a 'dead-end' host. Rickettsia are obligate intracellular organisms, which penetrate the host-cell plasma membrane and grow only within eukaryotic host cells; they multiply by binary fission. *Coxiella burnetii* produces endotoxins which are physiologically similar to those of Gram-negative bacilli.

With the exception of Q fever, a rash, usually maculopapular (and sometimes with a haemorrhagic component) is part of the clinical presentation. In some, an eschar—a lesion at the site of the bite which develops a black base, associated with local lymphadenopathy—is present also (Table 15.5). These rashes should be distinguished from several others including measles and meningococcaemia. Mild splenomegaly is common. DIC is a feature of several rickettsial diseases, notably Rocky Mountain spotted fever. Table 15.5 summarises some clinical features of the rickettsial diseases. Differentiation from typhoid (and other enteric) fever(s) is a frequent clinical problem; while laboratory results are awaited, chloramphenicol is sometimes started. A mild leucopenia (which is also consistent with typhoid fever) is a common haematological finding. While isolation of rickettsiae or their antigens from blood, urine and tissues is possible this is beyond the scope of a routine laboratory. Serological testing remains the usual method of laboratory diagnosis; however, this is nearly always retrospective because an antibody response rarely occurs before the end of the first week of the disease; the IFAT, which can be made group- and in some cases species-specific is the most widely used. The Weil–Felix reaction, agglutination against *Proteus* OX–19, and complement fixation tests are also used; ELISA tests are undergoing development. Species identification is often difficult. In south-east Asia, doxycycline (100 mg weekly or twice weekly) as a prophylactic has proved effective in British soldiers, especially in louse-borne typhus.

Treatment depends on prompt antibiotic administration; tetracyclines are most widely used but chloramphenicol is probably equally effective. Tetracycline 500 mg q.d.s. for 14 days is the usual treatment. Response within 24 h is usual and mortality rate should be zero. Rarely, tetracycline resistance in *C. burnetii* and chloramphenicol resistance in *R. prowazekii* have been reported. Single dose doxycycline treatment has also proved effective especially in scrub typhus, but it has not been widely used in some of the other rickettsial diseases. However, treatment is not *cidal* and the organisms remain within the body, being dealt with by an immunological response which is poorly understood. Fluid and electrolyte balance must be maintained, and cardiovascular and other complications should be treated on merit; occasionally

Table 15.5
SOME RICKETTSIAL DISEASES

Disease	Distribution	Life-cycle Arthropod vector	Life-cycle Reservoir	Basic lesion	Clinical Incubation period	Clinical Eschar
Typhus group						
Murine (*R. mooseri*)	Worldwide (scattered foci)	Flea	Rodents	Vasculitis	8–16	–
Epidemic (*R. prowazekii*)	Worldwide	Body louse	(man)	Vasculitis	10–14	–
Brill–Zinsser disease (*R. prowazekii*)	Worldwide	Louse	(man)	Vasculitis	?	–
Scrub typhus						
Tsutsugamushi disease (*R. tsutsugamushi*)	Asia, Papua New Guinea, Pacific, Australia	Chigger	Rodents	Vasculitis	9–18	+

Spotted fever group					
Tick typhus (*R. conorii*)	Africa (especially east and southern), Mediterranean littoral, India, Pakistan	Ixodid ticks	Rodents, dogs	Vasculitis	5–7	+
Rocky Mountain spotted fever (*R. rickettsii*)	Western hemisphere	Ixodid ticks	Small mammals	Vasculitis	3–14	−
Rickettsialpox (*R. akari*)	USA, USSR, Korea	Mouse mite	Mice	Vasculitis	9–21	+
Q fever (*Coxiella burnetii*)	Worldwide	(Ticks)	Mammals	Granulomas	10–26	−
Trench fever (*Rochalimaea quintana*)	North Africa, Mexico, eastern Europe	Body louse	(man)	Unknown	4–35	−

corticosteroids have apparently given beneficial results in some infections. There are no effective vaccines. Vector control should be a major line of attack.

Murine typhus

This is a common cause of acute febrile illness worldwide and is undoubtedly underdiagnosed. Although usually sporadic, local outbreaks are reported. A high fever (up to 41°C) and marked debilitation are usual features, but the mortality rate is very low; headache, generalised aches and pains and a rash appearing on the 5th or 6th day are characteristic. Murine typhus does not respond to ampicillin or co-trimoxazole; this makes clinical differentiation from typhoid fever possible.

Epidemic louse-borne typhus

Both the acute disease and its recrudescent form (Brill–Zinsser disease) are caused by *R. prowazekii* (*see* Table 15.5, pp. 246–7). The immunological basis for development of the latter is unknown. Clinically it is similar to murine typhus, the headache being especially severe; conjunctivitis and photophobia may be present. A cough is commonly present. Hypotension and renal failure contribute to a mortality rate of 10–60% in untreated cases. Tetracycline or doxycycline reduces the mortality almost to zero. Medical personnel who come into close contact with patients with this disease are at risk.

Scrub typhus

This disease is widely spread, but is especially common in southeast Asia and the Pacific; it was a major problem during the Pacific campaign of World War II (1939–45). There are multiple serotypes of *R. tsutsugamushi*; cross-immunity to another serotype is transient, probably lasting for no more than 1–2 months. In approximately 60–70% of cases an eschar develops. The systemic illness is similar to that of other rickettsial disease, and includes mild splenomegaly. Signs of meningoencephalitis, cranial nerve lesions, myocarditis, anuria and even gangrene may all develop during the second week of illness. Mortality rates vary between 0 and 30% in the untreated. Tetracycline produces a rapid recovery; doxycycline is of value, but relapses may occur after a single dose.

Tick typhus

Several species of rickettsiae are transmitted by ticks; these tend to differ from continent to continent. Probably the best known is that caused by *R. conorii* which occurs mainly in Africa but extending to the Mediterranean littoral and to India and Pakistan; it is also known as *fièvre boutonneuse*. After an incubation period of 5–7 days, a systemic febrile illness lasting from a few days to 2 weeks is rarely fatal except in the elderly and debilitated. Headache, myalgia and conjunctival injection are common. It is a zoonosis with man the accidental 'dead-end' host. An eschar (2–5 mm diameter) has a black base, and is accompanied by regional lymphadenopathy. The maculopapular rash appears on about the 4th day (*see* Chapter 13). The diagnosis is a clinical one and serology is confirmatory in the second week. Prognosis is good but is hastened by antibiotics. Response to tetracycline, doxycycline, and also chloramphenicol is rapid.

Rocky Mountain spotted fever

This is a more severe disease than tick typhus (*see* above) and carries a higher fatality rate. It is widely distributed in the USA and central and south America. The vasculitis is more severe than in most other rickettsial diseases. The characteristic rash begins on the wrists and ankles and spreads to involve the whole body; macules later become maculopapular, petechial and finally haemorrhagic; these lesions often coalesce. Widespread organ involvement may ensue and in 10–60% of untreated cases death occurs late in the second week; if initiation of treatment is delayed, mortality is still significant. Tetracycline, doxycycline or chloramphenicol should be started immediately there is a clinical suspicion of the disease.

Rickettsialpox (*see* Table 15.5, p. 246–7).

Rickettsialpox is a mild systemic disease with no mortality. The rash is initially maculopapular, and later vesiculopapular: it should be distinguished from chickenpox. When tetracycline is started response is rapid, but the disease resolves without chemotherapy.

Q fever

This infection, which is usually acquired by inhalation of airborne organisms (*Coxiella burnetii*) (usually from asymptomatic cattle, sheep and goats) consists of an acute febrile illness with headache, myalgia, malaise and rarely a rash; a pneumonitis may be present. The role of infected unpasteurised milk is controversial. Hepatitis and endocarditis are complications. It is distributed worldwide but is more common in dry climates. Widespread granulomas in liver, lungs and bone marrow are common. Radiological changes in the lungs consist of multiple rounded densities, usually in the lower zones. A granulomatous hepatitis with a tender liver and abnormal biochemical tests must be differentiated from other causes of acute hepatitis. Endocarditis (the most serious complication) may not be diagnosed until 2 to 20 years after the acute infection; it is sometimes superimposed on congenitally abnormal or prosthetic valves—vegetations contain *C. burnetii*. It is a cause of culture-negative endocarditis (*see* Chapter 8). There may be accompanying fever, anaemia, finger-clubbing, splenomegaly, embolic phenomena and a raised ESR; glomerulonephritis may also occur. Untreated, death usually occurs in about 3 years. Clinically this disease is difficult to diagnose and can mimic many other communicable diseases. Serology is however of value; phase II ('rough') complement-fixing antibodies are detected about 1 week after onset, reach a peak at 3–4 weeks, and subsequently fall slowly; persistence of phase I ('smooth') antibody suggests a chronic infection, leading either to hepatitis or endocarditis. The causative organism can occasionally be demonstrated in granulomas or vegetations.

Treatment with tetracycline, doxycycline or chloramphenicol is usually satisfactory; however, resistance to tetracycline is reported from Cyprus. A killed phase I vaccine is not commercially available. Treatment of endocarditis is difficult; although a prolonged course using a combination of doxycycline, and trimethoprim, rifampicin or lincomycin has been used, results are variable. Valve replacement may be necessary.

Trench fever

This is a short-lived febrile illness which is never fatal, occurs in epidemics and has a tendency to relapse; it was recognised in World Wars I and II. Aching muscles, joints and bones may be accompanied by a macular rash. Treatment is not usually necessary but the organism responds to tetracycline and chloramphenicol.

Bartonellosis

This is a sandfly-borne disease confined to south America and occurring in Andean valleys, which is caused by *Bartonella bacilliformis*. A severe illness ('Oroya fever') is often fatal; however, a chronic disease which causes verrucous skin eruptions is benign. The incubation period is usually about 3 weeks but can vary between 7 and 100 days. Untreated, the fatality rate for the acute disease is around 40%. It is frequently complicated by salmonellosis. Treatment is with chloramphenicol; penicillins, tetracyclines and streptomycin are also effective. Blood transfusion is often necessary in the acute disease.

BACTERIAL INFECTIONS

Septicaemia

In the UK, most septicaemias are caused by Gram-negative organisms. Non-sporing anaerobes (*see* p. 22) are also important and can cause a similar illness. The incidence of Gram-positive septicaemias (caused by streptococci and staphylococci) has declined over the past few decades; however, in 'Third World' countries, these are still very common. While in most cases only one organism is isolated, in some situations, e.g. drug-addicts, a polymicrobial cause frequently exists involving both Gram-negative and Gram-positive organisms. Table 15.6 summarises the more important aetiological agents. Release of endotoxin from Gram-negative organisms may result in toxic shock. Anaerobic bacteria (*Bacteroides fragilis* and *Bacteroides spp.*) are usually derived from abdominal or gynaecological sepsis; anaerobic streptococci, either from the female genital tract or from oral sepsis can also cause a bacteraemia. In addition to toxic shock, staphylococcal septicaemia can be associated with DIC; these complications may be caused by the effects of protein A of *Staph. aureus*. During the last decade, shock accompanied by a febrile reaction and rash has been shown to be caused by vaginal tampons which have become colonised with toxin-producing *Staph. aureus*; cure is usually spontaneous when the tampon is removed. Other causes of septicaemia include: arboviruses and viral haemorrhagic fevers, *Clostridium perfringens*, *Coxiella burnetii* and typhus, and *Candida spp.*, *Cryptococcus neoformans*, *Histoplasma capsulatum* and

Table 15.6
SOME CAUSES OF SEPTICAEMIA AND LIKELY SOURCES OF INFECTION

Gram-negative	Source of infection
Escherichia coli *Klebsiella spp.* *Proteus spp.* *Enterobacter spp.*	Abdominal sepsis Urinary tract infections Hepatobiliary infections Leukaemia
Salmonella typhi and other salmonellae	Typhoid fever, salmonellosis—especially in infants and elderly
Haemophilus influenzae *Neisseria meningitidis*	Respiratory and CNS infections—mostly in infants
Pseudomonas aeruginosa *Serratia marcescens*	Leukaemia Respiratory and urinary tract infections Burns
Neisseria gonorrhoeae	Pelvic inflammatory disease (*see* Chapter 12)
Gram-positive	
Streptococcus pneumoniae	Pneumonia and other respiratory infections, meningitis, splenectomy
Strep. pyogenes	Cellulitis Obstetric and neonatal infections Skin infections
Strep. faecalis	Urinary tract infections, endocarditis
Strep. milleri	Abdominal sepsis, liver abscess, empyema
'*Strep. viridans*' microaerophilic streptococci	Bacterial endocarditis (*see* Chapter 8)
Staphylococcus aureus	Skin, wound, bone and joint infections, pneumonia, lung abscess, pyomyositis, endocarditis, infected pacemaker, drug addicts
Staph. epidermidis	Joint prosthesis, heart or CNS infection; infected i.v. line
Listeria monocytogenes	Immunosuppression, reticuloses, splenectomy

Aspergillus spp. In many tropical countries, pyomyositis commonly predisposes to septicaemia. Clinically, fever, rigors, confusion, tachycardia and hypotension are prominent features; however, septic shock, DIC and acute renal failure may be present also. Mortality rate is often high, e.g. one-third of cases; however, this depends on age, the general underlying condition of the individual, and the efficacy of treatment. Immediately cultures have been set up, antibiotic treatment must be commenced; Table 15.7 summarises some appropriate regimens. These regimens are guidelines to initial treatment; they should be modified in the light of subsequent microbiological results. The treatment of

Table 15.7

TREATMENT OF SEPTICAEMIA

Underlying condition	Antibiotic combination (adult dose)
(i) No clues regarding cause or site of infection	Gentamicin (2 mg/kg t.d.s.) + cloxacillin (1·5 g q.d.s.) + benzylpenicillin (900 mg q.d.s.)*
(ii) Abdominal/pelvic sepsis (therefore probably Gram-negative)	Metronidazole (500 mg t.d.s.) + gentamicin (2 mg/kg t.d.s.)
(iii) Immunosuppression (or severe neutropenia)	Gentamicin (2·5 mg/kg t.d.s.) + carbenicillin (5 g q.d.s.)
(iv) Urinary tract infection (therefore probably Gram-negative)	Gentamicin (2 mg/kg t.d.s.) + ampicillin (1 g q.d.s.)
(v) Meningitis and purpuric rash (presumably meningococcal)	Benzylpenicillin (30 mg/kg 4-hourly)
(vi) Skin sepsis, acute osteomyelitis, etc (therefore probably Gram-positive)	Cloxacillin (2 g q.d.s.) + benzylpenicillin (1·8 g q.d.s.)
(vii) *Staph. aureus* strongly suspected	Cloxacillin (2 g q.d.s.) + gentamicin (2 mg/kg t.d.s.)
(viii) *Clostridium perfringens*	Benzylpenicillin (900 mg q.d.s.) + metronidazole (500 mg t.d.s.) + gentamicin (2 mg/kg t.d.s.)

*=This regimen covers some 80% of bacteria likely to be responsible for the septicaemia; in 5–10%, *Bacteroides fragilis* is responsible and this is *not* covered by this antibiotic combination.

septicaemia is also discussed in Chapter 16. In addition, localised pus, if present, must be evacuated.

Typhoid Fever

This is an acute systemic febrile illness which is caused by *Salmonella typhi*; it should not be confused with infection caused by the zoonotic salmonellae which give rise to symptoms and signs localised to the gastrointestinal tract. Paratyphoid fever is similar to typhoid but usually causes a less severe illness. Throughout the centuries, the disease has carried a high morbidity and mortality rate and only became treatable in 1948 when chloramphenicol was shown to be of value. Throughout the world, most cases are sporadic, but epidemics occasionally occur. Historically, typhoid was probably first differentiated from typhus (*see* p. 248) in the early or mid 19th century.

S. typhi is a Gram-negative, flagellated, non-encapsulated, non-sporulating, facultative anaerobic bacillus. Although it exists worldwide, most infections occur in 'Third World' countries where standards of sanitation and hygiene are defective and the disease is endemic. In England and Wales, approximately 200 cases are presently diagnosed annually of which some 80% are 'imported'. Contaminated food or water is the usual source of infection; *S. typhi* can survive for several weeks in water, dust, clothing, etc. The organisms are concentrated in shellfish. Epidemiologically, human carriers are important; this state increases in the elderly, in those with gall bladder disease, and in the presence of sickle-cell (SS) disease, urinary tract schistosomiasis, and bartonellosis. Hypochlorhydria is a predisposing factor to infection. After initial passage through the small intestinal mucosa with lymphatic and haematogenous carriage, *S. typhi* is taken up by the reticuloendothelial system (including the liver and spleen) in which it multiplies. Peyer's patches are involved in the first week of the disease (i.e. after an incubation period of 7–14 days); later, healing without residual lesions occurs, or ulcers with haemorrhage or perforation may complicate the disease. There is widespread involvement of other organs; the pathogenesis of the lesions of typhoid is unclear.

Clinically, presentation is variable but fever and headache are usual; many factors underlie the severity of disease: the size of infecting dose, nutritional and immunological status, etc. Other symptoms, including constipation (and rarely dysentery) are common; hepatosplenomegaly or splenomegaly, a relative bradycardia, 'rose spots' on the trunk, and other system involvement may be present. Untreated, fever usually resolves in the third week by lysis; it is then that ileal perforation and haemorrhage may occur. Neuropsychiatric symptoms, the pathogenesis of which is unknown, cardiovascular, hepatobiliary involvement, (with jaundice) and renal complications are rare occasional complications. Cholecystitis, osteomyelitis and soft tissue abscesses may also occur. Approximately 20% of patients excrete *S. typhi* for 2 months, and a small minority become carriers.

Diagnosis is from many other febrile illnesses and PUOs (*see* Chapter 1). Leucopenia and reduced platelet count is usual; transaminases are usually mildly elevated. *S. typhi* is most easily isolated from a bone marrow aspirate; blood culture is only second best. The 'Enterotest' (*see* p. 27) gives a high percentage of positive results; a rectal swab may be of value. Serological tests are frequently difficult to interpret; newer techniques for detecting *S. typhi* antigen in blood and urine seem promising. Prompt treatment should reduce the mortality rate to less than 1%; however, rates of up to 30% are still common in developing country hospitals.

Chloramphenicol (50 mg/kg) continued for 10 days after 'defervescence' which usually takes 4–5 days is the most effective and cheapest antibiotic. Courses of similar length with trimethoprim-sulphamethoxazole (6·5–10 mg/kg), amoxycillin (75–100 mg/kg) or ampicillin (100–150 mg/kg) also give good results but are inferior to chloramphenicol. Some *S. typhi* strains are resistant to multiple antibiotics. In severe cases, corticosteroids are of proven value. For the carrier state, high dose amoxycillin (100 mg/kg/day for at least 28 days) should be combined with probenecid. Complications must be treated on merit; ileal perforation should in most cases be managed surgically. Monovalent typhoid vaccination gives some protection to travellers in endemic areas (*see* Chapter 17); oral vaccines are undergoing clinical trials.

Brucellosis

This is a zoonosis (sheep, goats, cattle and pigs are affected) which is accompanied by sweating, muscle pains, arthritis and splenomegaly. The causative organism which occurs worldwide was first isolated by Sir David Bruce in 1886 in Malta. It is caused by several related bacteria (small Gram-negative, non-motile, non-spore forming rods), most importantly *Brucella melitensis*, *B. abortus* and *B. suis*. In the UK, *B. abortus* is the sole cause. Infected raw milk and milk products are the usual sources of human infection; person-to-person transmission is rare. It is an occupational disease. Rarely it is acquired by inhalation or inoculation. After lymphatic and haematogenous spread, bacteria localise in the reticuloendothelial system where granulomas form in many organs; further haematogenous spread results in symptomatic disease. Incubation period varies from a few days to many months; it frequently presents as a PUO (*see* Chapter 1), and causes intermittent febrile episodes with arthralgias and sweating. Splenomegaly, and occasionally lymphadenopathy and swollen joints may be present. Most cases recover spontaneously within 1 year. However, if chronic disease results, bone and joint complications, particularly spondylitis of the lumbar spine (with narrowing of the intervertebral spaces), are a major problem. Neurological and psychiatric sequelae may also occur and other system involvement includes: endocarditis, genitourinary complications, hepatitis and pneumonia.

Diagnosis is based on culture of the organism from blood or bone marrow; however, these may be negative in chronic disease. Leucopenia and a rising agglutination titre are rarely diagnostic. Detection of IgG antibodies is of value in chronic disease.

Oral tetracycline (500 mg q.d.s. for 21 days) is the treatment of choice, and in chronic and complicated disease, the addition of streptomycin (1 g daily for 10 days) usually produces a cure. In a minority, relapse occurs and further courses of antibiotic are necessary.

Spirochaetal diseases

Leptospirosis and syphilis are covered in Chapters 6 and 12 respectively. Yaws (caused by *Treponema pertenue*) and pinta (by *T. carateum*) are basically dermatological diseases (*see* Chapter 13).

Lyme disease

This occurs worldwide (including the UK) and is caused by the spirochaete *Borrelia burgdorferi* carried by ixodid ticks. Skin (erythema chronicum migrans), CNS, myocardium and joints are affected. The disease was first described in the USA (at Lyme, Connecticut) in 1977. Systemic symptoms and signs last from 2–10 weeks. The lesions can be divided into phase 1 (skin), phase 2 (neurological or cardiac) and phase 3 (established arthritis). An oligoarthritis involves the larger joints, and the most common neurological finding is a meningoencephalitis; conduction defects (usually an AV block) may sometimes be present in an ECG. Isolation of the organism from blood, skin and CSF, together with serological tests (specific IgM and IgG) are of value in diagnosis. Treatment is with penicillin and tetracycline; however, recurrent episodes of headache, and joint and muscle pains become chronic in about 50% of patients.

Relapsing fevers

These comprise two febrile illnesses: epidemic (louse-borne) which is caused by *Borrelia recurrentis*, and endemic (tick-borne) by *B. duttoni*. They are distributed worldwide in both temperate and tropical regions; Australia, New Zealand and Oceania are apparently not affected. The epidemic disease occurs most commonly in Africa, Asia and south America, while the endemic one is more widely spread. The incubation period is from 4–18 days, and symptoms begin while the spirochaetes, which are localised to the blood and reticuloendothelial systems, are dividing, having first achieved a sufficiently high concentration. The organisms themselves are pyrogenic. A Jarisch–Herxheimer reaction can occur spontaneously or during treatment (*see* p. 204); fatality rates are then at their highest.

Clinically, apart from an abrupt onset of intermittent fever lasting for 2–6 days and separated by 7–9 days, there is headache, generalised systemic symptoms, hepatosplenomegaly, a petechial rash and sometimes jaundice. Hypotension and jaundice are bad prognostic signs. Spirochaetes are visible in peripheral blood films; abnormal liver function tests, proteinuria and microscopic haematuria are frequently present. A thrombocytopenia results from sequestration of platelets in bone marrow. Although usually self-limiting, high mortality rates have occasionally been reported in epidemics of louse-borne disease.

Tetracycline and erythromycin are of value in treatment; a single oral dose of either antibiotic is probably adequate. Penicillin G produces a much slower reduction in the spirochaete concentration.

Rat-bite fevers

These are caused by *Streptobacillus moniliformis* and *Spirillum minor*; the consequent illnesses have been named Haverhill fever and Sodoku, respectively. They occur worldwide, are caused by bites, scratches or mere contact with rodents or their predators, and produce a febrile illness with regional lymphadenopathy, myalgia, arthropathy, and other systemic symptoms and signs. Treatment is with penicillin.

Plague

This has a reservoir in rodents, especially rats (*Rattus rattus*) and is caused by a Gram-negative cocco-bacillus, *Yersinia pestis*; it is spread from rat to rat by the flea *Xenopsylla cheopsis*. It is now a very rare disease although small epidemics occurred in south-east Asia in the 1970s. After an incubation period of 2–6 days, inguinal and other lymph glands may become tender and the patient febrile ('bubonic plague'); following a haemorrhagic illness, death ensues (the 'Black Death'). If lung infection occurs (pneumonic plague) transmission from person to person is by respiratory droplets—'atishu! atishu! we all fall down' in the words of the 17th century nursery rhyme. According to the *Oxford Dictionary of Nursery Rhymes** 'ring-a-ring-a roses' might refer to the rash, and 'a pocket full of poses' to the herbs carried as a 'protective' measure against the disease. Diagnosis is by lymph node aspiration; *Y. pestis* may be isolated after prolonged culture. Streptomycin (30 mg/kg b.d. for 10 days) is the antibiotic of choice; chloramphenicol is also of value. Strict public health measures, including quarantine, are necessary to prevent spread of the disease.

Tularaemia

This is largely a north American disease caused by *Francisella tularensis*; it has a reservoir in many mammals. It is most common

---

*Opie I., Opie P., eds (1951). *Oxford Dictionary of Nursery Rhymes*. Oxford: Oxford University Press.

in butchers and hunters. The disease can be acquired from animal bites and scratches, tick bites, inhalation or ingestion. Skin ulceration, followed by regional lymphadenopathy, fever, headache and hepatosplenomegaly may occur. However, clinical manifestations are very variable. Culture of a biopsy from a skin lesion, guinea-pig inoculation, or demonstration of a rising antibody titre confirms the diagnosis. Streptomycin (0.5 g intramuscularly b.d. for 10 days) should be given.

Anthrax

This is a disease of sheep and cattle. In man it is an occupational disease in workers handling contaminated hides, hair and other cattle products, sheep wool or bone meal. Although now almost unknown in developed countries, it is still a problem in Asia and parts of Africa. The causative organism, *Bacillus anthracis*, is a Gram-positive, spore-forming bacillus which survives for many years in contaminated soil; herbivores become infected by ingesting the spores. Cutaneous anthrax is characterised by the 'malignant pustule'; organisms can be cultured from a swab of the lesion. Pulmonary anthrax is very rare and is acquired by inhalation of spores ('woolsorter's disease'). Following a septicaemia, infection is widely disseminated. Parenteral penicillin (1.2 g daily) is of value in the cutaneous form. Pulmonary disease is associated with a very high mortality rate.

Nocardiosis

Actinomyces infections are caused by branching Gram-positive bacilli. *Nocardia spp.* are weakly acid-fast and possess a Gram-positive beaded cocco-bacillary branching appearance; they cause subcutaneous lesions including Madura foot (*see* p. 218) and respiratory, renal, intestinal and CNS infections in the immunocompromised. Co-trimoxazole and erythromycin are effective.

Actinomycosis

Actinomyces israelii is an anaerobic Gram-positive bacillus which is not acid-fast. It is present in normal buccal flora; most infections are therefore probably endogenous. Cervicofacial, pulmonary and abdominal forms of the disease exist. The first produces an ulcerated suppurative lesion with sulphur granules and sinus formation in the neck; the jaw and facial bones can be involved. Pulmonary disease may involve the chest wall and produce discharging sinuses. The abdominal form involves the caecum and/or appendix; there may be local sinuses and portal venous spread to the liver sometimes occurs. In women, local infection can follow pelvic inflammatory disease, sometimes resulting from the use of an intrauterine device. The organism can be isolated from swabs from affected sites; a 'sulphur granule' should be selected for Gram-staining and prolonged anaerobic culture. Prolonged penicillin treatment (e.g. 3.0–6.0 g daily intramuscularly for 6 weeks, followed by 1.2–3.0 g orally for 3–12 months) is indicated. Local surgery may be necessary.

FUNGAL INFECTIONS (INCLUDING THE DEEP MYCOSES)

The superficial mycoses are covered in Chapter 13. Subcutaneous mycoses are acquired by the percutaneous implantation of organisms; multiplication takes place in the skin. The principal forms are: mycetoma (maduramycosis), sporotrichosis and chromomycosis. Less common infections are: subcutaneous zygomycosis, rhinosporidiosis, and phaeohyphomycosis. If unchecked, local tissue destruction is extensive; only in chromomycosis does widespread dissemination occur. The natural habitat of these organisms is in soil or vegetation; man is a non-essential, accidental host. The best-known example is 'Madura foot', first described in India in the mid 19th century. Advanced tissue invasion with sinus formation progresses to bone involvement and later destruction. Diagnosis is from direct smears and culture; in advanced chronic cases, serology is of value. Many therapeutic agents have been used including amphotericin B and 5-fluorocytosine; ketoconazole has recently given encouraging results. Formerly, amputation was frequently necessary.

Systemic or Deep Mycoses

The systemic or deep mycoses are a group of infections involving internal organs, e.g. lung and brain; some occur as opportunistic infections in the presence of compromised immunity. Histoplasmosis comprises two major diseases and is caused by related organisms: classical (small form) (*Histoplasma capsulatum*) and African (*H. duboisii*) histoplasmosis. The classical disease is widespread geographically and is acquired from bird or bat excreta, often present in caves; pulmonary and reticuloendothelial involvement are usual. In the African form, the portal of entry is the respiratory tract and cutaneous and bone lesions predominate. In the classical disease, a chest radiograph may show: hilar lymphadenopathy, and consolidation and/or bilateral mottling which sometimes later calcifies.

Coccidioidomycosis, blastomycosis and paracoccidioidomycosis are confined to the American continent. The former is characterised by pulmonary, meningitic, bony and disseminated lesions. Blastomycosis can produce cutaneous, bone and respiratory lesions; consolidation, fibrosis and cavitation, and less commonly pleural effusion and hilar lymphadenopathy may result. Paracoccidioidomycosis causes microcutaneous, pulmonary, lymphatic and mixed manifestations; disseminated disease also occurs. Amphotericin B has formed the basis of management, but ketoconazole is increasingly used.

Systemic Opportunistic Mycoses

Although the respiratory system and CNS are usually involved, disseminated disease caused by *Cryptococcus neoformans* may occur in the presence of immunosuppression (*see* Chapters 9 and 11). Aspergillosis (*see* Chapter 7) and candidiasis also can result in disseminated disease in the immunosuppressed. Mucormycosis (*Rhizopus, Absidia* and *Mucor*) is a further example. Treatment is with amphotericin B, 5-fluorocytosine or the imidazole compounds (ketoconazole or miconazole).

PROTOZOAL DISEASES

Toxoplasmosis

Toxoplasmosis is a generalised (multisystem) infection of man and many other species of animal. It is caused by the sporozoan *Toxoplasma gondii*; clinically, infection ranges from the asymptomatic to overwhelming disease in the immunocompromised (e.g. AIDS). Human prevalence rates, estimated by serological testing, show an increase with age and a great variation in different geographical areas; it is, for example, very common in France. The definitive host is the cat; oocysts are shed in faeces. Moist soil can thus be contaminated. Tissue cysts are present in intermediate hosts (e.g. sheep and pigs); they can be ingested in undercooked, infected meat. After ingestion of the cysts, a mild febrile illness with gastroenteritis often goes unnoticed and is followed by invasion of many organs including the lungs, liver, myocardium, muscles and brain; lymphadenopathy (cervical lymphadenopathy is most common) and sometimes splenomegaly persisting for several months may be present. The incubation period is 7–17 days. EBV and CMV infections and lymphoma should be excluded. Transplacental infection also is important in man; congenitally, infection causes numerous congenital defects, including choroidoretinitis and fetal death. An initial infection during the first trimester of pregnancy should therefore be avoided, but if evidence of this exists termination should be considered; subsequent infants will be free of congenital toxoplasmosis. In the immunocompromised, cerebral involvement resulting from relapse of a chronic infection is most important. In these chronic infections, tiredness and malaise are frequent symptoms.

Investigations reveal high or rising IgG and IgM toxoplasma antibodies; the dye test (which depends on lysis of toxoplasma by the patient's antibody in the presence of complement) is of greater value. CT scan and brain biopsy of patients with AIDS are sometimes necessary to confirm the diagnosis.

Treatment is rarely necessary. However, spiramycin (500–750 mg q.d.s. for 4–6 weeks in the adult) is the most satisfactory agent. Alternatively, sulphadiazine (75 mg) + pyrimethamine (500 mg q.d.s.) can be used; the main drawback with this regimen is occasional bone marrow depression. When choroidoretinitis is present concurrently, the latter regimen should be accompanied by corticosteroids.

Leishmaniasis

The causative protozoa exist in man as intracellular non-flagellated amastigotes. There are three major clinical forms of this disease:

(i) Visceral (Kala azar).
(ii) Cutaneous.
(iii) Mucocutaneous.

The two latter conditions are covered in Chapter 13.

Visceral leishmaniasis

The term Kala azar is an Indian one meaning *black fever*. Fig. 15.3 summarises the geographical distribution of this disease; it exists in foci in Africa, the Mediterranean littoral, the Middle-east, the Indian subcontinent and southern America. The protozoan parasite *Leishmania donovani*, is transmitted by the bite of the sandflies *Phlebotomus*, *Lutzomyia* and *Psychodopygus*. The life-cycle is straightforward. The three subspecies are: *L. donovani donovani* (India), *L. donovani infantum* (Mediterranean littoral, Middle-east, Africa and China), and *L. donovani chagasi* (South America). There is often a reservoir in canines and rodents but the one in man is probably underestimated.

Promastigotes are injected from the proboscis of a female sandfly into human skin; these in turn invade reticuloendothelial (RE) cells and transform into amastigotes which invade other RE cells. Transmission can also occur via blood transfusion. Clinically, the disease usually presents with a febrile illness some 2–3 months after the initial infection; this can however be delayed for 2 years or more. Many infections remain subclinical; host immune response varies enormously. Tiredness and malaise, resulting from the accompanying anaemia, and weight-loss (which may be severe) may also lead to the initial presentation. The patient is often markedly wasted, with a high swinging fever (sometimes with a double rise within each 24 h), anaemia, hepatosplenomegaly; sometimes lymphadenopathy is present also. Tuberculosis may be a complication. The differential diagnoses include many febrile conditions with anaemia and hepatosplenomegaly: malaria, tropical splenomegaly syndrome, trypanosomiasis, schistosomiasis, cirrhosis, myelofibrosis, etc.

Leishman–Donovan bodies (amastigotes) are demonstrable in a smear and culture of splenic aspirate, and later in bone marrow and liver biopsy. Although splenic puncture gives a higher yield of positive results a risk of haemorrhage exists because platelets are depressed and prothrombin time prolonged; many physicians therefore begin with a bone marrow biopsy. Although in India, a

264 *Communicable and Tropical Diseases*

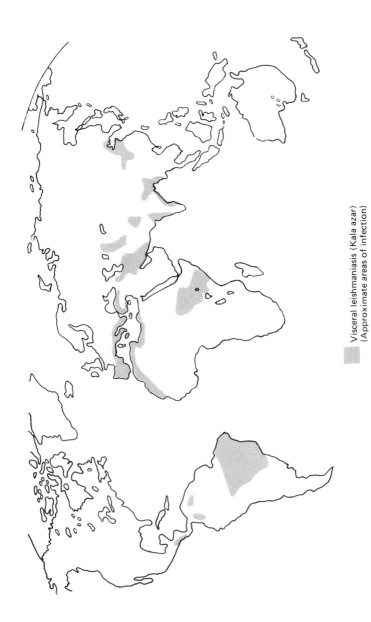

Fig. 15.3. Geographical distribution of visceral leishmaniasis (Kala azar).

buffy-coat smear from peripheral blood often yields amastigotes, this is unusual in other areas. Only rarely should treatment be started without a parasitological diagnosis. The serological tests using promastigote antigen (IFAT and ELISA) are strongly positive (titre > 1:256) in at least 95% of cases. A leishmanin skin test is negative in the acute disease but usually becomes positive 6 weeks to 1 year after recovery. Anaemia (often severe), leucopenia and impaired liver function tests are prominent features. A massive hypergammaglobulinaemia (consisting predominantly of IgG) is usually present. The serum albumin concentration may be depressed.

Untreated, the disease has a mortality rate of at least 70%. Recovery after starting treatment is usually rapid and the temperature falls within a week to 10 days; however, careful long-term follow-up is desirable. Treatment is with sodium stibogluconate ('Pentostam') (850 mg intravenously daily for 21 days in an adult of average weight). ECG changes are relatively common, but rarely serious; changes should be monitored twice weekly. The anaemia (usually predominantly iron-deficient) also requires treatment. Recovery is usually complete and relapse unusual, but should this occur, a second course of treatment is usually successful. Recently sodium stibogluconate has been combined with allopurinol, which inhibits *L. donovani* in *in vitro* studies. Targetted chemotherapy, using liposome-incorporated antimony compounds gives a higher concentration within the RE system. In resistant cases, splenectomy has rarely been carried out. Post Kala-azar dermal leishmaniasis is a complication which can last for up to 20 years; although common in India it is unusual in Africa and rare in China. Rashes appear on the face, extensor surfaces of the arms, trunk, and occasionally legs; nodules which sometimes resemble those of leprosy can be present.

South American Trypanosomiasis (Chagas' Disease)

Fig. 15.4 shows the geographical distribution of this disease which is confined to south, central and to a lesser extent north America. (For African trypanosomiasis *see* Chapter 9.) It is caused by *Trypanosoma cruzi* which is transmitted to man by the bite of the reduviid bug (*Triatoma infestans* and related species) which is found in the walls and roofs of rural houses. A large reservoir of infection is present in a wide range of mammals, including

266 *Communicable and Tropical Diseases*

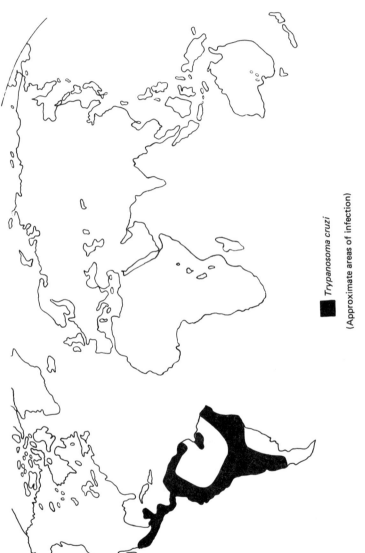

Fig. 15.4. Geographical distribution of *Trypanosoma cruzi* infection (Chagas' disease).

domestic dogs and cats. Congenital infection and transmission via breast milk occasionally occur. Accidental laboratory infection and via a contaminated blood transfusion are other possibilities.

The parasites multiply in the tissues, especially the heart and other muscles, in the amastigote phase. Cardiac damage probably results from an immune reaction, rather than a direct effect of the parasite; this also probably applies to autonomic nervous system damage. Clinically, an acute illness (usually before 10 years of age) often goes unnoticed; there may be a fever with hepatosplenomegaly and cardiac involvement. A classical sign which is not often seen in practice in the acute disease, is unilateral orbital oedema (Romaña's sign). Fever, tachycardia, hepatosplenomegaly and lymphadenopathy are frequently present; an arrhythmia and/or cardiac failure are bad prognostic signs. However, most cases manifest in adult life usually decades after the acute infection with chronic manifestations of the *mega* syndromes: megaoesophagus, megacolon (caused by abnormalities in the myogenic plexuses) and cardiomyopathy (often associated with conduction defects) (*see* Chapter 8). Dilatation of the stomach, gall bladder and urinary bladder has rarely been recorded.

Serological diagnosis (CFT) is valuable, although there is cross-reaction with African trypanosomiasis, leishmaniasis and mycobacterial infections. Xenodiagnosis, in which reduviid bugs are infected by the patient undergoing diagnosis is usually positive for several years after an acute infection; the diagnosis is established by demonstrating the organisms in the insect intestine after 25–30 days.

Treatment is unsatisfactory; nifurtimox ('Lampit') and benzonidazole ('Rochagan') have given encouraging results in the acute disease where parasitaemia is usually abolished, but xenodiagnostic tests often remain positive at follow-up. The value of these agents in the chronic disease is unclear. Conduction defects and arrhythmias are treated on merit; the megasyndromes occasionally require surgery. Control of infection is with insecticides; however, reduviid bugs are robust insects and are only eliminated with difficulty. Community participation is essential.

Babesiosis

This is a zoonotic protozoan infection which occurs rarely in Europe and northern America. The reservoir of infection is in both domestic and farm animals. Transmission of *Babesia spp.* is by *ixodid* ticks. It was the first organism shown to be transmitted by an arthropod, in Texas cattle fever in 1893. The protozoan is an intraerythrocytic one and therefore can be mistaken for one of the malaria parasites (*see* Chapter 4); there is no evidence of an exoerythrocytic cycle. Splenectomy predisposes to infection, as in malaria (and some other infections also, including pneumococcal disease), and contributes to a higher mortality rate. After an incubation period of 1–4 weeks, it causes a fever, haemolytic anaemia, haemoglobinuria and renal failure. The disease can continue for several months.

Diagnosis is by identification of parasites in blood films; serology is of value but there is some cross-reaction with malaria.

Quinine + clindamycin has been used in treatment but proper evaluation is required; in addition, exchange blood transfusion has been used.

HELMINTHIC DISEASES

Filariasis

There are four major filarial diseases of man, and they are all clinically very different:

(i) Lymphatic, which is caused by *Wuchereria bancrofti* and *Brugia malayi* (which is confined to Asia).
(ii) Onchocerciasis (or river blindness).
(iii) Dracontiasis (guinea-worm disease).
(iv) Loaiasis.

In addition, *Mansonella streptocerca* causes a chronic itching dermatitis associated with lymphadenopathy, and *M. perstans* and *M. ozzardi* a significant eosinophilia and only rarely significant symptoms. The adult worms do not replicate in man; therefore severe clinical manifestations usually occur only in indigenous people in endemic areas who are chronically and repeatedly infected.

Lymphatic filariasis

Fig. 15.5 summarises the world distribution of these diseases, which are transmitted by the bites of various species of mosquito

Systemic Infections 269

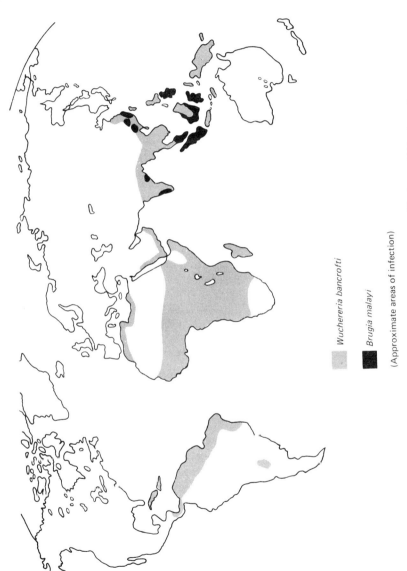

Fig. 15.5. Geographical distribution of the lymphatic filariases (*Wuchereria bancrofti* and *Brugia malayi*).

(including *Anopheles*). Larvae, which are introduced into the skin develop into adult worms within the lymphatics; here they produce microfilariae which enter the blood stream some 6 months to 1 year after the initial infection. Their presence may continue for 5–10 years. The life-cycle is completed by mosquitoes taking up microfilariae; these subsequently develop into larvae within this intermediate host. Progressive, chronic lymphatic obstruction gives rise to elephantiasis in the lower, and occasionally (especially with *B. malayi*) the upper limbs. Early on, recurrent episodes of adenolymphangitis and fever may be present, especially with a *B. malayi* infection. Similar obstruction to the ureteric and renal lymphatics diverts chyle to the urinary tract, and chyluria may be a significant (and impressive) clinical finding; although this gives rise to a substantial calorie loss, there are few other sequelae. Hydrocoele, orchitis and epididymitis are further complications. The tropical pulmonary eosinophilia (TPE) syndrome is a clinical manifestation which occurs especially in India and Sri Lanka (*see* Chapter 7); wheezing and breathlessness in the presence of a very high eosinophilia, raised IgE concentration, and mottled opacities on a chest radiograph, are the usual presenting features. This results either from a type-I allergic reaction to an occult filarial infection, or a more complex immunological reaction with immune-complex deposits and granuloma formation around dead microfilariae. Diagnosis of the lymphatic filariases is by identification of microfilariae in peripheral blood, usually at night (nocturnal periodicity); they are however absent in TPE.

The most sensitive technique for detecting microfilariae is by injection of peripheral blood directly through a nuclepore membrane (pore size 3–5 µm) filter. Serology (ELISA) is of great value in the active disease; however, by the time chronic sequelae have developed, this is usually negative.

Treatment is with oral diethylcarbamazine (DEC) (3 mg/kg body weight t.d.s. for 21 days). DEC reactions are caused either by direct toxicity of the drug or as a result of the rapid destruction of microfilariae, and can be reduced by starting with low dosage. Control depends on improved personal protection from mosquitoes, mass and/or selective treatment with DEC, and vector suppression.

Onchocerciasis

Onchocerciasis is transmitted by black flies (*Simulium*) which are commonly present beside fast flowing rivers especially in west Africa. Fig. 15.6 summarises the geographical distribution. Adult worms are present predominantly in the dermis and subcutaneous tissues of the pelvis. The initial lesion is a dermatitis. Pruritus and skin discoloration may result; dermal collagen is replaced by scar tissue ('hanging groins' may result from lymph node scarring). The formation of firm/hard nodules (containing a mass of adult worms) over a bony prominence is a further clinical manifestation. However, the most serious complications result from ophthalmic involvement, with punctate keratitis and pannus formation; blindness results in high percentages of affected individuals (15% or more) in villages where the disease is common. Corneal opacities, uveitis, choroidoretinal lesions, and optic neuritis, and atrophy can be produced. Eye lesions are directly and indirectly related to invasion by, and local death of microfilariae.

As in many other tropical infections, including leprosy, the immunological mechanisms involved are complex; cell-mediated immune (CMI) responses are present in those with active skin disease (who are actively killing their microfilariae), but absent in those in whom it is quiescent (but who also have a high peripheral microfilariae concentration). The mechanisms involved in the way in which adult worms are killed are poorly understood.

Diagnosis is by examination of skin snips from the scapula region and lower back (and also iliac crest and buttocks); occasionally, microfilariae are present in peripheral blood (especially after DEC treatment). A high eosinophil count and positive serology (ELISA) support the diagnosis. The Mazotti reaction consists of the production of transient dermal manifestations following 50 mg DEC given orally. Slit-lamp examination of the eyes is important and microfilariae may be visualised. A nodule may be removed for histological examination.

Treatment is also with DEC. Within minutes after taking DEC, an itchy rash with swollen lymph nodes and more importantly keratitis, iritis and retinopathy with permanent ocular damage, occasionally occur. On rare occasions, DEC is followed by peripheral circulatory collapse, breathlessness and coma; this is probably a result of a type-I allergic reaction to antigen released by the damaged microfilariae. Suramin (which is not without toxic properties) is necessary in addition if killing of the adult worms as well as the microfilariae is required. Long courses (3–4 weeks) of mebendazole and flubendazole have also given good results. Recently, ivermectin (0·2 mg/kg body weight as a single

272 Communicable and Tropical Diseases

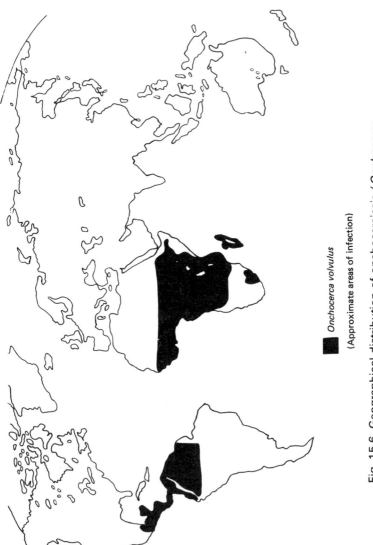

Fig. 15.6. Geographical distribution of onchocerciasis (*Onchocerca volvulus* infection).

■ *Onchocerca volvulus*
(Approximate areas of infection)

oral dose), which has few side-effects, has been used in west Africa; initial results are encouraging but further controlled trials are required. Vector control is of value.

Dracontiasis

This disease is confined to west Africa and India, with several minor foci in Africa and Asia (Fig. 15.7). The disease is contracted by ingestion of infected *Cyclops spp.* in contaminated drinking water; the WHO has recently launched water purification schemes to eradicate the disease. The adult female nematode *Dracunculus medinensis* (which is approximately 70 cm in length) grows in subcutaneous tissue, usually in the lower limbs. When mature, it presents with a painful blister usually on the foot, which gives rise to the emergence of approximately 5 cm of worm together with many thousands of larvae, which reinfect water. Secondary infection with cellulitis is common; this may affect one or more joints with the production of a septic arthropathy. Tetanus spores are occasionally introduced into the ulcer. Filarial serology may be positive, and there is usually an eosinophilia. The time-honoured method of treatment is slowly to remove the adult worm by winding it around a matchstick over several days thus drawing it out of the subcutaneous tissue. Thiabendazole is also of value, and metronidazole, niridazole and mebendazole have in addition been used. Provision of safe drinking water is the obvious prophylactic measure.

Loaiasis

This is the most benign of the four human filariases; it is confined to west and central Africa (Fig. 15.8). The vectors are tabanid flies of the genus *Chrysops*. Adult worms live in the subcutaneous tissues. Transitory subcutaneous (Calabar) swellings occur, especially over the dorsum of the hands. Generalised pruritus may be troublesome. Worms may occasionally wander across the eye subconjunctivally. Peripheral eosinophilia may be gross. Microfilariae are present in peripheral blood; maximum parasitaemia occurs at approximately mid-day. Treatment is with DEC (*see* p. 270). Dead worms may be outlined in subcutaneous tissue after treatment.

In all filarial infections, it is advisable to 'cover' the specific therapy with a short course of corticosteroid if the parasitaemia is very heavy.

274 Communicable and Tropical Diseases

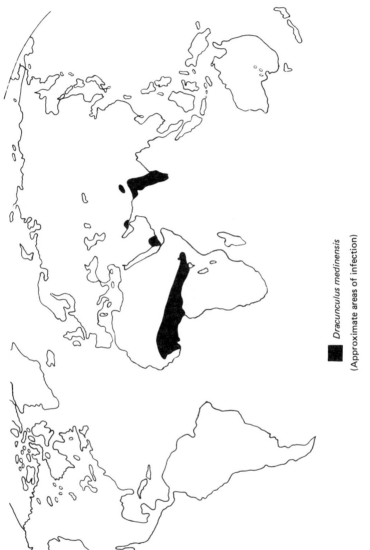

Fig. 15.7. Geographical distribution of dracontiasis (*Dracunculus medinensis* infection).

Systemic Infections 275

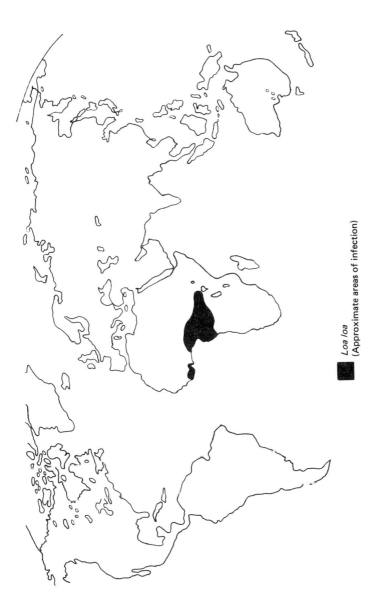

Fig. 5.8. Geographical distribution of loaiasis (*Loa loa* infection).

Toxocariasis

Toxocariasis is a common helminthic infection which is present worldwide, and is caused by *Toxocara canis* (acquired from dogs) and *T. cati* (from cats). The major importance of this disease is that it produces retinal lesions, which include choroidoretinitis and subsequent blindness. Adult nematodes live in the small intestine of infected animals; human infection occurs from ingestion of eggs in food and water contaminated by their faeces. Children are vulnerable to infection because eggs are ingested while sucking their fingers after playing in parks contaminated by dog faeces. After traversing the intestinal wall the migratory route is via the liver and thence to many other organs. Retinoblastoma is an important differential diagnosis of a retinal lesion. Hepatic, pulmonary and cerebral lesions are rarely encountered. The histological lesion is a granuloma which usually contains many eosinophils. An eosinophilia is frequently but not always present; serological tests usually include an ELISA and are positive. Both DEC and thiabendazole have been used in treatment, but neither has been adequately evaluated. Ophthalmic damage during treatment, caused by the larvae, can be minimised by local or systemic corticosteroids.

Trichinosis (Trichinellosis)

This is acquired by ingestion of *Trichinella spiralis* larvae which are present in the muscles of wild animals and domestic pigs. It is characterised by fever, gastrointestinal symptoms, myositis, swollen eyelids and a peripheral eosinophilia. Geographical distribution includes the USA and much of Africa and Asia. The larvae, which are resistant to gastric acid, mature to adults in the small intestinal wall. Production of larvae which are able to invade striated muscle throughout the body takes place here. During the intestinal phase, there may be a mild gastroenteritis; after some 7–9 days muscle invasion occurs. A febrile illness with myalgia, and sometimes associated with periorbital oedema, associated with an eosinophilia, following a meal of undercooked pork or game should suggest the diagnosis. 'Splinter haemorrhages', and muscle pain, and tenderness are accompanied by an eosinophilia. A myocarditis and respiratory muscle involvement may also occur. Neurological symptoms may also be present. Although unusual, a fatal outcome in heavy infections results usually from a myocarditis, encephalitis or pneumonitis. Larvae may be detected in small intestinal biopsy specimens during the intestinal phase. Skeletal muscle biopsy is of value later, but a negative result does not exclude the diagnosis. Serology using the ELISA technique is of value. Thiabendazole is of value in the initial stage; in the stage of muscle involvement, mebendazole + corticosteroids are usually combined. The disease is self-limiting and recovery usually occurs within a few months. Avoidance of undercooked meat, including pigs and warthogs in Africa, and polar and black bears in Arctica and the USA, respectively, forms the basis of prevention.

Other Helminths

Gnathostomiasis (caused by *Gnathostoma spinigerum*) and angiostrongyliasis (by *Angiostrongylus cantonensis*) can both cause systemic disease involving many organs. Involvement of the central nervous system can occur in both *G. spinigerum* and *A. cantonensis* infections. *A. costaricensis* causes ileocaecal disease. In both infections, an eosinophilia is frequently present.

FURTHER READING

Association of Clinical Pathologists, Symposium. (1980). Septic shock. *J. Clin. Path*; **33**: 888–96.
Al-Awadi A. R., Al-Kazemi N., Ezzat G., *et al.* (1982). Murine typhus in Kuwait in 1978. *Bull. WHO*; **60**: 283–9.
Banatvala J. E. (1986). Lassa fever. *Brit. Med. J*; **293**: 1256–7.
Burgdorfer W., Barbour A. G., Hayes S. F., *et al.* (1982). Lyme disease—a tick-borne spirochetosis? *Science*, **216**: 1317–19.
Cook G. C. (1985). Management of typhoid. *Tropical Doctor*; **15**: 154–9
Editorial. (1984). Tick-borne borrelia. *Lancet*; **2**. 1134–5.
Editorial. (1985). EBV and persistent malaise. *Lancet*; **1**: 1017–18.
Editorial. (1985). The lymphatic filariases. *Lancet*; **1**: 1135–6.
Editorial. (1986). Enervating illness in Epstein–Barr virus. *Lancet*; **2**: 141–2.
Editorial. (1986). Loa loa—a pathogenic parasite. *Lancet*; **2**: 554.
Editorial. (1986). Yellow fever in Africa. *Lancet*; **2**: 1315–16.
Editorial. (1987). Lymphatic filariasis—tropical medicine's origin will not go away. *Lancet*; **1**: 1409–10.
Editorial. (1987). Monkeypox in Africa: future health hazard or public health nuisance? *Lancet*; **1**: 369.
Editorial. (1987). The known and the unknown about dengue fever. *Lancet*; **1**: 488–9.

Emond R. T. D. (1986). Viral haemorrhagic fevers. *J. Infect*; **13**: 103–6.
Fergusson R. J., Shaw T. R. D., Kitchin A. H., *et al*. (1985). Subclinical chronic Q fever. *Q. J. Med*; **57**: 669–76.
Gajdusek D. C., Zigas V. (1959). Kuru: clinical, pathological and epidemiological study of an acute progressive degenerative disease of the central nervous system among natives of the Eastern Highlands in New Guinea. *Am. J. Med;* **26**: 442–69.
Giasuddin A. S. M., Idoko J. A., Lawande R. V. (1986). Tropical pyomyositis: is it an immunodeficiency disease? *Am. J. Trop. Med. Hyg*; **35**: 1231–4.
Glover S. C. (1987). Lyme disease—another spirochaetal mimicker? *J. Infect*; **14**: 99–102.
Greene B. M., Taylor H. R., Cupp E. W., *et al*. (1985). Comparison of ivermectin and diethylcarbamazine in the treatment of onchocerciasis. *N. Engl. J. Med*; **313**: 133–8.
Hausen H. zur. (1986). Intracellular surveillance of persisting viral infections. *Lancet*; **2**: 489–91.
Haywood A. M. (1986). Patterns of persistent viral infections. *N. Engl. J. Med*; **315**: 939–48.
Helmick C. G., Webb P. A., Scribner C. L., *et al*. (1986). No evidence for increased risk of Lassa fever infection in hospital staff. *Lancet*; **2**: 1202–5.
Matthews W. B. (1981). Slow virus infections. *J. R. Coll. Physns*; **15**: 109–12.
Muhlemann M. F., Wright D. J. M. (1987). Emerging pattern of Lyme disease in the United Kingdom and Irish Republic. *Lancet*; **1**: 260–62.
Palmer S. R., Young S. E. J. (1982). Q-fever endocarditis in England and Wales, 1975–81. *Lancet*; **2**: 1448–9.
Parke A. (1987). From New to old England: the progress of Lyme disease. *Brit. Med. J*; **294**: 525–6.
Rao L. S., Hardy J. G., Wilson C. G. (1983). Tissue distribution and fate of free and liposome-encapsulated (^{125}Sb) sodium stibogluconate by gamma scintigraphy. *Int. J. Pharmaceutics*; **17**: 283–90.
Spelman D. W. (1982). Q fever: A study of 111 consecutive cases. *Med. J. Aust*; **1**: 547–53.
Stuart F. A. (1982). Comparison of rifampicin and tetracycline based regimens in the treatment of experimental brucellosis. *J. Infect*; **5**: 27–34.
Teklu B., Habte-Michael A., Warrell D. A., *et al*. (1983). Meptazinol diminishes the Jarisch–Herxheimer reaction of relapsing fever. *Lancet*; **1**: 835–9.
Teutsch S. M., Juranek D. D., Sulzer A., Dubey J. P., Sikes R. K. (1979). Epidemic toxoplasmosis associated with infected cats, *N. Engl. J. Med*; **300**: 695–9.
Watts R. A., Hoffbrand B. I., Paton D. F., Davis J. C. (1987). Pyomyositis associated with human immunodeficiency virus infection. *Brit. Med. J*; **294**: 1524–5.
Wirth D. F., Rogers W. O., Barker R. (1986). Leishmaniasis and malaria: new tools for epidemiologic analysis. *Science*; **234**: 975–9.

Chapter Sixteen

Antibiotics and Other Antimicrobial Agents

A delicate balance of varying precision exists between the action of agents used in the prophylaxis and treatment of an infection, albeit it viral, bacterial, fungal, protozoan or helminthic, and their effect(s) on the human host. Therefore antimicrobial agents can ideally be administered to man with reasonable safety, but with severe 'toxic' effects on the infective organism. Only a well-conducted clinical trial can establish the exact nature of this balance. Whereas some therapeutic agents are *bactericidal*, many others are *bacteriostatic* and in this latter case the host's defence mechanisms are of crucial importance in the final elimination of the infective agent. Bactericidal activity is also dependent on the concentration of the drug achieved in human tissues. When host defence mechanisms are compromised, e.g. in the presence of immunosuppression and AIDS (*see* Chapter 11), it is essential that a *cidal* compound is used against the opportunistic infection(s); such an agent is also required in the chemotherapy of a life threatening disease, e.g. infective endocarditis.

Table 16.1 summarises some of the specific sites at which chemotherapeutic agents exert their major impact. Penicillin, for example, interrupts synthesis of the bacterial cell wall during division; it is therefore, ineffective against mycoplasmas, which do not possess a cell wall. Sulphonamides (which are not only used against bacteria but also, in combination with other agents, against malaria parasites) inhibit folic acid synthesis; although man can utilise dietary folic acid to synthesise purines and pyrimidines (which are necessary for nucleic acid synthesis), bacteria cannot. Many bacteria can actually synthesise folic acid by metabolising *p*-aminobenzoic acid to dihydrofolic and subsequently tetrafolic acid. Because sulphonamides are similar structurally to *p*-aminobenzoic acid, when present in excess they are taken up in preference to this compound and this results in a

Table 16.1
SITE OF ACTION OF SOME CHEMOTHERAPEUTIC AGENTS

Site of action	Example (bactericidal unless stated)	Mode of action—interference with:
Nucleic acid replication	Rifampicin	RNA replication
	Nalidixic acid, Ciprofloxacin	DNA replication
	Metronidazole	DNA replication
	5-Fluorocytosine, Griseofulvin	Nucleic acid synthesis in certain fungi
	Idoxuridine, Cytarabine	DNA synthesis in DNA viruses
Ribosomes	Tetracycline	Transfer RNA and protein synthesis
	Chloramphenicol*	Translocation
	Erythromycin†, Lincomycin†, Fusidic acid†	Translocation and protein synthesis
	Aminoglycosides	mRNA attachment to ribosome
Cytoplasmic membrane	Polymyxins	(Affinity for membrane of Gram-negative bacteria)
	Amphotericin B*, Nystatin*	(Affinity for 'sterol' in fungal membrane)
Cell wall	Bacitracin, Vancomycin	Peptidoglycan formation
	β-lactams (penicillin, ampicillin, cloxacillin, cephalosporins)	Cross-linkages of peptidoglycan molecules

* Static only; † Static at low, but cidal at high concentration

blocking of folic acid synthesis. In purine synthesis, dihydrofolate reductase is inhibited by trimethoprim; although a similar enzyme exists in man, trimethoprim has a far greater affinity for the bacterial enzyme.

Some chemotherapeutic agents (Table 16.2) have a 'narrow' spectrum of activity; penicillin is most active against Gram-positive bacteria, while streptomycin, gentamicin and the other aminoglycosides are very largely active against Gram-negative bacteria. Metronidazole is active against anaerobic bacteria and also some protozoa. However, 'broad' spectrum antibiotics (Table 16.3), which include tetracyclines, ampicillin and the cephalosporins, are active against a wide range of bacteria (both Gram-positive and Gram-negative).

Most parasitic infections come under the tropical 'umbrella' because this is where their major impact lies. Unfortunately the pharmaceutical industry (with certain exceptions) does not readily finance research into these agents because sales to 'Third World' countries are limited, and the field is unrewarding financially.

PHARMACODYNAMICS OF ANTIMICROBIAL AGENTS

It is important to understand those factors which determine the concentration of a therapeutic agent at any given site of infection. Age and weight of the individual, adequacy of hepatic and renal function and the possible coexistence of a dialysis procedure must all be taken into account. During pregnancy, those agents which can adversely influence fetal development must be clearly recognised.

The safest route of administration is always by mouth. Intestinal absorption is, however, influenced by many factors; some have not been fully elucidated. In severe disease, absorption is sometimes compromised, and it is then wise to initiate therapy by the parenteral route. Some agents, e.g. vancomycin and amphotericin B, can only be given intravenously. Serum concentration, plasma protein and tissue binding, half-life of the compound, and its concentration at the infection site are all important. Distribution and bioavailability are especially important in certain situations, e.g. whereas a lipid-soluble compound (e.g. chloramphenicol) is widely distributed and easily crosses the blood–brain barrier (BBB), a water-soluble one remains localised in the plasma and extracellular fluid. Penicillins and cephalosporins only penetrate the BBB when meningococcal irritation is present, or when potentially toxic doses are administered. Table 16.4 summarises some agents which are influenced by impaired renal and hepatic

Table 16.2

APPROXIMATE RANGE OF ANTIBACTERIAL ACTIVITY OF SOME 'NARROW' SPECTRUM ANTIMICROBIALS

Antibiotic	Cocci Gram +	Cocci Gram −	Bacilli Gram +	Bacilli Gram −	Others
Penicillin	Strep. pyogenes Strep. pneumoniae	N. meningitidis N. gonorrhoeae	C. diphtheriae L. monocytogenes	P. multocida Vincent's organisms	Treponemes
Phenethicillin (penicillinase-sensitive)	Strep. viridans Staph. aureus* Anaerobic cocci		Clostridium spp.	B. necrophorus	Leptospira spp.
Cloxacillin: Flucloxacillin Methicillin (penicillinase-resistant)	Staph. aureus				
Fusidic acid	Staph. aureus				
Macrolide: Erythromycin	Staph. aureus Strep. pyogenes Strep. pneumoniae Strep. viridans		C. diphtheriae Propionibacterium acnes	Campylobacer spp. Legionella spp.	Mycoplasma pneumoniae
Lincosamides: Clindamycin/ lincomycin	Staph. aureus Strep. pyogenes				
Novobiocin	Staph. aureus Streptococci				

Vancomycin	Staph. aureus Strep. viridans	Clostridium difficile
Aminoglycosides: Streptomycin Kanamycin Gentamicin Tobramycin Amikacin	Staph. aureus	E. coli Klebsiella spp. Proteus spp. Other coliforms Pseudomonas aeruginosa M. tuberculosis
Polymyxins		Pseudomonas aeruginosa Other coliforms
Quinolones: Nalidixic acid Ciprofloxacin		E. coli Other coliforms
Amidino-penicillin: Mecillinam		E. coli Klebsiella spp. Other coliforms Salmonella spp.
Nitroimidazole compounds: Metronidazole Tinidazole	Anaerobic cocci	Clostridium spp. Bacteroides fragilis Bacteroides necrophorus Bacteroides melaninogenicum Fusiforms

* = Active against a minority of strains only.

Table 16.3
APPROXIMATE RANGE OF ANTIBACTERIAL ACTIVITY OF SOME 'BROAD' SPECTRUM ANTIMICROBIALS

Antibiotic	Cocci Gram +	Cocci Gram −	Bacilli Gram +	Bacilli Gram −	Others
Tetracyclines	Strep. pneumoniae Strep. pyogenes Staph. aureus	N. gonorrhoeae	Clostridium spp. P. acnes	Haemophilus influenzae Other coliforms Brucella spp. Yersinia spp. Vibrio cholerae (El-tor)	Mycoplasma pneumoniae Coxiella burnettii Chlamydia trachomatis Chlamydia psittaci
Chloramphenicol	Staph. aureus Strep. pneumoniae	N. meningitidis		Haemophilus influenzae Salmonella typhi E. coli, Other coliforms Bacteroides fragilis	Rickettsia
Ampicillin Amoxycillin Pivampicillin	Strep. pneumoniae Strep. pyogenes Strep. faecalis Staph. aureus*	N. gonorrhoeae N. meningitidis	L. monocytogenes C. diphtheriae Clostridium spp.	Haemophilus influenzae E. coli Other coliforms*	
Antipseudomonal penicillin: Carbenicillin Azlocillin	Streptococci			Pseudomonas aeruginosa* Enterobacter spp. Proteus spp.	

Antibiotics and Other Antimicrobial Agents 285

Cephalosporins	Strep. pyogenes Strep. pneumoniae Staph. aureus	N. gonorrhoeae		E. coli Klebsiella spp. Other coliforms
Trimethoprim (used also in combination with sulphamethoxazole, as 'Co-trimoxazole')	Staph. aureus Streptococci	Neisseria spp.		Haemophilus influenzae E. coli Klebsiella spp. Other coliforms* Salmonella typhi
Sulphonamides	Staph. aureus Streptococci	N. meningitidis		E. coli Other coliforms*
Nitrofurantoin	Staph. saprophyticus			E. coli Other coliforms*
Rifampicin	Staphylococci Streptococci	N. meningitidis	Clostridium spp.	E. coli Other coliforms* Salmonella typhi	M. tuberculosis

* = Only some strains are sensitive

Table 16.4

SOME EXAMPLES OF ANTIMICROBIAL AGENTS THE CONCENTRATION OF WHICH IS INFLUENCED BY DEFECTIVE RENAL, HEPATIC AND BILIARY METABOLISM AND/OR EXCRETION

Renal excretion (dose must be reduced in the presence of renal insufficiency)	Sulphonamides Trimethoprim Penicillins Cloxacillin Mecillinam Aminoglycosides Cephalosporins Nitrofurantoin Nalidixic acid Polymyxin Amphotericin B
Hepatic metabolism (dose must be reduced in the presence of hepatic insufficiency)	Fusidic acid Lincomycin Chloramphenicol Metronidazole Rifampicin ⎫ De-acetylated Isoniazid ⎭
Biliary–faecal excretion (bile concentration is reduced in biliary obstruction)	Ampicillin* Erythromycin Novobiocin Rifampicin

* = This agent is partly excreted by the kidneys, also; this is important in treatment of the typhoid carrier-state.

function. Interaction between therapeutic agents is a further factor which requires careful evaluation. An unnecessarily long course of an antibiotic increases the likelihood of serious side-effects.

ANTIMICROBIAL SENSITIVITY AND RESISTANCE

The causes of antibiotic resistance include:

(i) Natural (innate) resistance for one or another reason.
(ii) Acquired resistance which can either be acquired as a result of drug-destroying enzymes or intrinsic mechanisms

(e.g. the development of an alternative metabolic pathway).
(iii) Gradual adaptation (or tolerance).
(iv) Chromosomal mutation and selection of drug-resistant mutants.
(v) Transmissible drug resistance, much of which is R factor (plasmid)-mediated. (Plasmids are extra-chromosomal DNA packets which can code for antibiotic resistance and are subsequently transferred from an antibiotic-resistant to an antibiotic-sensitive strain, thus conferring resistance on the latter.)

Antibiotic resistance tends to be more common in developing countries, where overall antibiotics are badly used. This is related to many factors: the occurrence of drug-resistance plasmids, the pattern(s) of use of antibiotics in the immediate environment (in farm animals as well as man) and the degree of cross-infection with antibiotic-resistant strains.

Disc diffusion techniques are used to determine *in vitro* antibiotic sensitivity. However, this does not always correlate well with *in vivo* sensitivity. A 'tube dilution technique' (using different concentrations of antibiotic) can be used to determine the minimum inhibitory concentration (MIC) of an antibiotic for a given organism. Similarly the concentration required to kill the organism(s), the minimum bacterial concentration (MBC) can also be determined. Synergism or antagonism between two antibiotics can be tested *in vitro*; in *Strep. faecalis* endocarditis, for example, a confirmation of synergy between penicillin and an aminoglycoside is important in successful management. Serum bactericidal assay tests are carried out *in vitro* by incubation of the bacterial isolate with fresh serum samples obtained before, and after the start of antibiotic treatment. Antibiotic assays may also be undertaken to ascertain whether an adequate (or possibly toxic) concentration of the agent is present in serum at any particular time; gentamicin assay is frequently used to assess safety and effectiveness.

Clinical failure of antibiotic therapy has several causes:

(i) The clinical situation is not susceptible to the prescribed treatment.
(ii) Use of the laboratory is incorrect, i.e. specimens have not been properly collected and/or transported.

(iii) Laboratory failure, e.g. failure to identify correctly the relevant organism(s).
(iv) Incorrect selection of the antibiotic(s), and/or suboptimal dose, and/or duration of therapy.
(v) An antagonistic combination of antibiotics has been chosen, e.g. a bactericidal combined with a bacteriostatic agent.
(vi) The route of administration is incorrect.
(vi) Antibiotic resistance has developed.

ANTIBIOTIC PROPHYLAXIS

This is frequently excessively used, especially in surgical practice. When it is indicated, 'narrow' rather than 'broad' spectrum prophylaxis is desirable. Acceptable indications include:

(i) Rheumatic fever (*see* Chapter 8)—phenoxymethyl penicillin.
(ii) Meningococcal meningitis (*see* Chapter 9)—a sulphonamide or rifampicin.
(iii) Recurrent urinary tract infection (*see* Chapter 10)—cotrimoxazole or trimethoprim.
(iv) Prevention of endocarditis during dental and other surgical procedures (*see* Chapter 8)—penicillin or amoxycillin.
(v) Preparation for colorectal surgery—metronidazole.
(vi) Specialist surgical operations, including orthopaedic, gynaecological, vascular, biliary tract and urological procedures.

ANTIBACTERIAL AGENTS

Mercury has been used in the treatment of syphilis since 1495, and salvarsan (an arsenical preparation) since 1911. However, it was not until 1935 that Domagk published the results of his experiments with prontosil (the first of the sulphonamides). Antibacterial properties of penicillin (a product of the mould *Penicillium notatum*) were first recognised in 1928 by Fleming; the compound was subsequently concentrated by Florey and Chain, and subjected to clinical trials in 1941. Later, the β-lactam formula was established. Streptomycin (which paved the way for antituberculosis treatment), was first isolated in 1944 by Waksman from the fungus *Streptomyces griseus* (*see* Chapter 3). This discovery was followed by the isolation and synthesis of chloramphenicol in 1947–49, and aureomycin in 1948. Dapsone was the first agent to be used against *Mycobacterium leprae*; it is still widely used in tropical countries (*see* Chapter 14). These early antibiotics and other antibacterials were the forerunners of many others (*see* p. 282–5).

Tables 16.2 and 16.3 (pp. 282–3, 284–5) summarise some clearcut indications for the use of various antibiotics. Benzylpenicillin and phenethicillin are readily hydrolysed by β-lactamases; they are therefore inactive against most strains of *Staph. aureus*. Cloxacillin and flucloxacillin are valuable against β-lactamase producing organisms but have less potent antibacterial properties. 'Broad' spectrum penicillin derivatives (e.g. ampicillin, amoxycillin and pivampicillin) are readily hydrolysed by β-lactamases, and are therefore ineffective against many skin and soft tissue infections. Clavulanic acid is a β-lactamase inhibitor, which when combined with a penicillinase-sensitive antibiotic covers a wider range of organisms. The oral cephalosporins (about 10% of individuals 'allergic' to penicillin are allergic to these agents) are valuable in urinary tract infections where the organisms are resistant to ampicillin, and against other penicillin and ampicillin resistant bacteria. The antibacterial range of erythromycin (a macrolide antibiotic) is similar to that of penicillin; it can, however, be given to 'penicillin-allergic' patients. The new quinolone compounds (e.g. ciprofloxacin) possess a wide spectrum of activity ranging from resistant staphylococci to *Pseudomonas*; they promise to be of value in a wide range of diseases which includes bronchitis, cystitis, gonorrhoea and typhoid fever. Furthermore, these compounds will be less susceptible than the earlier ones to plasmid-mediated resistance.

Several points should be established before an antibiotic is prescribed for a bacterial infection:

(i) The presence of sufficient *clinical* evidence of a bacterial infection.
(ii) The justification or necessity for administration of an antibiotic in this clinical situation.
(iii) The fact that all relevant specimens (blood, urine, faecal sample, etc) have been obtained for culture before initiation of treatment.
(iv) The correct decision on the most appropriate (ideally a

'narrow' spectrum) (Table 16.2, p. 282–3) antibiotic for this *clinical* situation has been made.

Previous antibiotic therapy should always be taken into account. Pharmacodynamic characteristics of the therapeutic agent (*see* p. 281) must also be considered: fusidic acid effectively penetrates bone or an abscess wall, while chloramphenicol crosses the BBB. Other facts should include: (i) antibiotic 'allergy' (e.g. penicillin), and (ii) whether the patient is a child or pregnant woman, when tetracycline and sulphonamides are in most circumstances contraindicated. Clearly, the antibiotic(s) may well have to be changed subsequently, in the light of results of sensitivity testing.

Although a 'narrow' spectrum antibiotic (Table 16.2, p. 282–3) should ideally be used for a Gram-negative bacillary infection, a 'broad' spectrum agent (Table 16.3, p. 284–5), e.g. ampicillin, cotrimoxazole or a cephalosporin, may be selected because the agent of choice, e.g. an aminoglycoside or polymyxin, is potentially toxic.

Certain combinations of antibiotics may exert special effects: e.g. two *cidal* agents may produce synergism, two *static* ones an additive effect, whereas a *cidal* + *static* combination is likely to be antagonistic. In certain situations, combinations of antibiotics are often used however; these include:

(i) An infection where the nature of the organism(s) is unknown, e.g. abdominal sepsis, where gentamicin + metronidazole may be used against coliforms and *Bacteroides spp.* respectively.

(ii) A *severe* infection, where a synergistic combination is desirable, e.g. infective carditis, where penicillin + gentamicin may be used for a *Strep. faecalis* infection.

(iii) A situation where prevention (or possibly only delay) in 'resistance' is sought, e.g. antituberculosis regimens; three or four agents are often used simultaneously (*see* Chapter 3).

Fusidic acid + erythromycin may be prescribed for a *Staph. aureus*, and gentamicin + azlocillin for a *Pseudomonas* infection.

It is always important to appreciate that *in vitro* sensitivity testing by no means always correlates well with *in vivo* results in antibiotic chemotherapy.

Side-effects of Antibiotics

Tetracyclines should be avoided in childhood and pregnancy because they are incorporated into growing bone and teeth (which can become stained); with the exception of doxycycline and minocycline they are also contraindicated in renal failure. Erythromycin occasionally causes a cholestatic hepatitis. Cotrimoxazole rarely produces marrow depression via its sulphonamide component; however, when trimethoprim is administered alone (e.g. in urinary tract infections), these side-effects are eliminated and there is no convincing evidence of increased bacterial 'resistance'. Aminoglycosides may cause ototoxicity and nephrotoxicity; doses should therefore be reduced in renal failure (Table 16.4, p. 286). Lincosamides (clindamycin and lincomycin) are the most common causes of pseudomembranous colitis, a result of the toxin of *Clostridium difficile*; vancomycin and metronidazole are of value in management. Chloramphenicol produces marrow depression, rarely.

ANTIVIRAL AGENTS

Viruses are dependent upon biosynthetic processes in the host-cell for their unique replicative mechanisms. Therefore, the development of specific chemotherapy presents difficulties. Adenine arabinoside (of value in herpes infections) and interferon, which is now synthesised by DNA recombinant technology, have opened new avenues of exploration.

Table 16.5 summarises some currently available antiviral agents. Acycloguanosine ('Acyclovir') is still undergoing evaluation but is clearly of value in severe herpes and varicella-zoster infections. It is also of value in zoster pneumonitis in the immunosuppressed. Amantadine is effective against the influenza A virus; it is of value both as a prophylactic agent (where a 75% success rate has been recorded) and also in treatment of infection. However, neurological, psychiatric, gastrointestinal and cardiovascular side-effects and rashes have been recorded; it is contraindicated in pregnancy and in patients with central nervous system disorders. Methisazone is effective against DNA viruses, including vaccinia; it is of particular value in association with vaccinia immunoglobulin if this virus is accidentally inoculated into the eye. A further use is in eczema vaccinatum, where it is combined

Table 16.5
SOME SYSTEMIC AND TOPICAL ANTIVIRAL AGENTS

Antiviral agent	Susceptible virus(es)
Cytarabine	Herpes simplex
Vidarabine	Herpes simplex
Acycloguanosine*	Herpes simplex; varicella-zoster
Amantadine	Influenza A
Methisazone	Vaccinia, variola
Adenine arabinoside	Herpes simplex, varicella-zoster, HBV
Interferon*	'Broad-spectrum' agent, HBV
9-(1,3-dihydroxy-2-propoxymethyl)-guanine	Cytomegalovirus (in presence of immunodeficiency)
Ribavirin	Lassa fever
Azidothymidine (AZT)	AIDS and *Pneumocystis carinii* pneumonia
Suramin	AIDS (?)
Phosphonoformate	AIDS (?)
Idoxuridine†	Herpes simplex

* = These agents can be given topically as well as systemically; † = While usually given topically, this agent is rarely administered by the intravenous route.

with vaccinia immunoglobulin. Toxic effects involve the skin, hair and liver.

Adenine arabinoside ('Ara–A') and interferon are of value in herpes (including herpes simplex encephalitis) and varicella-zoster infections in immunosuppressed patients. Recently, encouraging results have been obtained in HBV infections progressing to chronicity, including HB_sAg positive chronic active hepatitis. Adenine arabinoside is less toxic than cytarabine and idoxuridine. Idoxuridine which is usually administered topically interferes with DNA synthesis and is of value in herpes and vaccinia infections. Its main value is in conjunctival and corneal infections caused by herpes simplex; extensive skin and mucosal lesions caused by varicella-zoster, and herpes simplex in immunosuppressed individuals also respond. It is, however, contraindicated in pregnancy and is too toxic for systemic use. Ribavirin has been shown to exert clear beneficial properties in individuals infected with Lassa fever.

Various agents have been used against virus infections in AIDS (*see* Chapter 11); the most promising agent to date is azidothymidine (AZT); further evaluation is required. Suramin and phosphonoformate have proved disappointing.

ANTIFUNGAL AGENTS

Treatment for both superficial and deep mycoses was formerly unsatisfactory.

Topical amphotericin and nystatin are of use in *Candida albicans* infections of the mouth and genitourinary tract. Griseofulvin (produced from *Penicillium griseofulvin*) is of value in superficial mycoses when given orally for long periods, but is of no value in the deep varieties. Toxic effects are rare.

The toxic compounds amphotericin B (produced from *Streptomyces nodosus*) and 5-fluorocytosine are effective in systemic infections. Used systemically in gradually increasing intravenous dosage, opportunistic infections with *Aspergillus*, *Candida*, *Cryptococcus spp.* and *Torulopsis glabrata* are responsive to amphotericin. In the Americas, *Histoplasma*, *Blastomyces* and *Coccidioides spp.* are amenable to treatment with this agent. It is, however, nephrotoxic (glomerular filtration is reduced in most patients on intravenous treatment) and also causes phlebitis and febrile drug reactions. The fluorinated pyrimidine compound 5-fluorocytosine, usually given orally, but occasionally intravenously, is effective against *Cryptococcus neoformans*, *Candida spp.*, *Torulopsis glabrata* and the causative agent of chromomycosis. It is often used in combination with amphotericin B for systemic infections to diminish the likelihood of mutant strains emerging. It is hepatotoxic, and bone marrow depression is a further problem. Dosage should be reduced in the presence of renal impairment. A 'narrow' spectrum synthetic antifungal agent, 2-hydroxystilbamidine is of value in the treatment of blastomycosis; rashes and hepatotoxicity have been reported.

Recently the imidazole compounds (e.g. miconazole and ketoconazole) have proved encouraging (Table 16.6). Clotrimazole and econazole are effective topically in *Candida albicans* skin and vaginal, and dermatophyte skin infections. The same applies to miconazole; this agent can also be administered intravenously,

Table 16.6

SOME ANTIFUNGAL AGENTS

Antifungal agent	Susceptible fungal species	Mode of administration*
Polyenes:		
Amphotericin B	*Candida albicans, Cryptococcus, Aspergillus, Histoplasma*	S/T
Nystatin	*Candida albicans*	T
Natamycin	*Candida albicans*	T
Griseofulvin	*Candida albicans, Histoplasma,* dermatophytes	S
5-Fluorocytosine	*Candida albicans, Cryptococcus*	S
2-Hydroxystilbamidine	Blastomycosis	S
Imidazoles:		
Clotrimazole	*Candida albicans,* dermatophytes	T
Econazole	*Candida albicans,* dermatophytes	T
Miconazole	*Candida albicans,* dermatophytes	S/T
Ketoconazole	South American *Coccidioidomycosis,* dermatophytes	S

*S = Systemic; T = Topical.

and is often used as a 'reserve' for amphotericin B in cryptococcus infection and coccidioidomycosis, when this agent has for some reason to be discontinued. It occasionally produces a mild phlebitis. The most recent of the group is ketoconazole (which was introduced in 1977); it is of value as a 'broad' spectrum agent in superficial candida and dermatophyte infections, histoplasmosis (north America), coccidioidomycosis and paracoccidioidomycosis (south America). It seems less effective in opportunistic disseminated aspergillus infections. It is relatively non-toxic.

ANTIPROTOZOAN AGENTS

Historically, anti-protozoan agents preceded the introduction of specific antibacterial drugs by several centuries. Qinghaosu had been used for malaria chemotherapy in China for many hundreds of years, and cinchona in southern America for at least 300 years (certainly before 1630). Ipecacuanha had for long been used in the treatment of 'tropical dysentery'; the beneficial effect resulted from the action of the alkaloid emetine (which has only recently been superseded by the nitroimidazoles) against the trophozoite of *Entamoeba histolytica*. Use of arsenic in the treatment of trypanosomiasis dates back to Ehrlich; suramin was introduced for this disease in 1920. The development of synthetic antimalarials was initiated in Germany in 1926; subsequently proguanil was synthesised in the UK at the 4888th attempt!

Recently, metronidazole (first used in *Trichomonas vaginalis* infections (Table 16.7)) and tinidazole have proved to be major advances in the treatment of amoebiasis and giardiasis. Various regimens including sulphadiazine + pyrimethamine, and spiramycin have proved moderately effective in toxoplasma infections. Cryptosporidiosis and related intestinal protozoan infections often respond to spiramycin, sulphadiazine + pyrimethamine, trimethoprim + sulphamethoxazole, nitrofurantoin + furazolidone, and paromomycin. Balantidiasis responds to tetracycline.

With the continuing emergence of *Plasmodium falciparum* resistance to multiple chemoprophylactic and chemotherapeutic agents, the search for new agents has intensified (*see* Chapter 4). Further work on qinghaosu, the halofantrines and the broad spectrum antibiotics (including erythromycin, clindamycin, spiramycin and paromomycin) is underway. Amphotericin B (*see* p. 293) is of value in free-living amoebic infections, which are not responsive to the usual antiprotozoal agents.

The treatment of opportunistic infections in AIDS presents a challenge of vast proportion. The intestinal organisms: *Cryptosporidium spp.*, *Isospora belli* and *Sarcocystis hominis* show little response; spiramycin is the most effective agent. Similarly, *Pneumocystis carinii* and *Toxoplasma gondii* respond poorly in this situation.

However, in all forms of leishmaniasis, pentavalent antimony compounds (sodium stibogluconate, 'Pentostam') still form the basis of management. Arsenicals also are still widely used in the treatment of African trypanosomiasis; melarsoprol ('Mel–B') is one example.

Table 16.7

SOME AGENTS USED IN PROTOZOAN INFECTIONS

Antiprotozoan agent	Susceptible protozoa
Metronidazole Tinidazole	*Entamoeba histolytica* *Giardia lamblia* *Trichomonas vaginalis*
Chloroquine	*Plasmodium falciparum, P. vivax, P. ovale, P. malariae*
Quinine Mefloquine Qinghaosu Halofantrines Various antibiotics	*P. falciparum*
Primaquine	*P. vivax, P. ovale*
Pyrimethamine + sulphadiazine	*Toxoplasma gondii, Cryptosporidium spp.*
Pentamidine + co-trimoxazole	*Pneumocystis carinii*
Trimethoprim + sulphamethoxazole	*Cryptosporidium spp.*
Nitrofurantoin + furazolidone	*Cryptosporidium spp.*
Paromomycin	*Cryptosporidium spp.*
Tetracycline	*Balantidium coli*
Spiramycin	*Toxoplasma gondii* *Cryptosporidium spp.*
Nifurtimox	South American trypanosomiasis
Pentavalent antimony compounds	Visceral and cutaneous leishmaniasis
Arsenicals	African trypanosomiasis

ANTHELMINTIC AGENTS

The male fern extract *Dryopteris filix-mas* has for long been used for the expulsion of cestodes, piperazine for some nematodes (including *Ascaris lumbricoides*), and a multiplicity of compounds for hookworm infection. Trivalent antimony compounds, already established in trypanosomiasis and leishmaniasis (*see* p. 295), were introduced for the treatment of schistosomiasis immediately after

World War I (1914–1918); for the next 50 years they were the most effective therapeutic agents in all forms of schistosomiasis.

Recently, the benzimidazoles—albendazole, mebendazole and thiabendazole—have proved effective in several intestinal nematode infections. In schistosomiasis, praziquantel, oxamniquine and metriphonate have proved effective and relatively non-toxic (Table 16.8). Treatment of the filariases however, remains unsatisfactory; diethylcarbamazine (DEC) is still widely used, and suramin is occasionally added for 'resistant' cases of

Table 16.8

SOME AGENTS USED IN HELMINTHIC INFECTIONS

Antihelminthic agent	Helminth infections
Mebendazole } Albendazole	*Acaris lumbricoides*, hookworm, *Trichuris trichiura*, *Enterobius vermicularis*, *Capillaria philippinensis*, trichostrongyliasis, hydatid disease
Thiabendazole	*Strongyloides stercoralis*, *Dracunculus medinensis*, trichinosis, toxocariasis, larva migrans
Diethylcarbamazine (DEC)	Onchocerciasis, loaiasis, lymphatic filariasis, tropical pulmonary eosinophilia, toxocariasis
Ivermectin	Onchocerciasis
Suramin	Onchocerciasis
Metronidazole } Niridazole	*Dracunculus medinensis*
Niclosamide } Mepacrine } Praziquantel	*Taenia solium*, *T. saginata*
Praziquantel	*Schistosoma mansoni*, *S. haematobium*, *S. japonicum*, cysticercosis, clonorchiasis, opisthorchiasis, fascioliasis, taeniasis
Oxamniquine	*S. mansoni*
Metriphonate	*S. haematobium*
Bithionol	Fascioliasis

onchocerciasis. Ivermectin is currently undergoing clinical trials. Metronidazole and niridazole are most widely used for guinea-worm infections. Thiabendazole remains the best agent for strongyloidiasis, but it produces side-effects, and cure rates of only 60–70% are to be expected. There is little worthwhile controlled work on the treatment of *Toxocara canis* infection (*see* Chapter 15); DEC is probably the most effective agent. Hydatid disease (*see* Chapter 6) frequently responds to the benzimidazole compounds provided an adequate concentration can be achieved within the cysts. The trematode infections: clonorchiasis, opisthorchiasis and to a lesser extent fascioliasis, respond to praziquantel; in the latter infection bithionol remains however the treatment of choice.

FURTHER READING

Cook G. C. (1986). The clinical significance of gastrointestinal helminths—a review. *Trans. R. Soc. Trop. Med. Hyg*; **80:** 675–85.

Cook G. C. (1986). *Plasmodium falciparum* infection: problems in prophylaxis and treatment in 1986. *Q. J. Med*; **61:** 1091–1115.

Cook G. C. (1987). *Cryptosporidium sp.* and other intestinal coccidia. London: Bureau of Hygiene and Tropical Diseases.

Gilman A. G., Goodman L. S., Rall T. W., Murad F, eds. (1985). *Goodman and Gilman's The Pharmacological Basis of Therapeutics*, 7th ed., p. 1839. New York, Toronto, London: Macmillan.

Hay R. J. (1987). Recent advances in the management of fungal infections. *Q. J. Med*; **64:** 631–9.

McCormick J. B., King I. J., Webb P. A., *et al.* (1986). Lassa fever: effective therapy with ribavirin. *N. Engl. J. Med*; **314:** 20–6.

Thomas H. C., Scully L. J. (1985). Antiviral therapy in hepatitis B infection. *Brit. Med. Bull*; **41:** 374–80.

Van den Bosshe H., Thienpont D., Janssens P. G., eds. (1985). *Chemotherapy of Gastrointestinal Helminths*, p. 719. Berlin: Springer-Verlag.

Warhurst D. C. (1986). Antimalarial drugs: mode of action and resistance. *J. Antimicrob. Chemother*; **18** (Suppl B): 51–9.

Chapter Seventeen

Diseases Affecting Travellers

Travel from temperate, to tropical and sub-tropical countries has and still is increasing at a great rate; over 20 million holidays are currently taken abroad by people resident in Britain, and in addition, businessmen, academics, VSOs, missionaries, and others visit or serve in the tropics for varying periods, from a few days to many years. Many members of the minor ethnic groups resident in the UK also visit friends and relations in their countries of origin. In addition to insect bites and insect-borne diseases, changes in food and water supplies bring their problems; the skin and gastrointestinal tract are the major 'portals of entry' for infective agents. Whereas advice for prevention of the major diseases is often sought, seemingly unlikely problems, e.g. hepatitis A (and B in medical personnel), poliomyelitis and rabies for example, are frequently neglected. Realisation that hazards are relatively close at hand, e.g. malaria in Turkey, and visceral leishmaniasis (Kala azar) in Malta or Tunisia is often not appreciated.

GENERAL ADVICE TO THE TRAVELLER

General advice on travel (often not related to communicable diseases) is rarely sought. In the prophylaxis of jet-lag for example, alcohol avoidance seems of value, and a new preparation—melatonin might also help; a genetic factor is doubtless involved also. Exposure to excessive solar radiation can produce serious burns. Road accidents are common; therefore, care in driving is especially necessary and alcohol must be avoided. Accidents, apart from road accidents are common. Hazards associated with casual sexual activity have always been present but have been highlighted by the colossal problems resulting from

HIV infection (*see* Chapter 11); infection rates of 80% and more exist in prostitutes in parts of tropical Africa. Emotional problems constitute a source of illness. Overall, the more experienced traveller tends to experience far less medical problems than the occasional one. Two DHSS (London: HMSO) pamphlets are of value to the potential traveller: (i) 'Protect your health abroad' SA 35/1987 and (ii) 'Medical costs abroad' SA 30/1987.

The fact that many diseases actually present after return to the temperate country (of origin) is also frequently lost sight of; this applies to malaria, hepatitis, various diarrhoeal diseases, typhoid, dermatological problems and tuberculosis. Further possible hazards are viral haemorrhagic fevers, including Lassa fever, and the muroid nephropathies.

The following questions should be asked:

(i) Are routine immunisations up-to-date?
(ii) Have the legal requirements regarding immunisations for the country/countries being visited been satisfied?
(iii) Has good advice on malaria prophylaxis been sought?
(iv) Is the individual fit to travel in the first place?
(v) Are basic principles of personal hygiene, acclimatisation, food and water risks, and avoidance of insect bites, clearly understood?
(vi) Are the teeth and eyes in good condition before travelling to an under-developed country? Tooth care is especially important because HBV and HIV infections can be transmitted by dental injections.
(vii) If applicable, has advice been sought concerning facilities for the management of diabetes mellitus, and for the possible problems involving pregnancy and childbirth in the country to be visited?

Concerning point (iii), the following centres are available for advice on malaria prophylaxis:

London—The London School of Hygiene and Tropical Medicine (01 636 8636)
Liverpool—Liverpool School of Tropical Medicine (051 708 9393)
Birmingham—Department of Communicable and Tropical Diseases (021 772 4311)

Emergency surgery is often not available and where it is, blood used for transfusion is frequently infected (with malaria, trypanosomiasis, HBV or HIV for example). Hernias, haemorrhoids, etc, should therefore be dealt with before departing for the tropics. Respiratory diseases (including asthma) respond differently in different locations. While eczema is frequently exacerbated by tropical exposure, psoriasis often improves. It is well worth taking out health insurance before leaving for the tropics; health facilities are often inadequate and urgent repatriation is occasionally required.

It should again be stressed however that the most important advice which the potential traveller should seek is sensible up-to-date information on malaria prophylaxis (*see* Chapter 4).

IMMUNISATION AND PROPHYLAXIS REQUIREMENTS

Table 17.1 summarises those immunisation regimens which are either compulsory or strongly recommended. For the geographical distribution of these diseases the appropriate chapter should be consulted; cholera (*see* Chapter 5) and yellow fever (*see* Chapter 6) are examples of diseases with clearly delineated areas of distribution. Typhoid is present worldwide, but incidence rates and risks vary substantially; whether immunisation is worthwhile before a holiday in a Mediterranean country in southern Europe is controversial. Although oral vaccines are undergoing tests, they are not yet available commercially. Table 17.2 summarises various immunisation regimens which are occasionally recommended, especially in certain geographical areas.

In all cases a balance exists between: (i) risk and potential seriousness of the infection, and the protective value of the vaccine, and (ii) the possible side-effects of the vaccine together with its cost.

The only group of individuals still receiving smallpox vaccination is the USSR Army. This, together with other rarely used vaccines underlies plans for potential 'germ warfare' strategies.

PREVENTION OF DISEASE IN THE TROPICS AND SUB-TROPICS

Care with personal hygiene, water and food diminishes the incidence of disease significantly. Water used for cleaning teeth

Table 17.1

IMMUNISATION REQUIREMENTS FOR OVERSEAS TRAVEL

Vaccine	Dose*	Frequency (years)	Contraindications
Compulsory			
(Tropical Africa and south America only)			
Yellow fever — Live (17D)	0·5 ml (s.c.)	10	<9 months, pregnant, immunosuppressed, severe egg hypersensitivity
Recommended but not compulsory			
Cholera — Heat-killed	0·5 ml (s.c. or i.m.) + 1·0 ml (s.c. or i.m.) after 4–6 weeks	0·5	<6 months
Typhoid fever — Heat-killed (*Salmonella typhi*)	0·5 ml (s.c. or i.m.) + 0·1 ml (i.d.) after 4–6 weeks	3	<12 months
Poliomyelitis — Live attenuated	3 drops (oral); repeat after 4 and 8 weeks	10	For pregnant and immunosuppressed, inactivated vaccine must be used
Tetanus — Inactivated toxin	0·5 ml (s.c. or i.m.); repeat after 6 weeks	10	
Hepatitis A (HAV) — Pooled human Ig	500–750 mg i.m.	0·5	

*s.c. = Subcutaneous; i.m. = Intramuscular; i.d. = Intradermal.

Table 17.2

IMMUNISATION REGIMENS WHICH ARE NEITHER COMPULSORY NOR RECOMMENDED FOR ALL TRAVELLERS

Vaccine	Comments
BCG	Mantoux-negative children (from birth) travelling to any 'Third World' country
Hepatitis B (HBV)	Medical, nursing, laboratory staff working in 'Third World' countries. Course of 3 injections at 0, 1 and 6 months
Rabies	High risk groups, e.g. veterinarians travelling to enzoonotic areas; human diploid vaccine (*Note* post-exposure vaccine is also effective)
Diphtheria	Primary course in infancy; booster at school entry—booster every 10 years. In adults, Schick testing advised before vaccination
Plague	Only for prolonged stay in rural enzoonotic areas where close contact with rodents is likely
Tick-borne encephalitis	Exposure to forests in eastern Europe and Scandinavia; tick-borne infection. Course of 2 injections (12 week interval) with 12 month booster
Japanese B encephalitis	Exposure to rural areas in SE Asia, Nepal, northern India and Sri Lanka during high-risk period (August–December). Course of 3 injections with 10 day intervals
Meningococcal (A and C)	Only recommended for affected areas in northern and west Africa, the Middle East, and Asia

and making ice drinks is an important source of infection. Other general measures include: the avoidance of excess sunlight, excess alcohol and, where possible, situations in which accidents might occur.

Travellers' diarrhoea, *Escherichia coli* gastroenteritis, giardiasis, shigellosis, amoebic dysentery, hepatitis A, typhoid and cholera can all be water-borne. Boiling is the most effective way of sterilising drinking water; filtration and chlorination with tablets are alternative methods. Some protozoan cysts and the hepatitis A (HAV) virus are highly resistant however. Hot tea and coffee are usually safe. Breast-feeding is protective against the ingestion of intestinal pathogens; when bottle-feeding is substituted, all utensils and water used for mixing must be scrupulously clean. Swimming pools (unless well chlorinated) constitute a reservoir of infection. Sea water is frequently heavily contaminated with sewage and this is especially so in some parts of the Mediterranean sea.

Food also is an important source of infection. Poultry (especially when eaten cold and/or reheated) is a common source of *Salmonella spp.* and *Campylobacter spp.* infection; therefore, all meat should be thoroughly cooked and eaten hot whenever possible. Vegetables and fruit are often in contact with manure (in some countries, human night soil is used as a fertiliser); fruit should therefore whenever possible be peeled, and salad vegetables very carefully cleaned, or alternatively avoided altogether. Unpasteurised milk can convey tuberculosis, brucellosis, salmonellosis and *Campylobacter spp.* and Q-fever infection; boiling is therefore a wise precaution. Toxoplasmosis and tapeworms can also result from contaminated foodstuffs. Shellfish can concentrate bacteria, e.g. *Salmonella typhi*, in their filter system. Fish-toxin poisoning is an occasional problem in the Pacific; gastrointestinal and neurotoxic symptoms may result.

Gonorrhoea, syphilis, non-specific urethritis, and more importantly HBV and HIV infection can result from casual sexual intercourse especially with indigenous people in Africa; this should be totally avoided.

Showers and air-conditioning systems are occasionally infected with *Legionella pneumophila* (*see* Chapter 7); infection is most likely when an aerosol is inhaled. Hotels continue to constitute a source of infection in many parts of the world. Other respiratory infections are common in tropical countries, especially in the cooler months; they usually have a viral origin. A persisting cough should however suggest pulmonary tuberculosis. Tuberculosis and leprosy are widespread in virtually all 'Third World' countries, but infection of expatriates (most of whom are well-nourished) is an unusual event; hospital personnel are at greatest risk but this is still a relatively insignificant one.

The danger of contracting schistosomiasis from swimming, or from any exposure to infected water must be appreciated (*see*

Chapters 6 and 10). Satisfactory footwear is important; contact with water or damp soil may be followed by penetration of leptospires and hookworm larvae as well as schistosomal cercariae. Penetrating wounds involving the feet especially, can be the portal of entry for *Clostridium tetani*. Spider and snake-bites can also occur in the bare-footed. However, open sandals significantly reduce the chance of *Tinea pedis* infection. Sea snakes (and other sea creatures) are a common problem in Asia and the western Pacific.

Malaria, leishmaniasis and trypanosomiasis are conveyed by bites of mosquitoes, sandflies and tsetse flies, respectively. Ticks transmit rickettsial (e.g. tick typhus), viral and other infections. Covering the exposed parts of the body, especially the legs, which is especially important in the evenings, prevents many mosquito bites. Other insect bites can also be a problem, and a marked individual variation in susceptibility exists. Insect repellents, e.g. diethyltoluamide, are of some value. Conjunctivitis may also be transmitted by small flies. Local erythema and urticarial rashes can be induced by mites, caterpillars, blister-beetles, bed-bugs and jelly fish.

Snake bites and leeches (*see* Chapter 15) can produce significant health problems. Excess snake venom should immediately be wiped off. Reassurance, sedatives (or alcohol), and adequate analgesia are of value. Careful observation over a 12 h period is essential. Systemic absorption of toxin after a snake bite is usually along lymphatics; therefore compression with a firmly applied bandage is of value in preventing the spread of the venom. In *viper* bites, spread of a local swelling occurs within 1–2 h and is accompanied by shock and a haemorrhagic tendency. With *elapids*, if shock and neurological sequelae occur within 1 h of the bite, a severe illness can be anticipated. Scabies, head-lice and bed-bugs can also be a problem when travelling.

Household pets, especially dogs in 'Third World' countries are rarely infected with rabies. Stray animals should be strictly avoided, and this advice applies to all mammals. With all animal bites and licks, the possibility of rabies must be borne in mind. Lesions should immediately be washed copiously and iodine or spirit applied. Post-rabies vaccination must always be considered.

Skin lesions in tropical conditions often take a considerable period to heal, and secondary infection is a common sequel even if reasonable care is taken. Minor skin trauma should therefore be dealt with promptly; iodine or mercurochrome and a dry aerated dressing should be applied. Chronic ulceration resulting from *Staphylococcus aureus* and *Streptococcus pyogenes* infections are major problems which may necessitate removal to a temperate climate. Prickly heat (*miliaria rubra*) can be followed by staphylococcal infection in children especially; prophylaxis involves prevention of copious sweating, cool showers, talc dusting and the wearing of light, loose, cotton clothing; calamine lotion and oral antihistamines are of value for the pruritus.

Febrile episodes are common and should always be taken seriously especially if they last for 2 days or more; a wide range of diagnoses headed by *Plasmodium falciparum* infection should be considered.

SYMPTOM-ORIENTATED APPROACH TO INFECTION IN THE TROPICS

Because most diseases are transmitted by food or water, or by 'insect bites', gastrointestinal and systemic illnesses and/or febrile episodes dominate the list of infective causes. Most of these diseases have been covered in previous chapters; Table 17.3 summarises some of them according to the major presenting symptom.

IMPORTED INFECTIONS

Many infections can be transmitted to temperate countries by travellers (and others) from the tropics and sub-tropics. Table 17.4 summarises some major imported infections in the UK. The majority are of trivial importance, but some are associated with a significant mortality rate. Many of these diseases are notifiable under British law; a list of those which must legally be notified is given in Chapter 1. Seriously ill patients should be managed at a centre which has special expertise in these conditions.

INFECTIONS IN PREGNANCY, CHILDHOOD AND OTHER SPECIAL GROUPS

In pregnant women, *Plasmodium falciparum* malaria is a major problem and correct advice should centre on avoiding visits to

Table 17.3
SOME IMPORTANT INFECTIONS IN TROPICAL AND SUB-TROPICAL COUNTRIES CLASSIFIED UNDER MAJOR PRESENTING SYMPTOMS

Fever
  Malaria
  Tuberculosis
  Influenza
  EBV
  CMV
  Lassa fever
  Typhoid
  Brucellosis
  Legionnaire's disease
  Q fever (*Coxiella*)
  Typhus
  Entamoeba histolytica (liver abscess)
  Kala azar
  African trypanosomiasis

Diarrhoea
  Travellers' diarrhoea
  Salmonellosis
  Shigellosis
  Campylobacter enteritis
  Typhoid/paratyphoid
  Yersinia enterolitica
  Giardiasis
  Cholera
  Entamoeba histolytica
  Schistosomiasis (*S. mansoni*)
  Postinfective malabsorption
  (tropical sprue)
  Inflammatory bowel disease
  (usually ulcerative colitis)

Diarrhoea and vomiting
  'Food poisoning'

Rash
  Mycotic infections
  Typhus (tick)
  Cutaneous leishmaniasis
  African trypanosomiasis

Respiratory
  Pneumococcal pneumonia
  Tuberculosis
  Legionnaire's disease

Headache
  Dengue
  Meningococcal meningitis
  Malaria
  Typhoid
  Tuberculous meningitis
  Trypanosomiasis

Jaundice
  Viral hepatitis
  EBV
  CMV

Sore-throat
  EBV
  Diphtheria
  Lassa fever

Haematuria
  Schistosoma haematobium

Pruritus ani
  Threadworm

Tiredness/malaise
  Schistosomiasis

Worm phobias
  Tapeworm
  Ascaris lumbricoides

Table 17.4

SOME INFECTIONS IMPORTED INTO THE UK, WITH INCUBATION PERIODS*

Infection	Incubation period (days)
Malaria	
P. falciparum	10–28
P. vivax	(2–50 weeks)
Salmonella	1–2
Shigella	4–8
Campylobacter enteritis	2–11
Cholera	1–3
Yersinia enterocolitica	
Giardiasis	
Amoebiasis	
Typhoid and paratyphoid	10–14
Hepatitis A	(3–5 weeks)
Hepatitis B	(6–25 weeks)
Poliomyelitis	9–12
Viral haemorrhagic fevers (Lassa, muroid nephropathy)	3–21
Legionnaire's disease	2–10
Tuberculosis	
AIDS	
Q-fever	18–21
Tick typhus	4–14
Relapsing fever	(12–30 weeks)
Syphilis	(3–5 weeks)
Tetanus	(7–12 weeks)
Rabies	(4–30 weeks)
Diphtheria	1–3
Intestinal helminthic infections	
Postinfective malabsorption (tropical sprue)	
'Exotic' parasitic infections:	
Trypanosomiasis	
Leishmaniasis	
Visceral	
Cutaneous	
Filariasis	
Schistosomiasis	
'Tumbu' fly	
Skin infections (e.g. fungal, of feet and groins)	

*Where incubation period is not given see relevant chapter.

infected areas whenever possible (see Chapter 4). Regarding malaria prophylaxis, this *must* always be maintained throughout pregnancy. 'Fansidar' should not be prescribed during the last trimester or during breast-feeding. Proguanil and pyrimethamine seem safe despite a theoretical risk to the fetus with antifolate agents. *P. falciparum* infections are also a major potential problem in infants and children; prophylaxis should start at birth.

Walking bare-foot can cause hookworm and strongyloides infections; larvae penetrate intact skin. Scorpion and snake-bites are more common in children. Other mosquito-borne infections, e.g. dengue, occur when children remain largely unclothed; this disease can sometimes be severe (with haemorrhagic manifestations) in infancy and childhood.

In countries where they are widespread, immunisation against diphtheria, pertussis, tetanus and poliomyelitis must be given early, i.e. in the first or second month of life. Similarly, measles vaccine can be given at 9 and 15 months. BCG should be given at birth; this should prevent both miliary and meningitic tuberculosis. Yellow fever vaccination should not be given before 9 months of age. In pregnancy, live vaccines should *not* be administered. This applies to yellow fever, although if the theoretical risk of yellow fever is high the risk of disease might outweigh the hazard of inoculation. (A medical certificate can be produced indicating that vaccination is contraindicated.) Inactivated poliomyelitis vaccine can be used instead of oral live vaccine. A tetanus booster dose can be given during pregnancy; some protection will then be passed to the unborn infant. Immunoglobulin gives partial protection against hepatitis A (HAV), which is sometimes more severe in pregnancy.

In the immunosuppressed, live vaccines (including yellow fever) should not be given. Limited evidence exists that immunisations given to HIV infected individuals, hasten the onset of end-stage AIDS.

FURTHER READING

Baer G. M., Fishbein D. B. (1987). Rabies post-exposure prophylaxis. *N. Engl. J. Med*; **316:** 1270–2.

Cossar J. H., Reid D. (1987). Not all travellers need immunoglobulin for hepatitis A. *Brit. Med. J*; **294:** 1503.

Dawood R. (1986). *Travellers' Health*, p. 498. Oxford, New York, Tokyo: Oxford University Press.

Editorial. (1986). Jet lag and its pharmacology. *Lancet*; **2:** 493–4.
Editorial. (1986). Oral cholera vaccines. *Lancet*; **2:** 722–3.
Flewett T. H. (1986). Can we eradicate hepatitis B? *Brit. Med. J*; **293:** 404–5.
Walker E., Williams G. (1983). *ABC of Healthy Travel*, p. 39. London: British Medical Journal.

Chapter Eighteen

Prevention and Control of Communicable Diseases

In the so-called developed countries of the world, the 20th century has seen a remarkable decline in the prevalence of many communicable diseases. The reasons for this are multifactorial. Improved standards of living, diminution of poverty, and more sophisticated sanitation standards have probably been the dominant factors. Improvements in the quality and implementation of immunisation and vaccination techniques and programmes have led to a decline in the incidence of many diseases, especially some of those important in childhood (*see* Chapter 2); smallpox is a unique example. The discovery and introduction of antimicrobial agents, followed by penicillin and other antibiotics were also of immense importance, but the fact that some of the relevant diseases were already declining when these agents were introduced should not be dismissed lightly. The decline in many diseases, e.g. tuberculosis and 'scarlet fever' in the UK during the early 20th century, and the epidemic behaviour of poliomyelitis during the 1950s are examples where the precise cause of a decline is unclear.

In a world context, only very limited success has however so far been achieved in disease control. Here, the problems attributable to communicable disease achieve gigantic proportions. In Africa alone, 1 million children die of malaria each year. Also, 3 million new cases of tuberculosis occur worldwide every year. In parts of southern America, up to 20% of blood used for transfusions is infected with *Trypanosoma cruzi*! The acquired immune deficiency syndrome (AIDS) is spreading rapidly in Africa (and other continents also) and will shortly eliminate many millions from the world.

Successes involving control (some only relative) so far include: smallpox, yaws, onchocerciasis and malaria (in temperate areas only). Failures include some of those diseases mentioned above, but also African trypanosomiasis and leishmaniasis (both visceral and cutaneous). Leprosy, Chagas' disease and the lymphatic filariases can be cited as examples where efforts at prevention have not yet significantly altered the incidence rate.

The 17D vaccine (live and attenuated) for yellow fever provides at least 95% protection. While the implementation of immunisation programmes was effective, the disease assumed a low profile in the affected areas of Africa. But now, following widespread complacency, the disease is back in prominence and in west Africa, epidemics with substantial mortality are again reported.

Treatment of some diseases has advanced very slowly. As an example, leishmaniasis and African trypanosomiasis are still managed with arsenical and antimonial compounds.

STRATEGIES FOR DISEASE CONTROL

Efforts at prevention can be divided into: (i) *non-specific* approaches, aimed at improved sanitation, and efforts to improve hygienic standards, nutritional status, and health education, and (ii) *specific* approaches focusing on drugs (chemoprophylactics and chemotherapeutic agents), vaccines, and pesticides. Some preventive measures are more practical than others. The prevalence of hepatitis A and other enterovirus infections is not, for example, easily influenced by the environmental control of faecal contamination. Also, it is extremely difficult to eliminate all breeding sites of the malaria parasite. An enormous financial outlay would be required for the improvement of housing conditions to such a level that Chagas' disease could be eradicated. Ethical restrictions must also be borne in mind; as an example of this, in the 14th century, King Philippe of France ordered the burning of all lepers! This is an extreme example of a disease prevention technique, which is unlikely to be acceptable in the latter years of the 20th century.

Specific remedies must be: effective, safe, simple, affordable and compatible with local culture and health systems. Even when satisfactory prophylactic and therapeutic agents become readily available, problems frequently arise; 'resistance' is a major problem, and this drawback applies also in the context of pesticides. Also, significant control after the introduction of a new preventive technique is frequently not immediately forthcoming; smallpox vaccination was introduced by Jenner in 1796, but the ultimate eradication of this disease occurred only in 1977. Eradication of yaws from large areas of the tropics had to await the introduction of a long-acting penicillin; the discovery of penicillin in 1928 was not enough! Although newer therapeutic agents now exist in the treatment of schistosomiasis, these are of limited value in the control of this disease in affected countries; however, selective (targetted) chemotherapy could prove in the long-term, to be effective. The consequence on subsequent developments in the field of communicable diseases of eliminating a disease is not always clear; now that smallpox has been eliminated, will monkeypox (caused by a closely related member of the *Orthopoxvirus* genus) become a major problem in central and west Africa?

Construction of successful health-control systems in the 'Third World' is a highly complex matter. They involve:

(i)   Primary health care *versus* high technology medicine.
(ii) A vertical *versus* horizontal approach.
(iii) A selective *versus* comprehensive strategy.

Successes with regard to yaws and onchocerciasis have resulted from vertical rather than horizontal eradication methods. The problems involved in disease control in developing 'Third World' countries (*see* p. 311) are therefore enormous. Considerable confusion has arisen between disease prevention and primary health care. In the control (and ultimate elimination) of communicable diseases, three areas are important:

(i)   *Disease prevention.* This, in the main, should not lie within the area of the medical practitioner; it is not even covered in undergraduate medical training. Engineers, sanitation experts, nutritionists, agriculturalists and other basic scientists are able to control the environment and raise living standards; as this occurs, most infections diminish in prevalence *pari passu* (*see* p. 6).

(ii) *Primary health care.* This involves medical management of people in rural and semi-rural areas; although medical personnel must be involved, much can be delegated to paramedical staff provided they are adequately supervised.

(iii) *Clinical (bed-side) medicine.* This must clearly be carried out by experienced medical personnel and of necessity much will be based in the referral centre(s) where the best facilities and equipment for the country under consideration are located. It is here that the various complications of all kinds of infections and those presenting diagnostic and therapeutic difficulties will rightly be managed.

Primary health care, therefore, incorporates education (involving especially the nutritional aspects of health), improved water supplies and sanitation standards, family health (including looking after the elderly in the population), control of endemic disease, as well as implementation of curative services, and delivery of essential drugs. There is frequently an absence of an effective structure for the implementation of recent advances (especially in the preventive field)! For example, should diphtheria toxoid be more widely administered in the UK? Should all pregnant women in Sri Lanka be immunised against tetanus?

New strategies for the prevention of communicable diseases are necessary. Will dracontiasis (guinea-worm infection) be the next disease, after smallpox, to be eliminated? Building new reservoirs in Africa should be viewed critically, with schistosomiasis very much in mind. Integrated community development is required. An educated populace is essential. Operational research should include: adaptation of old and new, and testing of control strategies. Research and development in preventive techniques has so far taken place intermittently; wars have often been necessary to instigate significant progress—discovery of newer antimalarial agents is a good example of this. Major advances were made in World War II (1939–45), but since then work has not been carried out seriously and systematically. Also much muddled thinking resulted in unjustified complacency. The WHO Global Education policy for malaria in the 1960s undoubtedly led to a decline in research into new antimalarial agents; this also applied to insecticides active against the mosquito vectors of this disease. As a result, vast amounts of finance have been wasted on unsuccessful prevention campaigns; one estimate is that £500 million have been spent by 'Third World' countries for the unsuccessful control of malaria!

Many problems remain in bringing the current AIDS pandemic under control. Government publicity and educational campaigns are of value, but there are many unanswered epidemiological questions: what is the length of the incubation period, of the latent period and the infectivity period? And what proportion of HIV positive individuals develop end-stage AIDS?

For successful disease control, simple diagnostic tests are necessary. A simple test for the diagnosis of malaria, for example, is urgently required; few doctors working in the 'Third World' countries, and even fewer in the UK, are able to identify and differentiate *Plasmodium spp.* in blood films with any degree of competence.

WILL VACCINES SOLVE THE PROBLEM?

At present, the search for vaccines dominates the scene; molecular biology has come to the fore, and it is widely assumed (especially by individuals who have not worked for substantial periods in the 'Third World') that vaccines will soon be the answer to all of the major world scourges. A vaccine for malaria is on the horizon. Similarly work on schistosomal and leprosy vaccines is progressing. However, a very high vaccination rate is essential for the eradication of a disease: perhaps 90% in the case of the viral diseases of childhood, and a figure of 99% has been suggested for malaria (when a good vaccine is available). But will the ultimate cost be prohibitive for most 'Third World' countries? In a world context, vaccination will not and cannot be the answer for a very long time. There are in any case still many problems inherent in vaccine production: for example, trypanosomes rapidly change their surface antigens, schistosomes 'escape' from the body's immune response, while filariae release their toxins only when the young microfilariae die. If, therefore, complacency continues to escalate, other methods of control and prevention will fall by the wayside. It is essential that research into chemotherapy continues and it is equally vital that policies for *disease prevention* continue to expand unabated. The same applies to raising socioeconomic conditions.

FURTHER READING

Baker M. R., Bandaranayake R., Schweiger M. S. (1984). Differences in rate of uptake of immunisation among ethnic groups. *Brit. Med. J*; **288**: 1075–8.
Booth C. (1985). The conquest of smallpox. *Q. J. Med*; **57**: 811–23.
Bruce-Chwatt L. J. (1987). The challenge of malaria vaccine: trials and tribulations. *Lancet*; **1**: 371–3.
Cook G. C. (1987). Preventive medicine or disease prevention? *J. R. Soc. Med*; **80**: 258–9.
Editorial. (1983). After smallpox, guineaworm? *Lancet*; **1**: 161–2.

Epstein M. A. (1986). Vaccination against Epstein–Barr virus: current progress and future strategies. *Lancet*: **1:** 1425–27.

Kunitz S. J. (1987). Making a long story short: a note on men's height and mortality in England from the first through the nineteenth centuries. *Med. History*; **31:** 269–80.

Lucas A. O. (1985). The persistent challenge of tropical parasitic infections. *J. R. Coll. Physcns*; **19:** 205–9.

Tyrrell D. A. J., Burkitt D. P., Henderson W., eds. (1977). *Technologies for Rural Health*, p. 187. London: The Royal Society.

Tyrrell D. A. J., Henderson W., Elliott K., eds. (1980). *More Technologies for Rural Health*, p. 186. London: The Royal Society.

World Health Organization. (1987). Expanded programme on immunization. *WHO Weekly Epid. Record*; **62:** 5–9.

Index

acquired immune deficiency syndrome (AIDS), 185–94
  African, 191–4
  associated infections and other diseases, 189 (table)
  hospital acquired, 19
  investigations, 188 (table)
  north American/European, 186–91
  treatment, 191
Actinomyces israelii, 22, 259
actinomycosis, 216, 259–60
acycloguanosine (Acyclovir), 206, 213, 291, 292 (table)
Addison's disease, 52
adenine arabinoside (Ara–A), 113, 292 (table)
African tick typhus, 214–215, 247 (table), 249
African trypanosomiasis (sleeping sickness), 168–71
albendazole
  for: helminths, 86, 296, 297, (table)
    hookworm, 86
    hydatidosis, 111
    roundworm, 87
    strongyloidiasis, 88
allergic diseases transmitted by domestic pets, 10 (table)
allopurinol, 265
amantadine, 126, 291, 292 (table)
amikacin, 58, 283 (table)
aminoglycosides, 200, 283 (table)
amodiaquine, 66 (table); 66–8
amoebiasis, hepatic, 108–9
amoebic colitis, 88–90
amoebic liver abscess, 28, 108–9

amoebic lung abscess, 132
amoxycillin, 284 (table), 289
  for: bronchitis, 123
  gonorrhoea, 200
  pneumonia, 128 (table)
  typhoid fever, 255
amphotericin B, 293, 294 (table)
  for: fungal infections, 168, 219, 260, 261
  leishmaniasis, 221
ampicillin, 284 (table), 289
  blood–brain barrier, 156 (table)
  for: bronchitis, 123
  gonorrhoea, 200
  pelvic inflammatory disease, 203
  typhoid fever, 255
amyloidosis, renal, 181
anaerobes
  non-sporing, 22
  spore-forming, 22–3
anaerobic infections, 22–3
angiostrongyliasis, 277
Angiostrongylus cantonensis, 172, 277
Angiostrongylus costaricensis, 83 (table), 277
Anisakis spp., 83 (table), 87, 90 (table)
Ankylostoma braziliense, 221
Ankylostoma caninum, 221
Ankylostoma duodenale, 83 (table), 85–6
anthrax, 129, 216, 259
antibacterial agents, 288–90
antibiotics and antimicrobial agents, 279–98
  allergy, 290
  blood–brain barrier, 156 (table)
  broad spectrum, 284 (table), 290

318 Index

antibiotics—*contd*
  children, 290
  concentrations, factors influencing, 286 (table)
  for: chronic bronchitis, 123
    gonorrhoea, 200
    lymphogranuloma venereum, 208
    septicaemia, 253 (table)
    skin infections, 215–17
    urinary infection, 177
  narrow spectrum, 282–3 (table), 290
  pharmacodynamics, 281–6
  pregnancy, 290
  prophylaxis, 288
  resistance, 286–8
  sensitivity, 286–8
  side-effects, 291
  sites of action, 280 (table)
  travellers' diarrhoea, 74
antifungal agents, 293–4
anthelmintic agents, 296–8
antiprotozoan agents, 295–6
antivaricella zoster immunoglobulin (ZIg), 41
antiviral agents, 162, 291–3
Antrypol (suramin), 171, 271, 292 (table), 297
Argentine haemorrhagic fever, 235 (table), 240
arsenicals, 295, 296 (table)
Ascaris lumbricoides, 83 (table), 85 (fig.), 86
aspergilloma, 133
aspergillosis, 133–4
  allergic bronchopulmonary, 133
  disseminated, 134
aspirin, 140
athlete's foot, 218
atypical mycobacteria, 56–8
azidothymidine (AZT), 191, 292 (table)

babesiosis, 267–8
Bacille Calmette–Guérin (BCG) vaccination, 45–6, 303 (table)
bacterial endocarditis, 140–4
  antibiotic prophylaxis/treatment, 143 (table)

causative organisms, 142 (table)
bacteriuria
  covert, 175
  significant, 175
Bacteroides fragilis, 22
Bacteroides melaninogenicus, 22
Bacteroides necrophorus, 132
balantidiasis, 90
Balantidium coli, 89, 90
Bantu siderosis (haemosiderosis), 116
bartonellosis, 251
benzathine penicillin, 139–40
benzimidazole compounds, 111, 298
benzonidazole (Rochagan), 267
benzylpenicillin, 128 (table), 143 (table), 157
  blood–brain barrier, 156 (table)
bephenium hydroxynaphthoate, 86
biliary ascariasis, 111
biliary infections, 111
bismuth subsalicylate, 74, 75 (table)
bithionol, 111, 136, 297 (table)
blastomycosis, 219, 261
blood–brain barrier, antimicrobial agents, 156 (table), 281
Bolivian haemorrhagic fever, 235 (table), 240
bone marrow culture
  Salmonella typhi, 26
  visceral leishmaniasis, 27
Bordetella pertussis, 36–8
botulism, 80
Brill–Zinsser disease, 214, 246 (table), 248
Brock's syndrome, 47
bronchiectasis, 132–3
bronchitis, chronic, exacerbations, 123–4
brucellosis, 28, 255–6
bullous impetigo, 215
Burkitt's lymphoma, 233
Buruli ulcer, 58, 217

Calabar swellings, 222, 273
Campylobacter spp., 9, 10 (table), 73 (table), 80, 81
Campylobacter jejuni, 79
cancrum oris, 216
Candida albicans, 122
candidiasis, 261

oral (thrush), 122
Capillaria philippinensis, 83 (table), 88
carbenicillin, 128 (table), 284 (table)
cardiovascular infections, 138–51
carriers of infection, 1
cefamandole, 123
cefuroxime, 123, 128 (table)
cell-mediated immunity, depression of, 23–4
central nervous system infections, 152–73
cephalosporins, 123, 285 (table), 289
cerebral abscess, 165–6
cerebral space-occupying lesion, 165–6
cestodes, 83 (table), 87
Chagas' disease (South American trypanosomiasis), 89 (table), 147, 265–7
  meningoencephalitis, 171
chancre, 203, 216
  trypanosomal, 221
chancroid (soft chancre), 198 (table), 206–7
Chédiak–Higashi syndrome, 233
chickenpox (varicella), 32 (table), 41
Chilomastix mesnili, 89 (table)
Chikungunya fever, 214, 234 (table)
Chikungunya haemorrhagic fever, 235 (table)
children
  antibiotics, 290
  dangers, tropical/subtropical countries, 287
  infections, 31–42
Chlamydia psittaci, 128 (table), 244
Chlamydia trachomatis, 196, 197 (table), 244
chloramphenicol, 284 (table)
  blood–brain barrier, 156 (table), 290
  for: bartonellosis, 251
    gonorrhoea, 200
    granuloma inguinale, 209
    leptospirosis, 107
    plague, 258
    rickettsial infection, 245, 249
    typhoid fever, 255
chloroquine, 65, 66 (table), 68, 69 (table), 70, 71, 296 (table)

  resistance of malaria parasites to, 65, 67 (fig.), 68
cholera, 76–8, 302 (table)
chromomycosis, 218, 260
ciprofloxacin, 283 (table), 289
clavulanic acid, 289
clindmycin, 282 (table)
clofazimine (Lamprene), 230, 231 (table)
clonorchiasis, 111
clostridial septic abortion, 22
Clostridium botulinum, 80
Clostridium difficile, 22, 81
Clostridium perfringens, 22, 80
Clostridium tetani, 22, 164
cloxacillin, 126, 143 (table), 282 (table), 289
cocci, anaerobic, 22
coccidioidomycosis, 150, 261
colitis, antibiotic associated (pseudomembranous), 81
common cold (acute coryza), 120
Communicable Disease Surveillance Centre, 4
complement fixation, 28, 29 (table)
Congo–Crimean haemorrhagic fever, 235 (table), 240
corticosteroids, 113, 134, 147, 236, 255
Corynebacterium diphtheriae, 38–40
coryza, acute (common cold), 120
co-trimoxazole, 285 (table)
  for: bronchitis, 123, 124
    granuloma inguinale, 209
    influenza, 126
    nocardiosis, 259
    Pneumocystis carinii, 134–5
    protozoan infections, 296 (table)
counter current electrophoresis (CEP), 28–9
Coxiella burnetii, 214, 245
Coxsackie infection, 145 (table)
creeping eruption, 221
Creutzfeldt–Jakob disease, 163 (table), 167, 168
Cryptococcus neoformans, 26, 168, 261
Cryptosporidium spp., 9, 11, 82 (table), 84
cycloserine, 54 (table), 55
cysticercosis, 87, 172

Cysticercus cellulosae (Taenia solium), 83 (table), 87
cystitis
  abacterial (urethral syndrome), 175, 177, 199, 200
  bacterial, 175
cytarabine, 292 (table)
cytomegalovirus (CMV) infection, 28, 233, 243

dapsone, 230, 231 (table)
Daraprim (pyrimethamine), 65, 66 (table), 146, 262, 296 (table)
dengue fever, 234–6
dengue haemorrhagic fever, 214, 234–6
dengue shock syndrome, 234, 235–6
diagnostic techniques, 25–9
  microbiological, 26
  parasitological, 27–8
  serological, 28, 29 (table)
diethylcarbamazine (DEC)
  for: filarial hypereosinophilia, 135
  filariasis, 270, 297
  loaiasis, 273
  onchocerciasis, 271
  toxocariasis, 276, 298
diloxanide furoate (Furamide), 90, 108
diarrhoea, 307 (table)
  at weaning time, 24
  bacterial, 76–81
  parasitic causes, 82–91
  travellers', *see* travellers' diarrhoea
  viral, 75–6
dichlorodiphenyl-trichloroethane (DDT), resistance to, 68
Dientamoeba fragilis, 89
diphtheria, 32 (table), 38–40, 303 (table)
Diphylobothrium latum, 83 (table), 87
Dipylidium caninum, 14 (table), 83 (table)
domestic pets, diseases transmitted by, 10 (table)
doxycycline, 58, 123, 201
  for rickettsial infection, 245, 248, 249
dracontiasis (dracunculiasis), 172, 222, 273, 274 (fig.)

Ebola virus disease, 235 (table), 237 (fig.), 239–40
Echinococcus granulosus, 109–11
Echinostoma spp., 83 (table)
ecogenetics, 5
Echo infection, 214
econazole, 293, 294 (table)
empyema, 131
encephalitis
  acute, 160–2, 303 (table)
  severe necrotising, 162
encephalomyelitis, 160–1 (table)
endemic disease, 2
Endolimax nana, 89
endomyocardial fibrosis (EMF), 148–9
Entamoeba coli, 89 (table)
Entamoeba hartmanni, 89 (table)
Entamoeba histolytica, 88–90, 91 (fig.)
  cerebral abscess, 172
  cutaneous lesions, 221
  diagnostic techniques, 27, 28
Entamoeba polecki, 89 (table)
Enterobius vermicularis (threadworm), 27, 90 (table)
Enteromonas hominis, 89 (table)
Enterotest, 27, 84, 88
enzyme-linked immunosorbent assay (ELISA), 28, 29 (table)
epidemic disease, 2
epidemic polyarthritis, 234 (table)
epidemic typhus, 214, 246 (table), 248
epidemiology, 2
  clinical, 2–3
  communicable disease in UK, 7–9
Epstein–Barr virus (EBV) infection, 28, 214, 232–3, 243
erysipelas, 215
erythema infectiosum (fifth disease), 42
erythema multiforme, 213 (table)
erythema nodosum, 48, 211
erythema nodosum leprosum, 217, 227, 230
erythromycin, 286 (table), 289
  for: Legionnaire's disease, 128 (table), 131
  leptospirosis, 107

lymphogranuloma venereum, 208
nocardiosis, 259
non-specific urethritis, 201
relapsing fever, 257
rheumatic fever prophylaxis, 140
Escherichia coli infection, 79–80
espundia (mucocutaneous leishmaniasis), 219
ethambutol, 54 (table), 55
ethionamide, 54 (table), 55

Fansidar, 65–6, 66 (table), 68, 69 (table)
farmer's lung, 134
Fasciola hepatica (liver fluke), 111
Fasciolopsis buski, 83 (table), 87
fièvre boutonneuse, 249
fifth disease (erythema infectiosum), 42
filarial hypereosinophilia (tropical pulmonary eosinophilia), 135
filariasis, 268–75
  lymphatic, 27, 268–70
Fitz–Hugh–Curtis syndrome, 198, 202
fleas, 11, 223
flucloxacillin, 128 (table), 289
5-fluorocytosine, 168, 260, 293, 294 (table)
folic acid, 95, 279–80
fomite, 2
food-poisoning, *Clostridium perfringens*-induced, 22, 80
fortified benzathine penicillin, 143 (table)
frequency/dysuria syndrome, 174–5
fungal infections, 260–1
  central nervous system, 168
  skin, 218–19
Furamide (diloxanide furoate), 90, 108
furazolidone, 296 (table)
fusidic acid, 282 (table), 290
Fusiformis spp., 22

gas-gangrene, 22–3
Gastrodiscoides hominis, 83 (table)
gastrointestinal infections, 72–98

'gay-bowel' syndrome, 196
genital herpes, 205–6
genital ulceration, 196
gentamicin, 128 (table), 143 (table), 283 (table)
  blood–brain barrier, 156 (table)
Giardia lamblia, 27, 82–4, 89 (table)
glanders, 129
glandular fever (infectious mononucleosis), 233
glomerulonephritis
  immune complex, 180
  post-streptococcal, 178–9
glucose-6-phosphate dehydrogenase (G-6-PD), deficiency, 70, 107
gluten-induced enteropathy, 93 (table, note)
Gnathostoma spinigerum, 83 (table), 277
gnathostomiasis, 172, 277
gonorrhoea, 195, 198–200
granuloma inguinale, 198 (table), 208–9
griseofulvin, 293, 294 (table)
ground itch, 85
group C virus fevers, 234 (table)
Guillain-Barré syndrome (infective polyneuritis), 164–5
guinea-worm infection (dracontiasis, dracunculiasis), 222, 273–4

Haemophilus influenzae, 154 (table), 156, 157–8
haemosiderosis (Bantu siderosis), 116
halofantrines, 296 (table)
Haverhill fever, 258
Heaf test, 45
helminths, intestinal, 83 (table), 84–8, 90–1
hepatitis
  acute, in tropics/subtropics, 103 (table)
  chronic active, 113
  chronic persistent, 113
  'toxic', 107
  viral, *see* viral hepatitis
Herpes simiae, 9, 10 (table)
herpes simplex, 205–6, 211
herpes zoster, 213–14
Heterophyes heterophyes, 83 (table)
Histoplasma capsulatum, 150, 261

322   Index

histoplasmosis, 261
hookworms, 27, 85–6, 221–2
hospital acquired infection, 15–19
   acquired immune deficiency
      syndrome (AIDS), 19
   tuberculosis, 18–19
   viral hepatitis, 19
human immunodeficiency virus-1
   (HIV-1), 185–94
human immunodeficiency virus-2
   (HIV-2), 186, 192
hydatid cyst, 109–11, 135–6
   cerebral, 172
   pericardial, 150
hydatidosis, zoonotic infection, 10
   (table), 11
   hepatic, 109–11
2-hydroxystilbamidine, 293, 294
   (table)
Hymenolepis diminuta, 83 (table)
Hymenolepis nana, 83 (table)
hyperpigmentation, 211
hypertrophic ileocaecal disease, 50
hypolactasia, 93 (table)
hypopigmentation, 211, 227

idoxuridine, 206, 292
immune complex nephropathy, 180
immunocompromised patient,
   opportunist infection, 21
immunoelectrophoresis, 28, 29
   (table)
immunofluorescent antibody test
   (IFAT), 29 (table)
incubation period, 2, 32 (table), 314
Indian childhood cirrhosis, 116–17
indirect immunofluorescence, 28, 29
   (table)
infection
   anaerobic, 22–3
   in pregnancy, 19–20
   nutrition interactions, 23–4
   opportunist infection, in
      immunocompromised patient,
      21
   predisposing factors, 4–6
      environmental, 6, 306–9
      genetic, 5–6
   world distribution, 6–7

Infectious Diseases (Notification) Act
   1889, 3
infectious mononucleosis (glandular
   fever), 233
infective polyneuritis (Guillain–Barré
   syndrome), 164–5
inflammatory bowel disease, 81
influenza, 125–6
insect-transmitted diseases, 13–15
interferon, 113, 292
Iodamoeba bütschlii, 89 (table)
isoniazid, 53, 54 (table)
isonicotinic acid hydrazide (INAH),
   53, 54 (table)
   blood–brain barrier, 156
Isospora belli, 82 (table), 84, 189
   (table)
ivermectin, 297

Jarisch–Herxheimer reaction, 107,
   204
jaundice, acute bacterial
   infection-induced, 107
JC virus (papovavirus), 163 (table)
jigger flea *(Tunga penetrans)*, 223

Kala azar (visceral leishmaniasis),
   263–5
kanamycin, 283 (table)
Kaposi's sarcoma, 188, 189 (table),
   193, 214
   management, 191
Katayama fever (acute
   schistosomiasis), 28, 109, 222
ketoconazole, 260, 261, 293, 294
   (table)
Klebsiella spp., 132
Korean haemorrhagic fever, 235
   (table), 241
Kuru, 163 (table), 167, 243
Kwashiorkor, 93, 116
Kyasanur Forest disease, 235 (table),
   241

Lampit (nifurtimox), 267, 296
   (table)
Lamprene (clofazimine), 230, 231
   (table)
Larva currens, 222
Larva migrans, 221

Lassa fever, 235 (table), 236–8
Legionnaire's disease, 127, 129, 130–1
leishmaniasis, 219–21, 262–5
  cutaneous (Oriental sore), 219–21
  diffuse cutaneous, 219
  disseminated anergic, 221
  mucocutaneous (espundia), 219, 221
  post-Kala azar, 221
  recidivans, 219
  visceral (Kala azar), 263–5
leprosy, 225–31
  bacteriology, 225–7
  clinical aspects, 227–30
  differential diagnosis, 229 (table)
  immunology, 226
  skin lesions, 217, 227
  treatment, 230–1
Leptospira canicola, 106
Leptospira icterohaemorrhagiae, 106
leptospirosis, 106–7
levamisole, 86, 87
lincomycin, 282 (table)
liver
  alcoholic disease, 116
  biopsy, culture of, 26
  chronic disease, 112–17
    differential diagnosis, 112 (table)
    haemosiderosis (Bantu siderosis), 116
    hepatocellular carcinoma, 114–15
    Indian childhood cirrhosis, 116–17
    macronodular cirrhosis, 113
    malnutrition, effect on, 116
    parasitic infection, 107–11
    veno-occlusive disease, 117
liver fluke *(Fasciola hepatica)*, 111
Loa loa, blood film, 27
loaiasis, 222, 273, 275 (fig.)
Löffler's syndrome, 124, 135
lower respiratory tract infections
  acute, 122–31
    bacterial causes, 126–31, 128 (table)
    viral causes, 125–6
  chronic, 131–6
lumbar puncture, 26
lung
  abscess, 132

fungal disease, 133–4
Lyme disease, 256–7
Lymphogranuloma venereum, 197 (table), 207–8
lymphoma, Burkitt's, 233
lymphoma, Mediterranean, 93 (table)

Madura foot (maduromycosis, mycetoma), 218–19, 259, 260
MAIS complex, 58
malabsorption, causes of, in tropical/subtropical countries, 93 (table)
malaria, 60–71
  nephrotic syndrome of 'quartan' malaria, 70, 180–1
  Plasmodium falciparum, 61–9
    chloroquine resistance, geographical distribution, 67 (fig.)
    clinical aspects, 64–5
    complications, 64 (table)
    liver involvement, 107–8
    parasitology, 61–3
    pneumonia, 129
    prophylaxis, 65–8
    treatment, 68–9
    treatment of complications, 69
  Plasmodium malariae, 70–1
    nephrosis (quartan malarial nephropathy), 70, 180–1
  Plasmodium ovale, 69–70
  Plasmodium vivax, 69–70
male fern extract, 295
malnutrition, 23–4
  liver, effect on, 116
Maloprim, 65–6, 66 (table)
Mansonella ozzardi, 268
Mansonella perstans, 268
Mansonella streptocerca, 268
Mantoux test, 45
Marburg virus disease, 235 (table), 237 (fig.), 238–9
Mayaro fever, 234
measles (rubeola), 31–3
  cell-mediated immunity depressed, 24
  chest infections following, 122
  incubation period, 32 (table)

324 Index

measles (rubeola)—*contd*
  portal of entry of virus, 32 (table)
  see also subacute sclerosing
    panencephalitis
mebendazole, 297 (table)
  for: dracontiasis, 273
    helminths, 90, 297 (table)
    hookworm, 86
    nematodes, 296
    roundworm, 87
    strongyloidosis, 88
mecillinam, 283 (table)
mefloquine, 68, 69 (table), 296
  (table)
melarsoprol (Mel B), 171, 295
melioidosis, 132
meningitis, 152–9
  bacterial, 153–9, 155 (table)
  causal organisms, 153–9
  fungal, 155 (table)
  Haemophilus influenzae, 157–8
  leptospiral, 159
  meningococcal, 156–7, 303 (table)
    C5–9 deficiency, 5–6
  neonatal, 155 (table), 159
  pneumococcal, 158–9
  protozoal, 155 (table)
  'secondary', 154 (table), 159
  tuberculous, 51–2, 166–7
  viral, 154 (table)
mepacrine, 87, 297 (table)
Metagonimus yokogawai, 83 (table)
methisazone, 291–2
metriphonate, 183, 297, 297 (table)
metronidazole, 283 (table)
  for: amoebiasis, 90, 108, 295
    dracontiasis, 273, 298
    Entamoeba histolytica infection, 90,
      296 (table)
    Gardnerella vaginalis infection, 201
    giardiasis, 295, 296 (table)
    pneumonia, 128 (table)
    protozoan infections, 296 (table)
miconazole, 261, 293
microfilariae, blood film, 27, 270, 273
minocycline, 157
mite-transmitted diseases, 13
mollusc-transmitted diseases, 12–13
monkeypox, 214, 241, 242 (fig.)
mucormycosis, 261

mumps, 32 (table), 35–6
murine typhus, 214, 246 (table), 248
muroid nephropathies, 241
mycetoma (Madura foot,
  maduromycosis), 133, 134,
  218–19, 259, 260
Mycobacterium avium intracellulare, 57,
  58, 189 (table)
Mycobacterium bovis, 43, 49
  airborne transmission, 48
  gastrointestinal disease, 50, 93
  (table)
  lymphadenitis, 50
Mycobacterium chelonei, 58
Mycobacterium fortuitum, 58
Mycobacterium intracellulare, 56, 57, 58
Mycobacterium kansasii, 56, 57, 58
Mycobacterium leprae, 217, 225–31
Mycobacterium marinum, 58
Mycobacterium scrofulaceum, 58
Mycobacterium tuberculosis, 43, 56, 189
  (table)
Mycobacterium ulcerans, 57, 58, 217
mycoses
  systemic (deep), 260–1
  systemic opportunistic, 261
myiasis, 223–4
myocarditis, acute infective, 144–6

nalidixic acid, 283 (table)
natamycin, 294 (table)
Necator americanus, 83 (table), 85–6
necrotising jejunitis, 22
Neisseria meningitidis, 154 (table), 156,
  157
nematodes, 83 (table), 85–8, 90 (*see
  also*, filariasis)
nephritis
  chronic, 179, 181
  chronic interstitial, 175
nephropathica epidemica, 241
nephrotic syndrome, 180–1, 183
niclofolan, 111
niclosamide, 87, 297 (table)
nifurtimox (Lampit), 267, 296
  (table)
niridazole, 273, 298
nitrofurantoin, 285 (table), 296
  (table)

5-nitroimidazole compounds, *see* metronidazole, tinidazole
nocardiosis, 259
non-specific urethritis, 195, 200–1
notifiable diseases, England & Wales, 3–4
novobiocin, 282 (table)
nutrition-infection interactions, 23–4
nystatin, 293, 294 (table)

Oesophagostomum spp., 90 (table)
Omsk haemorrhagic fever, 235 (table)
onchocerciasis, 222, 270–3
Onchocerca volvulus, 27, 222, 272 (fig.)
O'nyong nyong fever, 214, 234 (table)
opisthorchiasis, 111
oral rehydration therapy, 95–6, 97 (fig.)
Oriental sore (cutaneous leishmaniasis), 219–21
ornithosis (psittacosis), 9, 10 (table), 128 (table)
Oropouche virus disease, 234 (table)
Oroya fever, 251
oxamniquine, 109, 297, 297 (table)
oxytetracycline, 123, 124

Paludrine (proguanil), 65, 66 (table)
pandemic disease, 2
para-aminosalicylic acid (PAS), 55 (table), 55
paracoccidioidomycosis, 219, 261
paragonimiasis, 136, 172
Paragonimus westermani, 27, 136
paramyxovirus, 31
parasites, diagnostic techniques, 27–8
paravertebral abscess, 51
paromomycin, 296 (table)
Paul–Bunnell test, 233
pellagra, 211
pelvic inflammatory disease, 201–2
penicillin, 279, 282 (table), 288
  for: actinomycosis, 260
    anthrax, 259
    bartonellosis, 251
    leptospirosis, 107
    Lyme disease, 257
    rat-bite fever, 258

pentamidine, 135, 171, 296 (table)
pentavalent antimony compounds, 221, 296 (table)
Pentostam (sodium stibogluconate), 265, 295
pericarditis, 149–50
pertussis (whooping cough), 32 (table), 36–8
phaeohyphomycosis, 260
phenanthene methanol compounds, 69
phenethicillin, 282 (table), 289
phlyctenular conjuctivitis, 48
phosphonoformate, 292 (table)
Picornaviridae, 34
pinta (endemic non-venereal treponematosis), 216–17
piperazine, 87, 295–6
pivampicillin, 284 (table), 289
plague, 216, 258, 303 (table)
  bubonic, 258
  pneumonic, 129, 258
Plasmodium falciparum, *see* malaria
pleural effusion, 48–9, 129, 130
pleurisy, 48–9, 129
pneumococci, antibiotic resistance, 127, 289
Pneumocystis carinii, 129, 134–5
pneumonia
  antibiotic therapy, 128 (table), 130
  atypical, 127
  bacterial, 126–31
  bronchial obstruction, 129
  causative organisms, 128 (table)
  investigations, 129–30
  Klebsiella pneumoniae, 127
  Legionella pneumophila, *see* Legionnaire's disease
  opportunistic, 124–5
  plague, 129, 258
  pneumococcal lobar, 127–8, 130
  Pneumocystis carinii, 129
  resolution slow/incomplete, 129
  Salmonella typhi, 128–9
  tuberculous, 48–9, 127
'pneumonitis', transient, 124
poliomyelitis, 32 (table), 34–5, 302 (table)
polymyxins, 283 (table)
postinfective malabsorption (tropical sprue), 92–5

Pott's disease, 51
praziquantel
  for: fluke infection, 111, 297 (table), 298
    helminthic infections, 297 (table)
    paragonimiasis, 136
    schistosomiasis, 109, 183, 297, 297 (table)
pregnancy
  antibiotisin, 290
  infections, 19–20
  precautions when travelling, 306–9
prevention (control of communicable disease), 311–16
primaquine, 70, 296 (table)
prion, 168
probenecid, 200
procaine penicillin, 200, 205
progressive multifocal leucoencephalopathy, 163 (table)
proguanil (Paludrine), 65, 66 (table)
protozoa, colorectal, 88–90, 89 (table)
protozoa, small-intestinal, 82–4
psittacosis (ornithosis), 9, 10 (table), 128 (table)
psoas abscess, 51
Pulex irritans, 11, 223
pyelonephritis, acute bacterial, 175, 179
pyoderma, 215
pyoderma gangrenosum, 211
pyrantel, 86, 87
pyrazinamide, 54 (table), 55, 166
  blood–brain barrier, 156 (table)
pyrexia of undetermined origin (PUO), 24–5, 26 (table)
pyrimethamine (Daraprim), 65, 66 (table), 146, 262, 296 (table)

Q fever, 28, 127, 214, 247 (table), 249–50
qinghaosu, 68, 69 (table), 294, 296 (table)
quartan malarial nephropathy (*Plasmodium malariae* nephrosis), 180
quinidine, 68, 69 (table)

quinine, 68, 69 (table), 268, 296 (table)
quinolones, 283 (table), 289

rabies, 6–7, 10 (table), 162–4, 303 (table), 305, 308 (table)
radioimmunoassay, 28
rat-bite fevers, 258
Reiter's syndrome, 81, 201
relapsing fevers, 257–8
renal amyloidosis, 181
renal failure, acute, 179
  antibiotics in, 286 (table)
Retortamonas intestinalis, 89 (table)
rheumatic fever, acute, 138–40
rhinosporidiosis, 260
ribavirin, 238, 292 (table)
rickettsia, 244–51, 246 (table)
rickettsial infection, 244–51
rickettsialpox, 214, 215, 247 (table), 249
rifampicin, 53, 54 (table), 285 (table)
  blood–brain barrier, 156 (table)
  for: bacterial endocarditis, 144
    Legionnaire's disease, 131
    leprosy, 230, 231 (table)
    lymphogranuloma venereum, 208
    meningitis prophylaxis, 157
    tuberculosis, 53, 54 (table), 128
Rift Valley fever, 234 (table), 235 (table)
ringworm, 10, 218
  of nails, 218
Rochagan (benzonidazole), 267
Rocky Mountain spotted fever, 214, 247 (table), 249
roundworm, 86–7
rotavirus infection, 79
rubella, 41-2

salicylates, 140
Salmonella spp. infection, 9, 10 (table), 79
Salmonella typhi, 128–9, 254–5
salmonellosis, urinary, 180
sandfly fevers, 234 (table)
Sarcocystis spp., 82 (table), 84
scabies, 223

scarlet fever, 32 (table), 40–1
Schistosoma haematobium, 27, 181–3, 182 (fig.)
  pyelonephritis, 175, 179
  urinary infection, 180
Schistosoma intercalatum, 90 (table)
Schistosoma japonicum, 27, 90 (table), 91, 109, 112 (table), 172
  geographical distribution, 110 (fig.)
Schistosoma mansoni, 27, 90 (table), 91, 109, 112 (table), 172
  geographical distribution, 110 (fig.)
  glomerulonephritis, 109
Schistosoma mattheei, 90 (table)
Schistosoma mekongi, 90 (table)
schistosomes, 90 (table), 112 (table)
schistosomiasis
  acute (Katayama fever), 28, 109, 222
  cardiac, 147–8
  colonic, 91
  hepatic, 109
  pulmonary, 136
  urinary, 181–3
scrapie, 167
scrub typhus (Tsutsugamushi fever), 7, 215, 246 (table)
septicaemia, 251–4
  treatment, 253 (table)
septicaemic shock, 16, 251
sexually transmitted diseases, 195–209
  organisms causing, 197 (table)
Shigella spp. infection, 9, 10 (table), 79, 81
Shigella boydii, 80
Shigella dysenteriae-1 (Shiga's bacillus), 80
Shigella flexneri, 80
Shigella sonnei, 80
shigellosis, 80–1
sickle-cell disease, 180, 211
sickle-cell gene, 6
Sindbis fever, 234
skin infections, 210–24
  arthropod borne, 223–4
  bacterial, 215–18
  fungal, 218–19
  helminthic, 221–2
  protozoan, 219–21
  rickettsial, 214–15
  viral, 211–14
skin-lightening cream, 180
sleeping sickness (African trypanosomiasis), 168–71
slow virus infections of CNS, 162, 163 (table), 167–8, 243–4
Snow, Dr. John, 2–3, 77
sodium stibogluconate (Pentostam), 265, 295
Sodoku, 258
soft chancre (chancroid), 198 (table), 206–7
sore throat, 120–1
South American trypanosomiasis, *see* Chagas' disease
spectinomycin, 200
spiramycin, 84, 146, 262, 296 (table)
sporadic disease, 2
sporotrichosis, 260
Sporotrichum schenckii, 218
Staphylococcus aureus
  carriers, 210
  enteritis, 80
  lung abscess, 132
  pneumonia, 127
Staphylococcus epidermidis, 142 (table), 210
Streptococcus pneumoniae, 127
  endocarditis, 141
  meningitis, 154 (table), 156, 158–9
Streptococcus pyogenes, Lancefield group A, 41, 215
streptomycin, 283 (table)
  blood–brain barrier, 156
  for: bartonellosis, 251
    brucellosis, 256
    leptospirosis, 107
    plague, 258
    tuberculosis, 54–5, 128 (table)
    tularaemia, 259
Strongyloides spp., 132
Strongyloides fülleborni, 88
Strongyloides stercoralis, 83 (table), 87–8, 90 (table), 222
  investigation of, 27, 88
subacute sclerosing panencephalitis, 33, 162, 163 (table), 167

sulphadiazine, 157, 262, 295 (table)
sulphamethoxazole, 58
sulphonamides, 208, 279–80, 285 (table)
  blood–brain barrier, 156 (table)
  long-acting, 219
  resistance to, 157
suramin (Antrypol), 171, 271, 292 (table), 297 (table)
Surinam, Dutch colonists in, 5
swimming pool granuloma, 58
syphilis, 202–5
  cardiac disease, 146
  congenital, 204
  incidence, 195
  investigations, 204
  primary, 198 (table), 203, 216
  secondary, 203, 216
  tertiary, 204
  treatment, 205

Taenia saginata, 83 (table), 87
Taenia solium (*Cysticercus cellulosae*), 83 (table), 87 (*see also*, cysticercosis)
Takayasu's disease, 147
tanapox, 214
tapeworm, 87
Ternidens deminutus, 83 (table), 90 (table)
tetanus, 164, 302 (table)
tetrachlorethylene, 86
tetracycline, 284 (table)
  for: balantidiasis, 295, 296 (table)
    bronchitis, 123
    brucellosis, 256
    gonorrhoea, 200
    infective endocarditis, 144
    infective myocarditis, 146
    leptospirosis, 107
    Lyme disease, 257
    lymphogranuloma venereum, 208
    non-specific urethritis, 201
    pneumonia, 128 (table)
    postinfective malabsorption, 95
    Q fever, 144, 250
    relapsing fevers, 257–8
    rickettsial infection, 245, 248, 249, 250

thiabendazole, 297, 297 (table)
  for: dracontiasis, 273
  strongyloidiasis, 88, 297
  toxocariasis, 276
  trichinosis, 277
thiacetazone, 55 (table), 55
threadworm (*Enterobius vermicularis*), 90
thrush (oral candidiasis), 122
tick-transmitted diseases, 13, 214–15, 247 (table), 249
tick typhus, 214, 247 (table), 249
tinea imbricata, 218
tinea infections, 218
tinea versicolor, 218
tinidazole, 84, 283 (table), 296 (table)
tobramycin, 128 (table), 283 (table)
tonsillitis, 120–1
toxic shock, 16, 251
toxocariasis, 10 (table), 10–11, 276
toxoplasmosis, 10 (table), 261–2
tracheobronchitis, acute, 122
trachoma, 244
transmissable (Aleutian) mink encephalopathy, 167
travellers, diseases affecting, 299–310
  advice to, 299–301
  children, 309
  immunisation/prophylaxis, 301, 302 (table), 303 (table)
  imported infections, 306, 308 (table)
  pregnant women, 306–9
  presenting symptoms of disease, 306, 307 (table)
travellers' diarrhoea, 72–5, 84
  treatment, 74–5, 75 (table)
  complications of treatment, 77 (table)
trematodes, 83 (table), 87, 90 (table)
trench fever, 214, 247 (table), 250
treponematosis, endemic non-venereal (pinta), 216–17
Trichinella spiralis, 83 (table) 276
trichinosis, (trichinellosis), 276
  muscle biopsy, 27–8
Trichomonas hominis, 89 (table)
Trichomonas vaginalis, 196, 197 (table)
Trichostrongylus spp., 83 (table)

Trichuris trichiuria (whipworm), 90
trimethoprim, 280, 285 (table)
  blood–brain barrier, 156 (table)
trimethoprim-sulphamethoxazole, *see* co-trimoxazole
trivalent antimony compounds, 296
tropical enteropathy, 92
tropical pulmonary eosinophilia (filarial hypereosinophilia), 135, 270
tropical splenomegaly syndrome, 70–1
tropical sprue (postinfective malabsorption), 92–5
tropical (phagedenic) ulcer, 215–16
Trypanosoma cruzi, 28, 265–7
Trypanosoma gambiense, 168–71
Trypanosoma rhodesiense, 168–71
trypanosomiasis
  African, 168–71, 221
  lymph node fluid, 27
  South American, 265–7
Tsutsugamushi fever (scrub typhus), 7, 215, 246 (table)
tuberculin test, 45–6
tuberculoma, 49, 166–7
tuberculosis, 43–59
  adrenal disease, 52
  arthritis, 51
  bacteraemia, 47
  BCG vaccination, 45–6
  Brock's syndrome, 47
  disseminated (miliary), 47–8, 52
  extrapulmonary, 49–52
  gastrointestinal disease, 50, 93 (table)
  genitourinary disease, 50–1, 179–80
  haematogenous spread, 47
  Heaf test, 45
  hilar lymphadenopathy, 129
  hospital-acquired, 18–19
  immunity, 46
    ethnic differences, 5, 46
  incidence, 43
  intradermal skin test, 45–6
  lymphadenitis, 50
  management, 52–6
  Mantoux test, 45
  meningitis, 47–8, 51–2, 166–7
  osteomyelitis, 51
  pericarditis, 51, 149–50
  pleurisy, 49
  pneumonia, 49, 127, 129
  primary (Ghon) focus, 44 (fig.), 47
  primary infection, 44 (fig.)
  pulmonary, 48–9
    investigation of, 49
  renal, 179–80
  susceptibility to, 5
  threat to medical personnel, 18–19, 43
  vertebral, 51, 152
tularaemia, 258–9
Tunga penetrans (jigger flea), 223
tungiasis, 223
typhoid fever, 254–5, 302 (table)
  Widal test, 28
typhus, 244–9
  epidemic, 214, 246 (table), 248
  murine, 214, 246 (table), 248
  scrub (Tsutsugamushi fever), 7, 215, 246 (table), 248
  tick, 214, 247 (table), 249

Ucinaria stenocephala, 221
ulcerative colitis, 81
upper respiratory flora, normal, 120 (table)
upper respiratory tract infections, acute, 119–20
urethral discharge, male, 199 (table)
  urethral syndrome (abacterial cystitis), 175, 177, 199, 200
urinary tract infection
  acute, 174–8
    causes, 175–7
    investigations, 176, 177
    treatment, 177–8
  chronic, 179–83

vaginal discharge, 196
vancomycin, 282 (table)
varicella (chickenpox), 32 (table), 41
veno-occlusive disease of liver, 117
Vibrio cholerae, 77–8
  El tor variant, 77–8
vidarabine, 213, 292 (table)
Vincent's infection, 121
viral febrile illness, 234 (table)

viral infections, 232–44
  diseases resulting from, 244 (table)
  persistent, 243–4
viral haemorrhagic fever, 7, 214, 235 (table), 236–41
viral hepatitis, 79, 99–103, 307, 312
  A, 99–100, 302 (table), 312
  B, 100–2, 214, 303 (table)
    hepatocellular carcinoma-related, 114–15
    vaccination, 115
  delta agent, 102
  hospital acquired, 19
  non-A non-B, 102–3

West Nile fever, 214, 234 (table)
whipworm (*Trichuris trichiura*), 90
whooping cough, *see* pertussis
Widal test, 28
Wuchereria bancrofti, blood film, 27, 270

X-linked lymphoproliferative syndrome, 233

yaws, 217
yellow fever, 104–6, 302 (table)
Yersinia enterocolitica, 81
Yersinia pestis, 129, 258
Yersinia pseudotuberculosis, 9–10, 81

zoonoses (zoonotic diseases), 1, 9–11
zygomycosis, subcutaneous, 260